DR. PS[ ]

SEASONAL ALLERGY

SOLUTION

The All-Natural 4-Week Plan to
Eliminate the Underlying Cause of
Allergies and Live Symptom-Free

JONATHAN PSENKA, ND

RODALE.

Rodale books may be purchased for business or promotional use or for special sales. For information, please write to:
Special Markets Department, Rodale Inc., 733 Third Avenue, New York, NY 10017

Printed in the United States of America

Rodale Inc. makes every effort to use acid-free , recycled paper.

Book design by Joanna Williams

Library of Congress Cataloging-in-Publication Data is on file with the publisher.

ISBN 978–1–62336–273–7

Distributed to the trade by Macmillan

2   4   6   8   10   9   7   5   3   1   paperback

⚜ RODALE.

We inspire and enable people to improve their lives and the world around them.
rodalebooks.com

I dedicate this book to my family, my friends, and my patients.
This book would not have been possible
without your love, companionship, and confidence.
Thank you.

Contents

Introduction

AS A NATUROPATHIC DOCTOR, I walk into my office each day armed with natural ways to help people help themselves and their loved ones lead happier, healthier lives. And I have to say, I love what I do.

In the midst of this labor of love, about 5 years ago, I started seeing more and more allergy patients in my Arizona practice. Many of them admitted to having moved to Arizona because they heard it was "the place to live" to ease allergies. But after a month or two of fewer sniffles and sneezes, just as these patients were getting used to their new desert environment, their allergies seemed to return and settle in full time. Many of them had tried various conventional allergy medications, but to no avail. Nothing their doctors prescribed worked.

What I noticed about these allergy pioneers was that, in addition to allergies, they frequently had other health concerns. They suffered from heart disease, were overweight, had diabetes, or struggled with other health problems that were well-established diseases of lifestyle. (Lifestyle diseases are conditions people develop when they eat unhealthy diets, don't exercise, or have too much stress.) I began to think that maybe there was more of a connection between allergies and general health than we'd previously thought.

So, I did some experimenting. I tried to treat these people's allergies using natural means. Modern medicine is all about using pills, sprays, drops, and even painful shots to treat allergy symptoms. But very few of these medications treat the *causes* of allergies, so symptoms continue to return. To try and break the cycle and pull folks out of these downward allergy spirals, so to speak, I treated them holistically.

My findings? Healthful eating and hydration practices, the right herbs and supplements, proper weight management, and avoidance of stress and anxiety all worked wonders. The people who took my advice got healthier—not just in terms of their allergy symptoms, but across the board.

Since then, equipped with what I've learned about treating allergies naturally, I have created an easy-to-follow plan that you, too, can use to ease your seasonal allergies—without having to make a single trip to your local drugstore. Using my three-pronged approach—foods, supplements, and exercise—you can say goodbye to the pesky runny nose, scratchy throat, and allergy shots for good! As a bonus, if you follow my advice, you'll be less likely to develop one of the chronic lifestyle diseases killing so many Americans today—cancer, diabetes, or heart disease.

As a result of my work, I have become known in the naturopathic community as an allergy guru. Everywhere I go, people ask me, "How can you help me with my allergies?" Using this book, I am spreading the word far and wide: With the right natural remedies, you can escape your allergy downward spiral, reverse your allergic tendencies, and ward off other lifestyle diseases at the same time.

THE PROBLEM OF RISING ALLERGIES

There are a ton of allergies out there, and it's only getting worse. Globally, 30 to 40 percent of people now suffer from allergies such as rhinitis, asthma, anaphylaxis, and food and drug allergies, and cases are increasing fastest in children. What's particularly scary is that we're not just becoming more allergic to respiratory allergens like pollens and grasses, we're also becoming more allergic to everyday things in our environment, from paint on the wall to new foods. Places like Arizona, once considered to be safe havens for people with allergies, now see sufferers in record numbers. And people who never before had seasonal allergies now find themselves filling prescriptions for allergy medications.

Why? There are multiple theories, from a too-sterile society to unhealthy diets to pollution. (This book will delve into these and other possible environmental causes in more detail). And then there's the role of what's going on *inside* your body. After all, it's not only environment, but also lifestyle, that predisposes you to becoming allergic.

One of the key inside-the-body factors is inflammation. So many of the diseases that plague people today—diabetes, obesity, heart disease, and cancer, just to name a few—are inflammatory in nature. Allergies are also the result of an inflammatory cycle. In fact, the allergic response and inflammation share some of the same chemical messengers; therefore, too much inflammation coupled with too much of an allergic response can cause an exaggerated response. In short, if your body is already in a state of inflammation when you enter allergy season, you're likely to be more miserable than the noninflamed guy. And on the flip side, by virtue of having allergies, you may suffer worse symptoms of other health conditions when allergy season hits.

WHY TREAT ALLERGIES NATURALLY?

As a naturopathic physician, of course I gravitate toward holistic, natural remedies. I have nothing against conventional medicine; it saves lives, undoubtedly. But I think there are some instances as well as certain conditions that people shouldn't—or would rather not—treat with conventional medicines. Based on my experience, I believe some allergies should be treated holistically.

Because we're becoming more allergic as a society, we'd be foolish to think that we're not going to see increases in the number of children and adults who are allergic to medications. When we throw medications at people who are highly allergic to other substances in their environments, there will likely be more allergic reactions and adverse drug reactions because these people are already allergy prone.

Also, I think it's best to save medications for when you or

someone you love is really sick—when, God forbid, you really need them. This will maximize the effectiveness of those medications when the need for them is most dire. Using an approach to treat your chronic allergies that doesn't rely on medical dosages gives you a real advantage.

HOW TO BREAK FREE FROM SEASONAL ALLERGIES FOR GOOD: INTRODUCING MY PLAN

Using the plan outlined in this book, you will be able to reverse negative cycles of allergy and inflammation with natural, nontoxic treatments. My plan is a core lifestyle program, fine-tuned for allergy sufferers like you. By "lifestyle program," I don't mean that you will have to live on wheatgrass. It's simply a holistic, healthy approach to living.

Here are the main components.

Good food. Eating well doesn't just mean eating lots of vegetables; it also means limiting junk food. A healthy diet includes foods that naturally reduce inflammation and/or the allergic response, such as watermelon, green tea, and dark chocolate.

Herbs and supplements. There are a number of natural herbs and supplements that can reduce the inflammation causing your allergies and lessen allergy symptoms' impact on your daily life. Examples include stinging nettle, bromelain, quercetin, and fatty acids.

Physical activity. Put simply, our bodies are meant to move. We're not designed to sit in front of our computer screens and type all day, but that's what many of us—myself included—do. And when we don't do what our bodies are intended to do, we see adverse effects. A healthy lifestyle means making exercise a priority nearly every single day.

Leading an easier life. In addition to the three components above, this book will help you examine the roles of anxiety, stress, and adequate sleep in allergies, as well as teach you the best ways to relax and sleep well for better health.

In short, with the help of this book, you will be able to:

- Discover which foods and supplements can eliminate the effects of your seasonal allergies
- Learn specific exercises to combat your allergy symptoms
- Gain the peace of mind of knowing that you will be a healthier person and won't be destined to a life on allergy medications.

Guided by my easy-to-follow plan, not only will you learn how to control your allergies naturally, without medications, but you'll also learn how to improve your lifestyle and become a happier, healthier person. I look forward to taking this journey with you.

Let's get started!

1

Allergies Are on the Rise

THERE'S NO QUESTION ABOUT IT: Allergies are skyrocketing across the world, especially in industrialized countries.

As I think about the increasing rate of allergies, a particular patient sticks out in my mind: About 2 years ago, I saw a young boy who would develop large, swollen eyes and very swollen lips whenever he was in his bedroom. His parents were smart people and had tried eliminating all of the common possible food allergens. I also did laboratory testing to see if maybe he was allergic to the family dog or cat or another common household allergen. All of the tests came back reporting the same thing: The boy's reactions could not be traced to a common allergy.

Puzzled, the boy's parents and I zeroed in on where the boy most frequently experienced symptoms. We determined that they most often occurred when he was sitting at his desk in his room, completing his homework. There was nothing unusual about this space; he had pens, paper, pencils, and erasers—all the normal stuff you would find on a school-aged boy's desk. But he also had a small fishbowl that contained one Siamese fighting fish. It was actually his brother who suggested that maybe the fish was causing the reaction. It was highly unlikely that this boy would be allergic to a fish, especially one swimming in a bowl; but the brother's theory did get the

1

ball rolling in the right direction. I eventually discovered that the boy had an allergy to the bloodworms he fed to his fish each night.

Granted, this was an unusual case. Nine times out of 10, it is the common allergens—pollen, dust mites, pet dander, ragweed—that cause reactions. But this boy's case highlights that you can also be allergic to the most unexpected things.

THE ORIGINS OF MY CLINICAL FOCUS ON ALLERGIES

Allergies have been around since the dawn of pollen itself, but they are undoubtedly becoming more common. (There are many theories as to why, which we will explore in Chapter 2.) The aeroallergens report recently released by the US Environmental Protection Agency (EPA) found that half of all Americans now suffer from some symptoms when exposed to airborne allergens such as ragweed, pollen, or dust.[1] According to the American College of Allergy, Asthma, and Immunology (ACAAI), each allergy season seems to be subsequently worse than the one before, an indication that seasonal allergies are on the rise.[2] And not only are we seeing more people allergic to common allergens, allergies to *uncommon* things—paint on the walls, foods not typically allergenic, and yes, bloodworms—are rising as well.

So it should come as no surprise that about 5 years ago, I started seeing a dramatic increase in the number of allergy patients coming into my office. Thanks to the dry climate, low mold levels, and shorter blooming periods, the Southwest was for a long time considered a safe haven for allergy sufferers; so many people moved here in hopes of easing their symptoms. (Of course, the picturesque scenery and bright sun didn't hurt, either.)[3]

From these patients, I repeatedly heard the same story: "When I first moved to Arizona, I was okay for a while. But then my allergies just took off. What was once a month or two block of time where I had allergic symptoms is now year-round. And my allergies don't seem to be improving. My doctor has put me on several medications, but nothing works."

After seeing more and more of these patients coming into my office, desperate for relief after their medications had failed them, I became very interested in treating allergies naturally. I tried using healthful eating, hydration, weight management, relaxation techniques, and herbs and supplements as treatment protocols. I was pleased to find that these treatments worked very well, not just to cure seasonal allergies, but also to help the patients become healthier individuals overall.

Today, about 60 percent of my patients have some sort of allergy or sensitivity, and most of them respond extremely well to the natural treatments and lifestyle interventions I prescribe. As you read on and start to follow the plan outlined in this book, you, too, can look forward to a healthier, happier life, with fewer sniffles, sneezes, and hives.

THE GROWING ALLERGY PROBLEM

Allergies are one of the fastest-growing chronic health problems in the world. According to the Asthma and Allergy Foundation of America (AAFA), about 50 million Americans—or 1 in 5—suffer from allergies. Broken down, the numbers look like this:

- About 8 percent of American adults have hay fever
- About 13 percent of adults have sinusitis
- About 8 percent of children have food allergies, and nearly 38 percent of those have a history of severe reactions[4]

Allergies also tend to occur in groups, hitting victims from multiple angles. Children with food allergies are two to four times more likely to have asthma or other allergies than those who do not have food allergies, for example. And the AAFA reports that 30 percent of the 15 million people with asthma can blame their wheezing and difficulty breathing on allergies.[5]

We will explore the physiology more deeply in Chapter 3, but put simply, allergies are an overreaction of the immune system to substances in the environment that don't cause a reaction in non-allergic people. These substances, which may include pollen, dust,

The Food Allergy Epidemic

One of the most alarming trends related to the rise in allergies is the growing threat of allergies to foods. According to Food Allergy Research and Education (FARE), a nonprofit organization formed in 2012 as a merger between the Food Allergy and Anaphylaxis Network and the Food Allergy Initiative, 1 in 13 children under age 18 has a food allergy. This equals 2 kids in every school classroom today.[6]

Food allergies are concerning because they can lead to the potentially life-threatening whole-body reaction called anaphylaxis. The biggest fear of every parent of a child with a food allergy, anaphylaxis involves difficulty breathing, swelling of the lips and throat, and, potentially, death.[7]

One of the most severe and potentially life-threatening food allergies—peanut allergy—is also on the rise. A study by Scott H. Sicherer, MD, professor of pediatrics and chief of the Division of Allergy and Immunology at the Jaffe Food Allergy Institute at Mount Sinai School of Medicine in New York City, found that peanut allergies had doubled in American kids between 1997 and 2002.[8] When they looked at the data again in 2008, peanut allergy rates had tripled![9] Research done in Canada, Australia, and the United Kingdom have shown similar increases. In the UK, for example, hospital admissions for food allergies have gone up 500 percent since 1990.[10]

mold, or other proteins, are called allergens.[14] Almost anything can cause an allergic reaction, and as evidenced by the alarming increase in allergy rates worldwide, we are becoming more and more allergic.

The most common allergies result from pollen, dust, food, insect stings, animal dander, mold, medications, and latex. Any of these offenders can spark a range of symptoms affecting numerous areas of your body: your nose, sinuses, ears, throat, skin, lungs, and stomach. Some allergic reactions, like occasional sneezing and runny nose, are just annoying. But more severe responses, such as swelling or itchy rashes, can interfere with work, sleep, and daily activities. And other reactions, such as anaphylaxis from food allergies, can be

And not only do more children have food allergies but also they tend to be allergic to more foods. In the past, a child with food allergies was typically allergic to one, maybe two foods. Today, kids are typically allergic to three or four different offenders.[11]

As a result, teachers, administrators, and school nurses carry devices to inject epinephrine so they can save an allergic child's life at any time.[12] Classroom walls display lists of kids' food allergies next to their artwork. Nonedible party favors have replaced cupcakes at birthday celebrations, out of fear of exposing an allergic child to even a trace of a peanut. And experts in the allergy field believe that food allergies are actually *underreported,* so the problem is probably even worse than we think.[13] Therefore, rising food allergies are a major health concern.

There are now blood tests available that can determine whether a child has an allergy to peanuts that will produce an anaphylactic-type reaction or one that will not be life threatening. The tests are widely available and are referred to as component testing. If you have a child with known or suspected allergies, you should ask your pediatrician about this type of testing. Knowing the severity of your child's allergy could really put your mind at ease and also potentially save your child's life.

life-threatening.[15] No matter what the cause or the specific reaction, no one who suffers from allergies will deny that they can take a real toll on your quality of life.

RISING ALLERGIES: THE NUMBERS SPEAK FOR THEMSELVES

The number of allergy sufferers has been steadily rising for decades worldwide. According to the American Academy of Allergy, Asthma, and Immunology (AAAAI), allergies have been on the rise in industrialized countries for more than 50 years.[16] And allergy rates aren't just increasing, they are *accelerating*. A major study by Quest Diagnostics found that overall sensitization rates for allergies rose by 6 percent between 2005 and 2008. Increases in some individual allergies are even more dramatic. Mold sensitivities, for example, rose by 12 percent, and ragweed sensitivities increased by 15 percent during the same 3 years.[17]

What's particularly troubling is the rate at which allergies are increasing in children. Worldwide, 40 to 50 percent of schoolchildren now have sensitivities to at least one allergen. That's nearly one out of every two kids! As an important note, I see more adults than children in my practice, but I think that it's important to raise the issue of allergies in children. A lot of the research on increasing allergies has been done on children, but these study findings reflect similar increases in adults. Plus, allergic children are much more likely than nonallergic children to become allergic adults, so the rising rates in children are a concern for people of all ages. Recognizing the seriousness of rising allergies in children, the U.S. Centers for Disease Control and Prevention (CDC) recently took a careful look at the numbers. Their National Health Interview Survey found that between 1997 and 2011, both food and skin allergies increased in children under age 18. And although there was no increase in respiratory allergies in children, they remained the most common types of allergies, at a high 17 percent between 2009 and 2011.[18]

Breaking it down further, the CDC also found that skin allergies rose from 7.4 percent between 1997 and 1999 to 12.5 percent between 2009 and 2011. And in children up to age 17, food allergies increased from 3.4 percent between 1997 and 1999 to 5.1 percent between 2009 and 2011.[19]

Researchers also discovered that while some allergies fade with age, others get worse. As children get older, skin allergy rates go down (from 14.2 percent in children from birth to 4 years old to 13.1 percent in children 5 to 9 and finally to 10.9 percent in children 10 to 17). Respiratory allergies, on the other hand, get worse with age, increasing from 10.8 percent in children from birth to 4 years old to 17.4 percent in children 5 to 9 and to 20.8 percent in children 10 to 17.[20] So the sooner in life we nip these allergies in the bud, the better.

Are Allergy Rates Rising with Income?

Interestingly, when you look at allergy statistics, as income levels rise, so do allergies. Children with family incomes greater than or equal to 200 percent of the poverty level have the highest rates of food and respiratory allergies. Here's a breakdown.

- In children with household incomes that are less than 100 percent of the poverty level, 14.9 percent have respiratory allergies and 4.4 percent have food allergies.
- When the income level rises to between 100 and 200 percent of the poverty level, 15.8 have respiratory allergies and 5 percent have food allergies.
- In families with income levels greater than 200 percent of the poverty level, 18.3 percent of children have respiratory allergies and 5.4 percent have food allergies.[21]

Race also seems to play a role, but no one is sure why. Hispanic children have lower rates of food, skin, and respiratory allergies than kids of all other races and ethnicities. Black children are more likely to have skin allergies than white children (17.4 percent in blacks, compared to 12 percent in whites). However, black children are less likely than white children to have respiratory allergies (15.6 percent in blacks, compared to 19.1 percent in whites).[22]

These numbers may make it look like income, race, and allergy risk are related, but I don't think money or race are truly causing these disparities. For one thing, the study done by Quest Diagnostics found that economically disadvantaged children are 18 percent less likely to be tested for allergies by the age of 5 than children whose parents have a higher income. Therefore, these children may not actually have fewer allergies—they just have fewer allergies that have been *diagnosed*.[23]

I think the real reason behind these differences is more a matter of better protection in people who live a more agrarian lifestyle, where agriculture is a focus. After all, scientists have found that children who grow up on a farm or who live in a family with at least one other sibling are less likely to have allergies.[24] As income level goes up, people are less likely to live on farms or to have large families. They are more likely to have a housekeeper who comes in and scrubs the entire house and to send their kids to a day care where they provide hand sanitizer four times a day. Clearly, besides income and race, there are other things at play, which we will explore more in Chapter 2.

Why Are Allergies Such a Problem?

On a day-to-day level, an allergy may force you to carry extra tissues or an EpiPen in case of an emergency. But allergies wreak havoc on a broader scale as well, both on our bodies and on our society as a whole.

Perhaps most importantly, and this is one of my biggest reasons for writing this book, I believe allergies are linked to some of the biggest health threats in the United States—obesity, diabetes, and heart disease. Many of my patients who come in complaining of allergies also have one or more of these lifestyle diseases, which are currently the leading causes of death in America. A major culprit behind all of these chronic conditions, allergies included, is inflammation in the body. When people eat unhealthy diets full of processed foods, avoid exercise, and live a stressed life, they are setting the stage for excessive inflammation. The more inflammation someone has in his or her body, the greater the potential for allergies and the greater the likelihood of developing other chronic health conditions.

There's also a strong connection between allergies and asthma, a chronic disease that causes inflammation in the airways. If you have asthma, airborne allergens are likely triggers for an attack.[25]

In addition to the toll they take on health, allergies also cost billions of dollars per year in medical treatments and lost productivity. The three most common allergic conditions—hay fever, asthma, and eczema—rank sixth among expenditures for chronic health conditions, and allergy treatment as a whole costs $21 billion a year.[26] Employees with allergies miss an average of 1.7 days of work due to their symptoms and deal with these symptoms for nearly 10 weeks each year. This equals a total of 4 million sick days and more than $700 million in lost wages and profits.[27] With these tolls in mind, it's in all of our best interests to eliminate allergies, once and for all.

Common Theories Behind the Allergy Explosion

With all of these numbers and facts in mind, the big question looms: *Why* the increase in allergies? We know that inflammation plays a role, but we don't know exactly what's fueling that inflammation. Scientists haven't uncovered any definitive answers, but there are lots of theories.

I believe the answer is two-pronged, with one cause being our environment and the other being our lifestyles. Here's a brief overview of the theories surrounding these two prongs. We will explore these in more detail in Chapter 2.

CAUSE 1: ENVIRONMENT

Pollution. Experts subscribing to this theory think that pollution is a major contributor to increasing allergies worldwide.[28] In Arizona and the Southwest United States in general, the air used to be much cleaner, but that's no longer the case. I recently read an article that linked children playing outside in the state of California (where air pollution is a big problem) to a higher risk of developing allergies. It sounds totally insane, but it's probably true.

That said, I'm not sure those kids would be any better off playing *inside*. "Pollution" is a very broad term. It's not just the smog in the air you breathe on your daily commute but also what you're eating in your food, what you're ingesting with your cosmetics and personal hygiene products, and what you're inhaling from the materials used to build your house that put you at an increased risk for illness and allergy.

Globalization. Our horizons are expanding too far: The world is getting smaller. As a result, environments are changing. So the theory here is that globalization is bringing foreign diets and more exotic products into our stores and kitchens, and this may contribute to allergies.[29] A century ago, my fish-owning young patient most likely wouldn't have had access to the bloodworms he feeds his fish, and therefore, he never would have reacted to them.

Arizona is a prime example of this shrinking-world phenomenon. Phoenix is still dry and hot with beautiful scenery, but it's a different place than it was a few decades ago. Where there used to be just desert and sand, people now have plants from all over the world growing in their gardens. There are golf courses on every other block, with sprinklers constantly keeping the greens lush. Also, air pollution levels are extremely high.[30] As a result, "the place to go" for allergy sufferers now has one of the fastest-growing allergy rates in the country.[31]

The hygiene hypothesis. For most of our evolution, we have had a close relationship with dirt, pollen, and microbes. Now that we've emphasized removing ourselves from the natural world, we've eliminated a lot of these background germs with antibiotics, hand sanitizers, and cleaning products. Consequently, when exposure does occur, the immune system doesn't know quite how to respond appropriately. As a result, your body can produce an inflammatory response, which in turn can heighten your chances of developing an allergy.[32] Research has shown that the years up to age 5 are very important for immune system development. Until children reach that point, it's important to find the right balance between clean living and healthy living. (In my opinion, kids are meant to get dirty.)

Climate change. This theory states that global warming and resulting increases in carbon dioxide and precipitation create more pollen. Plants use carbon dioxide to produce energy through photosynthesis, so carbon dioxide acts like a plant fertilizer. Warmer temperatures cause plants to grow faster, bloom earlier, and produce more pollen. More pollen, in turn, can lead to more seasonal allergies.[33,34]

CAUSE 2: LIFESTYLE

Stress. Too much stress destroys our immune systems. Our bodies aren't built for long-term, unrelenting stress. Instead, we're wired for short bursts of stress followed by long periods of rest and relaxation.

Imagine being a human 5,000 years ago. Most of your time is spent looking for food and picking fleas off your family members. Every now and then, as you walk through the woods, a big bear pops out and starts chasing you. At this point, you have two choices—run or fight (i.e., the fight-or-flight response). The stress hormones start flowing; epinephrine puts your body on high alert. All available resources are directed toward running or fighting. Digestion and assimilation, immune function, and all other nonessential operations are suspended until the coast is clear. In most cases, escaping from the bear took a relatively short period of time, and pretty soon you were back to picking fleas off your sister.

Now think about our fast-paced society. We've flip-flopped our stress and relaxation times; you now have long periods of sustained stress more frequently than you don't. As a result, your body feels like it's constantly running from a bear in the woods (or reacting to a cell phone ringing in your pocket). According to this theory, your body is almost constantly in a state of high alert, expending resources reacting toward the perceived emergencies. This sustained stress response can deplete your body's resources. When you combine this with the unhealthy diets we tend to eat and our poor sleep habits and lack of rest, we're much more vulnerable to developing allergies and other health problems.

Unhealthy diet. The Standard American Diet, or SAD, is not a health-promoting diet—it is sad in the true sense of the word. It's too high in sugar, saturated fat, and processed ingredients such as trans fats—all the things that can create excess inflammation in your body and make you more vulnerable to allergies. The SAD also robs your body of the vitamins, minerals, and antioxidants it needs to protect itself. For all of these reasons, an unhealthy diet increases your risk of allergies.

Additionally, there is a theory in the medical community—and some studies to back it up—that the foods and drinks a woman consumes during pregnancy help determine whether or not her child will have allergies, both in childhood and later in life. Studies show that some foods, such as margarine and diet soda, increase the risk of allergies in the unborn child. Other foods, such as fish rich in omega-3 fatty acids, help protect the child against allergies.[35,36]

Nutrient deficiency. The theory here is that we're undernourished and literally starving for good nutrition. For example, over the past 15 to 20 years, lack of vitamin D has been increasingly recognized as a risk factor for allergies and other conditions.[37] I test most of my patients to evaluate their vitamin D levels, and most of them are suboptimal. Many people think that they are getting enough from being in the sun or from taking multivitamins, but this is apparently not the case. People need more of it, for sure.

For example, a 2013 study published in the *American Journal of Rhinology & Allergy* found that Taiwanese patients with chronic rhinosinusitis and nasal polyposis were more likely to have low vitamin D than those without the condition. This shows a potential link between allergic rhinitis and low vitamin D.[38]

All of the aforementioned theories have some merit. But we still lack a definitive explanation for the rise in allergies at this point. The true reason is likely a combination of our overly sterile environments, constant exposure to the toxins in our increasingly polluted world, our habit of eating unhealthy foods, and our overly stressful lives that ultimately subtract from our good health.

The explanations surrounding allergies may be in part theoretical, but the lifestyle changes you can use to prevent and treat allergies—the changes I've seen make such an amazing difference in my patients, and the ones I will give you in the chapters that follow—are not. They are based on sound medical research, and even better, they are achievable by everyone. So let the ultimate seasonal allergy solution—and your journey to better health—begin.

Carlo's Story

Before seeing Dr. Psenka for his allergies, Carlo, a 32-year-old hairstylist, couldn't be near his cat without developing an itchy neck, itchy eyes, sneezing, and shortness of breath. "I am very allergic to cats," he says.

Carlo tried taking Benadryl to control his symptoms. "But I didn't like how I felt when I took it," he says. Not wanting to give up his pet, Carlo decided to see Dr. Psenka—and today he is very happy he did.

In the middle of his treatment with Dr. Psenka's all-natural plan, Carlo started noticing a marked improvement in his allergy. "When I am around the cat, even when he is sitting right next to me on the couch, I am not sneezing or itching nearly as much as I was, if at all," he says.

Carlo has been vegan since 2010, so his eating habits didn't change much under Dr. Psenka's guidance. But the sublingual immunotherapy (SLIT) Dr. Psenka prescribed has made a big difference. "I wish I would have known about SLIT earlier," he says.

He has also lost a few pounds. "Overall, I've been feeling much better since starting the treatment," Carlo says. And because he doesn't worry about the cat being around, Carlo says his stress level has gone down.

Overall, after seeing his cat allergy clear up right before his eyes, Carlo says he would refer anyone with seasonal or other allergies to Dr. Psenka.

2 What's Causing Your Allergies

THE FIRST RECORDED ALLERGY appeared in an ancient Egyptian publication in 3500 BC. Fast-forward a few thousand years to 1906, when an Austrian pediatrician named Clemens von Pirquet noticed some odd symptoms in his patients that he couldn't attribute to any particular disease. He named these symptoms "allergy," which is derived from two Greek words: *allos,* meaning "other," and *ergon,* meaning "reaction."

Despite knowing of their existence for literally thousands of years, modern medicine hasn't been able to eradicate allergies. In fact, they're more prevalent than ever. Study after study clearly shows that more and more people are allergic to more and more things. What's not so clear, however, are the reasons *why* people throughout the world—especially those in developing nations—are so much more allergic than they were only decades ago.

THEORIES BEHIND THE RISE IN ALLERGIES: A DETAILED LOOK

In Chapter 1, you got an overview of some of the theories on what's driving the increase in allergies, including pollution, the hygiene hypothesis, unhealthy diets, poor lifestyle choices, and climate change. In this chapter, you'll get more comprehensive information on the science fueling these theories.

Whether or not you choose to support these theories, one theme is common throughout: the rapid shift away from the conditions in which our human species evolved. Consider this: For the grand majority of human evolution, our diets were much different than they are today. Our ancestors weren't exposed to the levels of synthetic and toxic chemicals that we are today. They also had *a lot* less stress and anxiety. Quite simply, the human body was not designed to run efficiently in the manner most humans do today—with high levels of anxiety combined with a nutritionally deficient diet.

Because of the chemicals we ingest, the anxiety we feel, our poor nutritional status, and the unnatural shields we put around ourselves (think antibacterial soaps and hand sanitizers), our bodies have become confused, overwhelmed, and—as a result—chronically inflamed. Many of the diseases plaguing people today—heart disease, cancer, and diabetes, just to name a few—are largely diseases of lifestyle and are promoted by exaggerated levels of inflammation.

The inflammatory process is a trigger for allergies, as well. In fact, allergies and inflammation share some of the same chemical messaging pathways within your body. When your body is chronically in a state of heightened inflammation, your immune system can become agitated and hyperreactive, promoting an amplified allergic response to new antigen exposures, potentially even developing an allergy to a substance that would not have elicited this response if the inflammation wasn't present.

This explanation aside, the scientific theories behind an increase in allergies may help you better understand the possible reasons for the increased potential for inflammation in your body and your potential to experience allergy symptoms. Here's a more detailed look at these theories.

Pollution

As mentioned in Chapter 1, pollution may be the single largest contributor to the increase in allergies. Over the past 25 years, researchers have become increasingly more interested in the effects of air pollution on health, and they've uncovered some compelling links between pollution and increases in both allergies and asthma.[1]

One study published in the *Journal of Allergy and Clinical Immunology*, for example, found that children exposed to high levels of air pollution as infants were about two times more likely to develop respiratory and food allergies later in life.[2,3]

The most common air pollutants—ozone, sulfur dioxide, and nitrogen dioxide—are proven hazards to people with allergies and asthma. Not only do these pollutants reduce lung function but also they irritate the airways and aggravate established allergy symptoms.[4]

Other pollutants, called diesel exhaust particles (DEPs), actually have the power to elicit allergic reactions, and there are a few reasons why. For one, DEPs are very tiny; more than 80 percent are classified as "ultrafine." Due to their small size, you can easily inhale them deeply into your lungs. Diesel exhaust also seems to spark allergies by stimulating your body's production of immunoglobulin E (IgE), one of the antibodies produced by your immune system in response to allergens. (IgE is what triggers the release of histamine and other chemicals that ultimately cause allergic symptoms).[5] Through the actions of IgE, DEPs can make allergens more powerful by enhancing a process called *mast cell granulation*, through which mast cells release histamine. Because of this, pollens in areas heavily polluted with DEPs may have more allergic potential than pollens floating in areas with less air pollution.[6]

One study found that DEPs can make an allergen 18 times more potent when it crosses the lung membranes—and this is at levels that are considered within the range of acceptable for health in the United States. In cities like Phoenix and Los Angeles, which have high pollution rates, people breathe in diesel pollution every day, and it is making their allergies nearly 20 times more severe.[7]

Air pollution containing DEPs is worst in industrialized, heavily populated areas. Research shows that the more developed a nation, the higher its levels of these pollutants and the higher its allergy rates. Hay fever was rare in Japan before World War II, for example.

But today, as the country has become more industrialized, hay fever is now common, especially in people who live near cities and high-ways.[8] North America and Europe also have much bigger allergy problems than third-world countries, and within these developed nations, people who live in cities have higher rates of allergy symptoms than those who live in more agrarian areas.[9] So clearly cities, and all the pollution they produce, are a big part of the problem.

Beyond DEP and other outdoor pollutants, the definition of pollution also includes indoor toxins. The additives and preservatives in food, the chemicals (such as parabens and methylparabens) in toothpaste and personal-care products, and the carcinogens in second-hand smoke can be just as health-damaging as the environmental pollutants produced by cars and factories.

The worst indoor pollutant is tobacco smoke; it has been shown to make allergy and asthma symptoms worse in those who are exposed to it. Pregnant mothers who smoke are more likely to have children with allergic eczema. Additionally, kids who have one or more smoking parents are at a higher risk for respiratory illnesses such as asthma, bronchitis, and chronic cough.[10]

Even if you don't smoke, but you live with a smoker—or if you're just casually exposed—you can breathe in enough toxins from cigarettes to make you sick. The particles in tobacco smoke stick to clothing and hair, producing that smoker smell. Keep in mind that if you can smell cigarette smoke, either in the air or on someone, you're breathing in its toxins.[11]

Besides the obvious cigarette smoke, there's a host of other health-detracting pollutants hiding inside our homes. If you can smell that new carpeting when you walk into your bedroom, for example, you are slowly poisoning yourself as you breathe it in at night. If you smell the "ocean breeze" coming out of a plug-in air freshener, the story's the same. (This pleasant smell can hide one or more of a variety of unhealthy chemicals, including alcohols, esters, formaldehyde, limonene, and petroleum distillates.) To make matters worse, many houses are tightly sealed these days, making it impossible for toxins to escape they way they do in older homes. This leads to an unhealthy toxic buildup.

In addition to smaller-scale indoor pollution troubles, there's something called sick building syndrome. This is a situation in which occupants of a building become ill, and the illness seems to be correlated with time spent in the building but no specific illness or cause can be identified. People affected may experience a variety of symptoms, including headaches, dizziness, cough, irritated throats, and breathing problems. I recently met a man in his forties who had been a professional bodybuilder who never smoked or drank and who ate a very healthy diet. He came into my office complaining of a recent onset of headaches, cough, and poor sleep. I discovered that he had recently rented a new home and his symptoms had developed within just a few weeks of moving in. He has no other known health problems, and it is likely his new living space is making him ill.

The take-home message is that when it comes to pollution and allergy risk, both outdoor and indoor pollutants are a threat.

The Hygiene Hypothesis

According to the hygiene hypothesis, a person's immune system needs to "toughen up" early in life by being exposed to a variety of antigens (microbes, bacteria, dander, etc.). In the past, most children lived in caves or ran around with animals on farms, which allowed their immune systems to develop in an environment filled with dust, dander, pollens, and so on. As a result of this high level of exposure to many different things in the environment, a person's immune system was able to develop a tolerance to many things. In a sense, it learned that it didn't need to react to everything it was exposed to. But today, kids in first-world countries grow up in ultra-clean environments full of antibacterial soaps and bleach wipes. Granted, these modern advances in cleanliness have saved many people from bouts of the common cold and even some deadly infections. But the trade-off comes in the form of confused, underexposed, hyperreactive immune systems that trigger allergic responses to otherwise innocent substances around us.[12]

There's research to support the hygiene hypothesis. In a study done at Brigham and Women's Hospital in Boston and published online in the journal *Science* in 2012, scientists tested the theory by comparing "germ-free mice," or mice lacking bacteria or any other microbes, to mice living in a normal environment, complete with normal bacteria and microbes. The researchers uncovered a few important findings. For one, they found that the germ-free mice had inflammation in their lungs and colons that looked like asthma and colitis. This inflammation was caused by abnormal activity of a special class of immune cells previously linked to both asthma and colitis in mice and humans. Second, the researchers found that when they introduced microbes to the germ-free mice during the first few weeks of their lives, those mice developed normal immune systems and were able to prevent disease. This effect was not seen if researchers introduced the microbes to the mice later during their adult years. Therefore, the study results show that microbe exposure is important early in life and can provide long-lasting protection, which is what the hygiene hypothesis predicts.[13]

I agree with the hygiene hypothesis in that I do think our overly sterile society contributes to increasing allergies. But I also think that timing is important, with "the earlier, the better" being a good motto for bolstering your immune system.

Here's how I look at it: When your mother was pregnant with you, you were in a nice, protected environment. A few of mom's microbes may have gotten into your environment via the cord blood, but for the most part, it was pretty sterile in there. Then all of a sudden, you came flying out into the world. Even before the moment you left your mother's body, you were exposed to new microbes. As you traveled through your mother's birth canal, you encountered all kinds of beneficial and sometimes pathogenic bacteria and yeasts. Then you met all of the microbes flying around in the delivery room air. Although sterile by medical standards, the doctor and nurse were also covered with bacteria. Nature intended for infants to meet all of these new microbes from the day they were born. And this onslaught of exposure is not just limited to newborns, but continues as a child ages. Consider how often young children put things into their mouths. All of this exposure helps to develop and teach your immune system how to operate. In our society today, we're fairly sheltered and germaphobic, so our exposure is pretty limited compared to that of our ancestors.

Compare that to most of our evolution, where people lived out-side and rolled around in the dirt—especially as children—and encountered microbes and pollens constantly. In these "dirtier" times, the body saw lots of different germs, so the immune system developed a tolerance to them. But today, we've eliminated so many background allergens and microbes that when they do show up, your immune system doesn't quite know how to react.

I believe exposure to background microbes is *most* important during the first 5 years of life, when your immune system is feeling out the world and trying to adjust. Consider how many small children pick their noses and taste it, despite their parents' attempts to stop them. Nearly every small child seems to do it, and nobody has to show them how; it just happens. What children find in their noses is dried mucus, which has trapped airborne particles such as dust and microbes. So, in essence, they are inoculating themselves.

In addition to nose-picking, another favorite topic among children—poop—may help bolster the immune system against allergies as well. One theory links low exposure to endotoxins, which consist of a family of molecules called lipopolysaccharides (LPS), with higher rates of allergies. LPSs are molecules on the outer membrane of gram-negative bacteria. Kids who live on farms or around animals get exposed to these endotoxins, which are con-tained in feces and which seem to then offer protection against allergies. Research has shown that children with the highest con-centration of endotoxins in their mattress dust have the lowest rates of hay fever, asthma, and allergen sensitivity. Similarly, kids who live in rural areas in southern Germany and Switzerland—where samples from kitchen floors and mattresses are teeming with endotoxins—have relatively low allergy rates.[14]

Fewer childhood infections may also be at play in rising allergy rates. Studies from a few different countries show that exposure to viral infections early in life may be protective against allergies later on. Young kids who are frequently around other sick kids—either older siblings or classmates in daycare—have lower rates of allergies and asthma once they reach school age. Chil-dren who have suffered through an actual measles infection have half the rate of dust mite allergies as kids protected by the measles vaccine. Another interesting fact is that babies born preterm, which is often the result of a bacterial infection in the mother,[15] tend to have lower rates of eczema than full-term babies, which may mean that the bacteria exposure they got so early in life helped protect them against skin allergies later on.[16]

In addition to a lack of infections, another element to the hygiene hypothesis is our use—or overuse—of antibiotics to combat these infections. It's true—antibiotics have saved many lives since they were first developed in 1929.[17] But we use them far too much. Some doctors in this country hand out antibiotic prescriptions to every desiring individual who walks in, regardless of whether or not the prescription is medically indicated. The problem with antibiotics is that, in addition to killing potentially deadly bacteria, they also kill the "good guys"—the probiotics, which are microbes that hang out in your gastrointestinal system and help your immune system fight off invaders. Because disease-causing bacteria have been exposed to antibiotics so often, they are developing a resistance to these drugs and creating new "superbugs" that antibiotics can't eradicate.[18]

There are some researchers who support the hygiene hypothesis when it comes to explaining the rise of allergies, and there are others who do not.[19] I agree with the notion that we are way too sterile. There needs to be a balance between healthy living and clean living. In some places, it's prudent to use hand sanitizer—in public restrooms, for example. But scrubbing down with the stuff every 15 minutes is likely taking it too far. We all need to get a little dirty now and then. And we need to let our kids get a little dirty now and then as well. So don't be afraid to let your kids or grandkids play in the dirt—both for the sake of their happiness and for their eventual immunity.

The Standard American Diet

As more people move away from farms and into cities, not only are they encountering fewer endotoxins but also they're eating fewer fresh foods. Out of sight, out of mind.[20] And in place of these nutrient- and antioxidant-rich fruits and vegetables, many people eat the Standard American Diet (SAD).

Sad but true, the Standard American Diet is *horrible*. It's terribly low in nutrients and high in sugar, trans fats, processed ingredients, and other chemicals that can promote inflammation in your body and potentially lead to higher levels of allergies.[21] Here are some of the most important elements (and pitfalls) of the SAD when it comes to allergy risk and overall health.

- **Omega-3 Essential Fatty Acids.** One thing that's well established in the health community is the importance of the right balance between omega-3 and omega-6 fatty acids in the diet. Omega-3 fatty acids are polyunsaturated fatty acids. Your body needs these omega-3s for important functions, and because they fight inflammation, they also offer protection against heart disease, cancer, and other diseases. Your body can't make omega-3s on its own (hence their "essential" designation), so you must get them from food. Good sources include oily fish, walnuts, some green vegetables (such as spinach and Brussels sprouts), and soybean and flaxseed oils.[22]

  Omega-6 fatty acids are also polyunsaturated fatty acids that your body gets from food. Food sources of omega-6s include soybean, safflower, corn, cottonseed oils, and red meat.[23] The problem with omega-6 fatty acids is that they are the backbone of *pro*inflammatory cytokines. In other words, they increase inflammation in your body. Omega-6s aren't bad in and of themselves, but when you eat them out of proportion to omega-3s, they can have bad effects. Most experts suggest eating a 1:1 or 1:2 ratio of omega-6s to omega-3s. Too great a proportion of omega-6s can lead to increased inflammation and all of the negativity and allergy risk that goes along with it.

  To illustrate the importance of a good omega-6 to omega-3 ratio, researchers at the American Society for Biochemistry and Molecular Biology fed 27 healthy adults a diet that provided the goal 2:1 ratio of omega-6 to omega-3 fatty acids for 5 weeks. After 5 weeks of eating this way, they found that the levels of key genes that promote inflammation were significantly lower than in people eating a normal American diet. The researchers also found that levels of a signaling gene for a protein called Pl3K—which is important for autoimmune and allergic reactions—were markedly lower in the people eating the higher omega-6 to omega-3 ratio as well.[24]

- **Sugar.** Most Americans eat massive amounts of sugar. In fact, according to the American Heart Association, the average American consumes more than twice the amount of recommended sugar—about 22.2 teaspoons, or 355 calories from sugar—per day. (The recommendation is 100 calories from sugar per day for women and 150 calories for men.[25])

  Sugar is tough to avoid. It is seemingly in everything these days, from the obvious sources like soda and candy to the sneakier ones like pasta sauce and energy bars. The problem with sugar is that, over time, large quantities of it can damage your pancreas and inflame your body.[26] I am also seeing nonalcoholic fatty liver disease in my practice more and more commonly. As the name implies, this condition causes fat marbling in the liver that is sometimes accompanied by metabolic dysregulation and impaired liver function. Eating too much fat and sugar contributes to nonalcoholic fatty liver disease, which in its most severe form can cause a person's liver to fail.

  As if sugar in its pure form weren't bad enough, the substitutes people use for sugar may be even worse. The coal tar derivative aspartame, for example, turns into formaldehyde in your brain. In fact, it is suspected that many health problems are caused by aspartame, including an imbalance in the antioxidant/pro-oxidant status in the brain.[27] Imbalances in certain brain antioxidants have been linked to Alzheimer's disease and other age-related diseases.[28]

- **Processed foods.** Sure, they're convenient. You can pop a frozen block of food in the microwave and have a hot meal in 3 minutes. But this convenience comes at a big health cost. I have to say, I think processed foods are the absolute worst foods people can eat. For one, they contain all sorts of chemicals meant to increase their shelf life and make them taste better, including sulfites, monosodium glutamate (MSG), and nitrites. These additives can cause allergic reactions, and they also contribute to inflammation and a higher risk of allergies.[29] Some of the chemicals added to processed foods will absolutely astound you. Recently, it has come to light that a major fast-food company serves bread that contains a chemical used to make yoga mats.[30]

Sulfites, found in wine, dried fruits, and frozen potatoes (among other foods), cause mild to life-threatening reactions in about 5 percent of people with asthma. Butylated hydroxytoluene (BHT), an additive found in some cereals and grain products, has been linked to chronic hives and other reactions. Tartrazine, a dye used in candy, desserts, salad dressings, beverages, and processed cheese, has been shown to cause hives and swelling. Nitrites in hot dogs, bacon, and other processed meats and fish can cause headaches and hives. MSG can cause Chinese restaurant syndrome—headache, chest tightness, nausea, and diarrhea.[31] It's not just synthetic food chemicals that cause problems. While being natural, red (carmine) and yellow (annatto) food colorings have been linked to the serious, potentially deadly allergic reaction anaphylaxis.[32]

Processed foods are also loaded with trans fats—by far the worst fat type. Also known as trans fatty acids or partially hydrogenated oils, trans fats are man-made fats created by adding hydrogen to liquid vegetable oil to make it solid.[33] These trans fats do all sorts of terrible things in your body, including promoting allergy and asthma. In a 2011 study published in the *Journal of Allergy and Clinical Immunology,* nonobese asthmatic individuals ate three types of meals—a low-fat meal, a high-fat meal, and a high–trans fatty acid meal. Researchers then measured their airway inflammation 4 hours after they finished eating each meal. The results: Asthma sufferers were more likely to have airway inflammation after the high-fat meals, and that airway inflammation was significantly worse after the high–trans fat meal than it was after the trans fat–free meal.[34]

- **Lack of nutrients.** In addition to all of the unhealthy elements it provides, a lot of what is so bad about the SAD is what it lacks in terms of basic nutrition. Much of the American diet is taken up by processed foods and sugar, so there's not much room left for the nutrients your body needs to protect itself. If you eat the SAD, you don't get the necessary vitamins, minerals, and antioxidants from fresh fruits and vegetables and lean meats, so you lack the resources you need to fend off allergies and other conditions.

DIET IN PREGNANCY

The role of diet in expectant mothers is extremely important, but the advice on what pregnant women should or shouldn't be eating isn't always very clear (see "The Ever-Changing Dietary Guidelines for Expectant Mothers" on page 26). There are all sorts of things that can happen to a baby in utero to predetermine his or her allergic profile later in life. (As I mentioned before, this book is for adults, but because so many of the things that can set people up for a lifetime of allergies happen in childhood, I want to educate parents to be aware of how they can minimize allergic risk in their children.)

Some foods and ingredients seem to be protective against future allergies in the developing fetus, and other foods and ingredients appear to be potentially harmful. In a 2007 German study published in the *American Journal of Clinical Nutrition*, researchers looked at the diets of 2,541 pregnant women during their last 4 weeks of pregnancy and then analyzed their children for allergies when they reached age 2.[35]

Interestingly, the researchers found that women who ate a lot of margarine and vegetable oils were more likely to have kids with eczema. On the other hand, those who ate plenty of fish were *less* likely to have kids with eczema. Pregnant moms who ate a lot of

The Ever-Changing Dietary Guidelines for Expectant Mothers

When it comes to what expectant mothers should eat and what they should avoid during pregnancy, the advice has been all over the map. Back in 2000, the American Academy of Pediatrics released guidelines suggesting that pregnant women should avoid potentially allergenic foods, use only soy-based formula, and wait to give their babies solid foods until they were at least 6 months old. If they had kids who were at risk for allergies, breast-feeding moms were advised to avoid eggs, fish, peanuts, tree nuts, and milk.[36]

But times have changed. The latest study, published in the December 2013 issue of the *Journal of the American Medical Association*, tells women to eat one of the most allergenic foods—peanuts—without restraint. The study looked at the eating habits of 8,200 pregnant women and found that expectant mothers who ate the most peanuts or tree nuts—five servings or more a week—had the lowest risk of having a child who was allergic to these nuts. In fact, these peanut-eating moms were 69 percent less likely to have a child with nut allergies than the mothers who ate one or fewer servings of peanuts a month while they were pregnant. The explanation: Early nut exposure may protect kids from developing a nut allergy.[37]

As a naturopathic doctor, I tend to take a more conservative stance when it comes to diet during pregnancy and the food introduction schedule once a baby is born. There's a high potential for allergies to eggs, bananas, avocados, tropical fruits, and nuts, so I think parents should hold off on giving their kids these foods until they are a little older. Start with bland foods with a lower allergenic potential and work your way into more complex foods.

citrus fruits and celery were more likely to have children with allergies to foods. And women who ate a lot of deep-fried vegetable fat, raw sweet peppers, and citrus fruits were more likely to have kids with respiratory allergies. Some of these findings parallel the theory regarding omega-3 versus omega-6 fatty acids. Eating margarine, which is made from proinflammatory omega-6 fatty acids, increased allergy risk in offspring; eating oily fish, which is rich in anti-inflammatory omega-3s, was protective.[38]

Another offender, both in terms of allergy risk and overall health, is artificial sweetener. If a mom-to-be drinks a lot of diet beverages, studies show that her child is more likely to develop allergies. A 2013 study published in the scientific journal *PLOS ONE* looked at the relationship between pregnant mothers' consumption of artificially sweetened beverages and their children's rates of asthma and allergic rhinitis at 18 months and 7 years of age. After looking at 60,466 pregnant women and their intake of artificially sweetened drinks, researchers found that the moms who drank diet drinks were 1.23 times more likely to have children with asthma at 18 months and 1.3 times more likely to have children who developed allergic rhinitis in the first 7 years of life than those who abstained.[39]

Vitamin D Deficiency

Vitamin D deficiency is quickly becoming recognized as a major health problem. Vitamin D is a fat-soluble vitamin responsible for many different actions in the human body, from maintaining proper immune function to inhibiting depression and building healthy teeth and bones. Vitamin D deficiency is also a risk factor for many chronic diseases and conditions, including cancer, heart disease, diabetes, and allergies.[40]

I frequently see vitamin D deficiency in my patients. Because this vitamin is so important, I have begun testing nearly all of my patients to assess their vitamin D levels. Most of the time, I find that patients are deficient, and some have levels that are very low. To give you an idea, the normal reference range for blood levels of vitamin D_3 is 30 to 100 ng/mL in the blood (depending on the laboratory). I've seen levels as low as 9, and I routinely see numbers less than 20. These low levels can put you at a greater risk for many different health problems, in addition to increasing your allergic potential.

Why are so many people deficient in vitamin D? Perhaps the biggest reason is lack of sunlight. Your body needs sunlight to make vitamin D. But these days, we spend most of our time indoors basking in the glow of computer screens instead of outdoors basking in the sun's rays. When we do venture outside, most of us coat ourselves with sunscreen.[41] As a result, we're not getting anywhere near the recommended daily allowance (RDA) of 800 international units (IU) of vitamin D per day. To reach this amount, you would have to expose 30 percent of your body to the sun at a moderate latitude for 30 minutes per day. Unless you work as a lifeguard, this just isn't practical. Most research says that 800 IU is much lower than what we actually need, anyway. Additionally, most Americans' diets don't include enough of the foods that are good sources of vitamin D, such as fish-liver oil, sardines, and shrimp. (Fortified foods like milk contain roughly 100 IU per 1-cup serving, which is not enough.)

Research substantiates the link between low vitamin D and increased allergy risk. A recent study published in the journal *Annals of Allergy, Asthma, and Immunology* found a link between low vitamin D levels and risk for allergic rhinitis in Korean adults.[42] And an earlier study published in *Allergy and Asthma Proceedings* looked at data from the National Health and Nutrition Examination Survey 2005–2006, done by the Centers for Disease Control and Prevention National Center for Health Statistics. The study found that people with vitamin D deficiency were more likely to suffer from allergies, including specific allergy symptoms like rashes, sneezing, and sinus infections.[43]

You can try to boost your vitamin D levels by eating D-rich foods—egg yolks, fortified milk, and fish-liver oils—or by taking supplements. And I recommend having your levels tested as part of your yearly comprehensive health exam (along with other vitamin and mineral levels and markers of nutrition and overall health, including omega-3 fatty acids) to see where you stand.

Stress

I think diet is the most important part of a healthy lifestyle. The second most important part is your level of stress. People are *way* too stressed-out these days. Our bodies are not designed for the weeks-to-months-on-end of stress and anxiety we put them through. We're not meant to be attached to cell phones constantly, with deadlines and money troubles dangling over our heads. Instead, as a species, we were originally designed to experience short bursts of anxiety—caused by, say, a wolf at the mouth of our cave—followed by much longer stretches spent picking berries or fetching water from the river. Our fight-or-flight response, as it is called, was designed for short responses to acute problems—for instance, until you escaped from the wolf. But these days, the wolf (let's call it a wolf in dysfunctional lifestyle's clothing) never really goes away, so we're in this unhealthy, high-adrenaline mode most of the time.

Let me explain how stress takes its toll. On the outside, stress looks like a frantic person racing from place to place, coffee in hand. On the inside, stress looks like an increasingly exhausted adrenal gland being asked to continuously secrete hormones in response to the perceived emergency. These hormones, often referred to as the fight-or-flight hormones, are named epinephrine and norepineph-rine. Your body's response doesn't really differentiate between the stress of having several must-be-met work deadlines, a parent-teacher conference, and 150 unchecked emails and the stress of a large predator trying to eat you; your stress response is essentially the same.

Your adrenal glands fire off the fight-or-flight hormones, which shift your body into a state of high alert. When your body is reacting this way, it directs all available resources to the matter at hand. Non-essential activities take a backseat. For example, gastrointestinal function is inhibited during the fight-or-flight response, because properly absorbing that last meal isn't going to save you. On the other hand, increases in heart rate and respiration, as well as having more avail-able sugar in your bloodstream, may provide you with the energy and oxygen to successfully fight off or run away from the danger.

To remain in this heightened, stressed-out state requires a lot of bodily resources. Eventually, your adrenal gland's ability to keep up the production of hormones can run dry, and when it does, your body has to look for energy in other places. Your thyroid gland may be able to keep things going temporarily, but eventually it also

becomes unable to meet your body's demands. Excitatory neurotransmitters may then be called to duty, providing your depleted
and exhausted body with a final crutch for meeting its energy
requirements. It is at this point that a person complains of being
completely exhausted but also of suffering from insomnia because
his or her brain can't "shut off" due to the excitatory neurotransmitters. Over time, this extended fight-or-flight mode takes a toll on
your entire body.

Think of it as being like driving your Ferrari at 190 miles per
hour with no oil in the engine. Eventually, the engine will blow. I see
people in this state in my practice far too often. The good news is,
there are things people can do to get back on track. We will explore
these tactics later in this book.

Focusing back on allergies, the hormone cortisol, which has
been shown to be one of the biomarkers of stress and which is also
secreted via your adrenal gland, can alter the functioning of your
immune system, possibly making you more sensitive to allergens.
Cortisol has also been correlated with specific types of allergic diseases, including atopic dermatitis.[44]

Research also supports the link between allergies and stress. A
study published in the journal *Psychosomatic Medicine* found a correlation between a person's score on the Minnesota Multiphasic Personality Inventory distress-related scale, a test that measures stress
levels resulting from previous trauma, and their reactivity in
response to an allergen.[45]

A newer study done at Ohio State University and published in
the journal *Psychoneuroendocrinology* found that even low levels of
stress and anxiety made people more sensitive to common allergens.
They also found that the stress lingered and made the second day
of an allergy attack even worse.[46] Researchers looked at 28 men and
women with a history of hay fever and seasonal allergies. They
started by asking the participants to complete a psychological ques-
tionnaire to determine their baseline anxiety levels. Then half of the
participants performed a low-stress task—reading aloud from a
magazine—while the other half had to give a 10-minute speech in
front of a panel of evaluators and then watch their videotaped per-
formances. After their tasks, participants took a skin prick test to

measure their response to an allergen. Researchers found that those with higher baseline anxiety had higher inflammatory responses to allergy tests, especially those who had to perform the high-stress speech. The participants with higher baseline anxiety who performed the speech task had continued inflammation the next day, which shows that stress and anxiety can also prolong allergic reactions.[47]

How and why did stress and anxiety combine to make allergies worse and lingering? The study authors propose that stress hormones such as cortisol might stimulate IgE, the protein that causes allergic reactions.[48]

Cortisol is indeed an important stress hormone, and I believe it contributes to allergies. However, it is not the only stress hormone (I mentioned epinephrine and norepinephrine as well), nor is it the only chemical in your body that can promote an allergic predisposition. Inflammatory cytokines and interleukins, which we will explore, have an influence, as well.

Climate Change

Scientists have given us lots of reasons to fear climate change and global warming, and now we have yet another: increased risk of allergies. By burning oil, coal, and other fossil fuels, industry has released tons of carbon dioxide into the atmosphere. People may not like the effects of all this carbon dioxide, but plants do; carbon dioxide helps them to grow faster and taller, and as a result, to produce more pollen. More pollen flying through the air equals more pollen in our lungs—and more sniffles, sneezes, and watery eyes in people with seasonal allergies.[49]

Aside from increasing the pollen count, a warmer temperature in and of itself can also make allergies worse. High summertime ozone levels can trigger reactions like chest pain, congestion, and throat irritation, and it can make it harder for all people, especially allergy and asthma sufferers, to breathe. (Depending on where in the country you live, you've probably seen "poor air quality" or "stay indoors" warnings from your local weatherman when things get particularly hot and sticky outside.) High temperatures and humidity during the summer months also create a breeding ground for indoor fungi and molds.[50]

Large fluctuations in temperature also seem to play a role. The greater the variation in temperature in a single day (called diurnal temperature range, or DTR), the more likely an asthma sufferer is to experience a flare. A 2014 Australian study published in the *Annals of Allergy, Asthma, and Immunology* found that children with asthma who were exposed to unstable weather and a greater DTR had worse lung function and more respiratory symptoms than those who were exposed to more stable daily temps.[51]

Another issue related to climate change is globalization. Not only are we changing the climate of our world, but that world is also getting smaller. People from all over the globe are coming to the United States, and with them they're bringing foreign diets and exotic products, which we take into our stores and homes. On the one hand, these new people and products are wonderful for our culture, making it more rich and diverse. On the other hand, the new products are changing our environment and possibly contributing to allergies. Remember my young patient from Chapter 1 who was allergic to the bloodworms he fed his Siamese fighting fish? His allergy provides good support for the globalization explanation for increasing allergies. We have exposure to things we never previously saw.[52] One hundred years ago, the boy would not have had access to a Siamese fighting fish, much less to bloodworms to give the pet as food.

We also bring outside things into our homes to make our living rooms more pleasant and homey. Houseplants make good decorating pieces and can help clean indoor air, but they can also change your indoor environment and promote allergies. A Belgian study found that more than 75 percent of people with hay fever are allergic to at least one common houseplant. The reason may not just be the sap on these plants, which gets into the air and into your airways; it may be that these "common" houseplants are actually pretty foreign to your immune system. The study showed ficus, yucca, ivy, and palm tree were most likely to cause sniffles and sneezes.[53]

From houseplants to hygiene, there are many theories surrounding the problem of increasing allergies, all of which share a common theme: The shift away from the lifestyle and environments in which we evolved. Within this shift, there is stress, poor diet and lifestyle choices, and exposure to environmental toxins. It's not a single thing causing allergies to rise, but a combination of factors that go along with our industrialized world.

Because there is no single allergy cause, there is also no single allergy treatment or medication. We need to get away from quick-fix drugs and come at the complex problem of allergy relief from all angles, by adopting a healthy lifestyle in all facets of our lives.

3 What's Happening Behind the Sneezes: The Physiology of Allergies

WHEN I THINK OF THE PHYSIOLOGY OF ALLERGIES, a particular patient comes to mind. Years ago, I met a young, college-age woman who had been suffering from a severe skin rash for many years. It would appear on her legs, arms, or face and seemed to come and go for no particular reason. She had tried all kinds of medications, seen several dermatologists, and even tried an exhaustive number of home remedies, but to no avail.

She was a great kid, and I could tell that having this condition was really bothering her. I suggested we do some food allergy and sensitivity testing to see if we could determine whether she had any issues with her diet, as there is an interesting correlation between the health of your gastrointestinal (GI) system and the health of your skin. If people suffer from some sort of GI disturbance, whether it be chronic diarrhea, constipation, or gas and bloating, addressing the underlying causes of these problems may help to clear up skin problems.

When I see a patient with a skin complaint, one of my first thoughts is to consider a food allergy or intolerance. As my college student with the skin rash proved, food allergies or sensitivities are often to blame. When this patient's testing came back, we discovered that she did in fact have several food allergies. Like most people with food allergies, she knew that certain foods caused her to experience GI issues, and the test results showed that she did have allergies to some of these suspect foods. We developed a diet plan that helped her avoid the foods that her lab results had shown she had an allergy. Her skin gradually cleared and her rash became less and less severe. Today, the rash is resolved most of the time and only comes back when she eats the foods she knows will cause problems. And now, when it does come back, it is generally short-lived and much less severe.

This girl's experience illustrates that allergies are not simply localized reactions that affect only one area of your body. My patient's skin reaction was not limited to just her skin or her gastrointestinal tract; instead, it resulted from a complex chain of events that affected her inside and out.

Whether you suffer from a pesky, embarrassing rash like my patient or your respiratory allergies are so bad that you're forced to stay inside for the entire spring season, you would probably be happy if your allergy symptoms went away. When it comes to allergies, the first step in winning the war is knowing your enemy. To best rid yourself of allergies once and for all, you first have to understand how they operate.

ALLERGIES 101: A CRASH COURSE IN THE PHYSIOLOGY

Simply put, allergies are hypersensitivity disorders of the immune system. Allergic reactions occur when a person's immune system reacts to normally harmless substances in their environment. The substance that triggers the allergic reaction is called an allergen. An allergen is a type of antigen, and antigens are substances capable of inducing an antibody response by the immune system. (Antibodies are proteins that the immune system produces in response to a foreign substance, or antigen.)

In people with allergies, the immune system becomes overreactive,

The Relationship Between Gastrointestinal Health and Skin Health

It should come as no surprise that the digestive system is one of the most important systems in your body, and it has an impact on many other systems in your body.

Conventional medicine has linked skin health to gastrointestinal health. In a 2013 study done at the University of Alberta, researchers looked at the connection between gastrointestinal diseases and dermatologic symptoms. They found a connection between skin manifestations and more than 30 different gastrointestinal diseases, including pancreatitis, hepatitis, and Crohn's disease.[1]

Because of the importance the naturopathic community places on digestive health, naturopathic doctors are well versed in treating digestive disorders such as irritable bowel syndrome, autoimmune diseases, and food allergies as well as in recognizing the connection between digestive upset and other health problems.

One particularly strong connection is between the gastrointestinal system and the skin. Many times, when a patient has a skin problem, such as acne or a rash, that person turns out to have a problem related to his or her GI tract, and it's often a sensitivity to a food.

A common food sensitivity that can manifest as skin problems is gluten or wheat intolerance. Wheat gluten, a type of protein found in pastas, breads, cereals, and other wheat products, is one of the most common causes of inflammation in the GI system, and it can lead to rashes and other types of skin irritation. Other symptoms of gluten sensitivity include low energy and weight gain or loss.

so in addition to viruses, bacteria, and other microbes that pose a genuine threat, it attacks innocent substances in its environment—allergens. Through a fairly complex process that we will explore in more detail below, the misguided immune system launches an attack against allergens and unleashes some unpleasant—and in some cases, potentially life-threatening—allergy symptoms.[2]

As we learned in Chapter 1, allergies can result from something as unlikely as bloodworms or as common as pollens, animal dander, house dust, dust mites, molds, medications, and foods such as nuts, milk, eggs, and fish. Reactions to these allergens may take a variety of different forms in your body, including:[3]

1. *Respiratory symptoms,* which can range from a mild runny or stuffy nose to severe asthma attacks with sneezing, coughing, and wheezing.
2. *Skin symptoms,* which may take the form of rashes (hives), swelling in the mouth, oral itching, facial swelling, or redness.
3. *Gastrointestinal symptoms,* which can show up as nausea, vomiting, cramps, diarrhea, or constipation.
4. *Cardiovascular symptoms,* which may leave you feeling lightheaded and faint.
5. *Anaphylaxis,* which is a severe and sometimes fatal reaction involving difficulty breathing, lowered blood pressure, constriction of airways, and loss of consciousness. (This is usually the result of a food or chemical allergy.)

These symptoms are what a person could experience when having an allergic reaction. Symptoms such as sneezing, blowing your nose, or scratching your itchy hives are the result of an extremely complex set of reactions happening within your body.

These reactions begin innocently enough. For instance, you may take a deep breath and lay your head down on your pillow. What you don't know is that a tiny dust mite has walked across your pillow, shedding a microscopic particle along the way: the allergen. Your deep breath causes you to inhale the dust mite allergen, where it is carried into the mucous membranes of your mouth, nose, or lungs. Once there, the allergen is found by an immune cell called an antigen-presenting cell. This antigen-presenting cell then carries the dust mite allergen to the nearest lymph nodes, where it is shown to the T cells. The T cells react to the dust mite allergen by releasing proinflammatory chemicals, which prompt another type of immune cell, the B cells, to begin producing an antibody called immunoglobulin E (IgE).

The IgE antibody triggers the mast cells to take on water,

swell, and burst, releasing chemicals into your bloodstream. These chemicals include cytokines, leukotrienes, and a chemical called histamine, which causes the annoying reactions in your eyes, skin, throat, lungs, nose, or gastrointestinal tract.[4] The release of these proinflammatory chemicals causes you to begin experiencing labored breathing, sneezing, and other symptoms of the allergic response.

Not even the most well-educated allergy experts fully understand why certain people react to particular substances and others do not. Obviously, not all people react to a particular allergen. For example, some people are allergic to cats and others are not. The lucky nonallergic people can handle large and repeated exposures to potential allergens such as pollen or peanut butter and never have a hypersensitive immune reaction.

The production of IgE plays an important role in the development of allergic symptoms, and it works in concert with mast cells.[5] You have mast cells throughout your body, and they are concentrated in certain places, such as your skin, eyes, trachea, lungs, and gastrointestinal tract. It's in these places, with concentrated numbers of mast cells, that allergic symptoms are the strongest. On the surface of these mast cells, there are special receptors designed for bonding with IgE. Like a key that fits into the right lock, these receptors are specially designed to match up with corresponding IgE antibodies. Pollen IgE receptors will only fit together with pollen IgE antibodies, dust mite IgE receptors will only fit together with dust mite IgE antibodies, and so on. Some unfortunate people have many IgE antibodies, so they react to multiple allergens.[6]

Regardless of the type of allergen, there are three main phases to the allergic response—sensitization to an allergen, early-phase response, and late-phase response.

Phase 1: Sensitization to an Allergen

In order to become sensitive to an allergen, you must first be exposed to it. You may initially come into contact with an allergen through one of the following:[7]

- **Touch.** You encounter some allergens when you touch them with your skin. These include poison ivy, latex, or an allergenic metal such as nickel.
- **Inhalation.** Some allergens cause reactions after you breathe them in. These include pollen, mold, dander, and dust mites.
- **Consumption.** There are allergens that cause a reaction when you swallow them. These include some foods and oral medications.
- **Injection.** Certain allergens only cause reactions once they get under your skin. These include some medications, venom from insect stings, and drugs.

Your first exposure to an allergen through one of these portals doesn't typically result in an outward reaction. In all likelihood, you probably had no idea you were exposed to an allergen. But inside your body, your immune system noticed the allergen and, through the series of reactions described above, produced antibodies against it. This process is similar to how your immune system reacts to a virus or bacteria in a vaccine: As a response to the allergen, it created specific IgE antibodies to defend against it the next time that allergen came around.

More specifically, when your immune system first encounters an allergen, the following chain reaction occurs:

1. The immune system "sees" the allergen—let's say pollen. It identifies the pollen as an invader. Antigen-presenting cells internalize, process, and express the allergens on their surface.
2. The allergens are presented to other immune cells, particularly T cells.
3. The T cells jump into action. The pollen sparks the T cells to activate B cells, which then turn into cells called plasma cells, which secrete antibodies.
4. Plasma cells release IgE antibodies that specifically target the pollen. Different allergens spark production of corresponding specially targeted IgE antibodies, so pollen stimulates the release of IgE antibodies that specifically target pollen,

mold stimulates the release of IgE antibodies that specifically target mold, and so on.

5. Once formed and released into your body, the IgE binds to special receptors on mast cells. Once the IgE has bound with a mast cell, the allergen receptor is left open so it is primed for subsequent exposures to that allergen.

6. The immune system is now sensitized. The mast cells are now ready and waiting like little bombs, prepared to detonate the next time the pollen appears.[8]

Phase 2: Early-Phase Response

The next time your body encounters an allergen—again, let's say pollen—the early-phase response kicks in. Each time your immune system encounters an allergen, it produces more antibodies than it did the time before—and it produces them more quickly. That's why, over time, allergic reactions can become more severe. In the early-phase response, within an hour of encountering the allergen, your immune system goes through the following:[9]

1. The pollen bonds to its corresponding IgE antibodies on the mast cells, cross-linking the IgE. Cross-linking means that when it comes to an allergic reaction, mast cells—much like protesters at a rally—need to join forces with other mast cells to make things happen. As mentioned, IgE antibodies on mast cells are like keys designed to fit perfectly with the allergen (lock) they are ready to attack. Once the pollen finds the IgE key with which it fits, the two bond together and then link up with a neighboring IgE antibody and pollen pair. This pattern continues, and the rally grows.

2. Once enough of this cross-linking takes place and the number of cross-linked IgEs reaches critical mass, the mast cells degranulate (explode) and release histamine and other inflammatory substances called mediators.

3. Mediators race through your body and cause the unpleasant symptoms of the allergic reaction—sneezing, sniffling, wheezing, hives, and so on.

Phase 3: Late-Phase Response

In some cases, there is an additional phase, called the late-phase allergic response. This response involves immune cells called eosinophils and occurs hours after the first early-phase allergic response—usually between 3 and 10 hours later—and it can last for 24 hours or more before subsiding. During this later phase, symptoms can actually be worse than those during the first phase.[10] I used to get this sort of late-phase, delayed allergic reaction when I cut the Bermuda grass in my yard. The night after I mowed, I would wake up and have difficulty breathing. But of course that was before I started taking my own advice.

THE PHYSIOLOGY OF FOOD ALLERGIES

Food allergy symptoms result from a similar physiological response to the one I just described, but they are important to address separately because the symptoms they cause can be much more severe.

Classic food allergies are IgE mediated and involve characteristics of type 1 hypersensitivity reactions. Type 1 hypersensitivity reactions develop rapidly—usually within a few minutes of the allergen binding with the correct IgE antibody on the mast cells. Symptoms of this type of reaction include urticaria (hives), angioedema (swelling similar to hives, but under the skin), and anaphylaxis. As a reminder, anaphylaxis is a very severe type of allergic reaction that can cause constriction of airways, difficulty breathing, lowered blood pressure, loss of consciousness and, potentially, death.[11]

Type 1 hypersensitivity reactions can be either local or systemic. Local reactions depend on the portal of entry. Generally, the reaction takes place on the area of the body that encountered the allergen. For example, if you breathe in mold spores and are allergic to mold, you will experience swelling and irritation in your respiratory tract.

As we discussed in Chapter 1, more and more people throughout the United States and the world are developing food allergies. The most common food allergens are milk, eggs, peanuts, soy, wheat, tree nuts (such as cashews and walnuts), fish, and shellfish. Within

What's the Difference Between an Allergy and a Sensitivity?

In my practice and beyond, the phrase "I'm allergic to . . . " gets used far too often. People frequently confuse allergies and sensitivities, particularly when it comes to foods. They'll say, "I'm allergic to wheat," when really, they're just sensitive to wheat and get gassy and bloated shortly after eating a doughy bagel.

What complicates things is that allergic reactions are difficult to differentiate from similar nonallergic symptoms. The sneezing and runny nose of hay fever, for example, can look very much like the common cold. Other allergic reactions, such as the swelling and difficulty breathing of anaphylaxis, are much easier to recognize.

I will use the example of lactose intolerance, which is a sensitivity, not an allergy. People with lactose intolerance suffer from diarrhea and gas when they eat dairy products. Specifically, they are sensitive to the lactose, or sugars, in milk. Lactose intolerance is not an allergy to milk and dairy. Rather, it is an enzyme deficiency that can either be genetic or acquired. Because a lactose-intolerant person cannot break down lactose, when he gives in to an ice cream craving, he experiences an influx of water into his intestines via osmosis. Soon after, he pays the price for his splurge—the diarrhea and gas kick in. One basic difference between allergies and sensitivities is this: *An allergic reaction is mediated by the immune system, and a sensitivity or intolerance is not.*

Unlike lactose intolerance, food allergies are mediated by the immune system. Also called hypersensitivities, food allergies occur when allergic substances, mostly proteins, make their way through the defenses of your digestive tract and end up in your blood or lymph, where they can elicit antibody responses.[12]

this list, the foods most likely to cause severe anaphylaxis are tree nuts, peanuts, fish, and shellfish (such as lobster and shrimp). People who have food allergies *and* asthma tend to be at risk for the most severe reactions.[13]

Most food allergies develop during childhood, but they can begin at any age. Some childhood food allergies are likely to go

There is also a gray area between allergies and sensitivities. When people undergo food allergy testing, some doctors look for levels of IgG. IgG is a substance your body releases in order to block and reduce levels of IgE. If someone shows a high level of IgG, some physicians will say he or she has a sensitivity, not an allergy. The thinking is that if it were an allergy, there would be high levels of IgE. But the problem is that IgG is not a single molecule—it is a family of molecules with different subpopulations. There is IgG1, IgG2, IgG3, and so on, and each of these subclasses has a different action in your body. So IgG1 could be something produced when someone is having a sensitivity or intolerance, but IgG4, which is thought of as a blocking antibody, could be produced in order to lower levels of IgE produced in response to an allergen. But unless the physician measures specific types of IgG, the level will simply come back as high.

Here's a practical example: When kids have an allergy to the proteins in egg white, the reaction is often so mild that parents don't even notice it. So they keep giving the child eggs. Then, when we test the child down the road, his IgG levels may be quite high, but when we investigate the subpopulations, we see that there is actually a lot more IgG4 (the type that blocks IgE) than any other type. This shows that the child has built up a tolerance to eggs. Basically, the parents have done home-grown immunotherapy. So, when trying to differentiate between allergies and sensitivities, the lesson is, relying simply on IgG levels without looking at subtypes is really not very effective.

away on their own. For example, most children who are allergic to milk outgrow their allergy by the time they reach age 5. Other food allergies, such as peanut allergies, are more stubborn; only about 20 percent of people with peanut allergies ever outgrow them.[14]

Food allergies can also manifest as a condition called food protein-induced enterocolitis syndrome (FPIES). Generally first seen in young children, FPIES is a non-IgE-mediated immune reaction that takes place in the GI system and causes profuse vomiting and diarrhea. As a result, it is often mistaken for a stomach bug. Any food can trigger FPIES, but the most likely culprits are cow's milk and soy. Other possibilities include oats, barley, rice, peas, green beans, squash, sweet potatoes, turkey, and chicken.[15]

As we discuss the physiology of all allergy types, a critical message—and one of the most important points in this book—is the connection between allergy and inflammation. Without inflammatory signals there would be no allergies. It is an inflammatory response that triggers your body's immune cells to begin producing the substances responsible for allergic symptoms, which are themselves proinflammatory. In essence, inflammation causes more inflammation.

In today's society, our bodies are chronically inflamed. This is largely due to unhealthy habits, such as consuming nutrient-deficient and highly processed diets, a lack of physical activity, and an epidemic of excess anxiety. All in all, this adds up to poor lifestyle habits. This inflammation often plays a leading role in the development of the diseases of modern society, such as heart disease, cancer, and diabetes, all of which are considered lifestyle diseases. It is likely that this excessive state of inflammation is a causative factor in the rise in the number of allergic people worldwide. By adopting a healthy lifestyle plan, people may reduce not only their potential for becoming more allergic, but also their potential for developing the other diseases of lifestyle.

A LESSON IN ALLERGY DIAGNOSIS

One of the reasons it's so important to understand the physiology behind your allergy symptoms is that it is often the physiological response to an allergen that is measured during the allergy diagnostic process. When it comes to diagnosing allergies—and determining which specific allergens are at play—there is some overlap between naturopathic medicine and conventional practices.

In the conventional medical world, the process may go like this:

Beth thinks she may have a ragweed allergy because she's been miserable for the last two fall seasons. So she talks to her primary care doctor, who refers her to his favorite allergist or immunologist. (Allergists and immunologists are medical doctors—usually pediatricians or internists—who have gone through at least 2 years of extra training. They specialize in treating patients with allergies, asthma, autoimmune diseases, and other immune system problems.) At Beth's first appointment with the allergist, he conducts a physical exam and performs allergy testing, which may involve skin tests, blood tests, or both.[16] The tests used for allergy screening include the following:

Scratch testing. During a scratch test, a doctor scratches your skin and drops in a tiny dose of the allergen in question. (Alternatively, the doctor may inject a small amount of the allergen into the skin on your back.) After 15 to 20 minutes, the doctor checks your skin to see if a round wheal with a flare (a red, angry-looking welt) has formed around the area. If there's no wheal, there's likely no IgE sensitization, and likely no allergy. If the wheal appears, you are indeed allergic to the particular allergen that was put in place.[17] Based on the degree of the reaction, the doctor may then rate you as slightly allergic or severely allergic. Scratch testing can also be used as a way to monitor the effectiveness of a treatment. This is done by comparing the sizes of the wheals formed before and after treatment. If the wheal got smaller with the second test, then presumably the treatment is working.

Scratch testing has been used for a long time, but it is not without certain limitations. It's fairly subjective, as providers must not only interpret the degree of your allergic response based on the wheal, they must also later compare the size of the first reaction with the size of the second one to determine whether a treatment is working.

Blood testing. In my practice, I prefer to use blood tests to help diagnose allergies. Blood tests for allergies look for antibodies—IgE or IgG—to determine the type of reaction a person is having.[18] They can also look for the total amount of antibodies in the blood. In other words, blood tests can tell you not only whether or not you are allergic, but also what you are allergic to and even how allergic you may be.[19] These tests are very precise, and I like them because I can get quantitative results and then come back and check levels again to see if levels of antibodies to specific allergens are dropping.

For example, if Beth comes in because she thinks she is allergic to ragweed, we can use blood tests to measure the specific amount of ragweed IgE in her blood. Then, after some treatment and lifestyle interventions, we can retest her in the future to see if her levels of ragweed IgE have indeed gone down. That means we can track the effectiveness of a treatment with blood tests like these. It's important to note that these tests can be used for both food and respiratory allergies.

Food challenge. To test for food allergies, the gold standard test—especially for nonanaphylactic food allergies, such as those experienced by people who come in with complaints of gastrointestinal problems—is a food challenge. In practice, I generally recommend the rotation elimination diet. This diet, which involves eating biologically related foods during a single day and then waiting at least 4 days before eating them again, is one of the most effective ways to identify which of the food allergens in question is causing your symptoms.[20]

Component testing. There's also a newer type of testing available, called component testing, which may help determine whether a person will have a mild or severe reaction to a particular allergen. Component testing works by looking for specific proteins within an allergic substance. Certain proteins are associated with mild reactions and others are known to cause more severe reactions, such as anaphylaxis.

To put the test into practical perspective, let's say that you're the parent of a kid with a peanut allergy. Your child may be required to sit at a special table at school and wear a medical alert bracelet wherever he goes. Naturally, as his parent, you are always afraid that he will be exposed to a peanut or that someone will bring a cupcake that contains peanuts to school. Component testing can help determine exactly how your child would react if accidental peanut exposure did occur. If you found out the reaction to peanuts would only be mild, it would take away a lot of unnecessary anxiety, wouldn't it? Component testing is becoming more and more commonplace, and if you think you may benefit from this type of testing, I encourage you to ask your doctor about it.

AN OVERVIEW OF STANDARD ALLERGY TREATMENT

I'd like to reiterate that I am by no means against conventional medications. (The decision of whether or not to take medications is a personal one.) There have been many times when conventional treatment methods have successfully treated a patient's condition. However, these medications are overused. If you can live a health-promoting lifestyle instead of a health-detracting one, then there is the potential for a reduction in or even elimination of the medications in your life.

When it comes to allergy medications, I appreciate their ability to control potentially life-threatening symptoms, but I am dismayed that they are really only able to treat symptoms. The vast majority of medications really do not improve overall health. It would be fantastic if we had medications that could actually cure diseases, but unfortunately, this is not the case. There are simply no magic medications for allergies. What these medications do is reduce the discomfort of allergies by easing their symptoms. They may offer a temporary solution, but beneath them, the wound is deepening. And too often, patients require multiple allergy medications at once to control their symptoms, which can be extremely taxing to the body.

For example, antihistamines work to block the histamine that unleashes allergic reactions. They're designed to treat isolated allergic symptoms, such as runny nose, sneezing, hives, or abdominal pain.[21] Antihistamines should not be routinely prescribed as the only treatment for allergies because they do not prevent allergy; they only prevent histamine from being released from mast cells once the allergic process has already gotten started. They do not help a person become less allergic in the long run, nor do they help move the person toward a better state of health. There are other things that can be used alongside antihistamines that may be able to reduce a person's dependence on those medications. My plan will discuss some of these options.

Another popular conventional treatment for allergies is allergy vaccination, or subcutaneous immunotherapy (SCIT). SCIT involves injecting a patient with increasing amounts of an allergen to help her

Tired of Allergy Shots? There's Finally a Good Alternative!

As a naturopathic doctor, in addition to the lifestyle interventions I present in my plan, one of my favorite treatments for respiratory allergies is what's called sublingual immunotherapy (SLIT). Sublingual immunotherapy works in much the same way that allergy shots do: It combats allergies by giving the allergic person a small dose of what he or she is allergic to. If a person is allergic to pollen, you give her a very small amount of pollen so her immune system gets used to it (i.e., builds a tolerance). But unlike injection immunotherapy (allergy shots), patients take SLIT painlessly administered under their tongues. Over time, SLIT retrains the immune system not to be allergic to that specific allergen.[22]

One of the reasons I recommend SLIT is that it lines up with my professional philosophy. There are certain principles that guide the naturopathic profession as we see patients, and one of those principles is to make sure to always treat the *cause* of the disease. I truly feel that SLIT fits this bill. It treats the immune system dysfunction that leads to the development of allergy symptoms, and it does so in a way that is completely natural—there's no medication involved.

immune system build resistance, and therefore lessen the allergic response. For example, if you're allergic to pollen, a doctor may inject you with pollen in increasing doses to stimulate your immune system's protective mechanisms against pollen exposure until he or she determines the right maintenance dose. The eventual goal is to reduce the number of allergy attacks or stop them altogether.[23]

My problem with allergy shots is not the philosophy behind them—in fact, I think in some patients, immunotherapy can work quite well. However, let's face it: No one really likes needles or pain.

For food allergies, conventional treatment usually involves avoiding the offending foods. This is sound advice. In my practice, once I identify a food allergy in one of my patients, I help them create a plan to avoid the offender. People with food allergies often become experts at scanning food labels. Allergenic foods frequently aren't listed by their common names; for example, peanuts may take the form of "hydrolyzed vegetable protein," and the ingredient "albumin" comes from eggs. People with allergies to these foods learn to recognize them behind these disguises.[24]

If you have a food allergy, you should also work with your health-care professional to develop an emergency action plan you can put in place in the event that you accidentally encounter the food to which you are allergic. I encourage patients with severe allergies with the potential for anaphylaxis to carry an EpiPen with them in the event of an emergency reaction. Epinephrine works to offset the anaphylactic response by relaxing narrowed airways and constricting small blood vessels to increase blood pressure.

To sum up, allergy medications only treat the symptoms of the disease; they do not improve the patient's health. In my practice, I have seen far too many allergic people who are fed up and desperate for a treatment that works, and you're probably in the same boat. After all, if your allergies were well controlled, you wouldn't be reading this book. So read on, and we will explore effective alternative treatments together.

Marie's Story

In addition to pumpkin carving and hayrides, each fall, Marie used to expect itchy eyes, sneezing, and a stuffy nose.

"My seasonal allergies were miserable, especially when it came time for the fall rye grass," says the 37-year-old accountant.

As is the case with many of Dr. Psenka's seasonal allergy patients, Marie's allergies first appeared when she moved to Arizona 13 years ago. Not wanting to take medications, she made an appointment with Dr. Psenka, who prescribed sublingual immunotherapy (SLIT), some supplements, and a healthier eating plan.

"Before I went to see Dr. Psenka, I ate lots of meat and potatoes and drank diet soda. Now, I eat more fruits and vegetables and drink less soda and more water," she says.

About six weeks into the program, Marie began to notice improvements in her allergy symptoms and overall vitality. Today, she feels wonderful.

"I feel like I have much more energy, and I've lost weight—about eight pounds so far," she says, adding she would encourage anyone with seasonal allergies to try SLIT.

"Not only has Dr. Psenka treated my allergy symptoms with natural methods, he has taught me how to lead a healthier life," she says. "He is great."

4 On the Origin of Sneezes: Common Allergies

A FEW YEARS AGO, I treated a 12-year-old boy who came to me complaining of constant nasal congestion. He was a seasonal resident of Arizona and spent the other half of the year in Minnesota. His mother told me that whenever they would leave Arizona and head back up north, the boy would "seize up," meaning his allergies got so bad they prevented him from participating in school or other activities.

I tested the boy for both food and respiratory allergies and found that he had a number of different allergies and sensitivities. I then tested his respiratory allergies using two respiratory allergy test panels specific to the geographic areas in which this boy lived. Respiratory allergy test panels are frequently organized into regional panels that contain the most commonly encountered allergens in that area—in this case, the Southwest and the Midwest. I also suggested that he try a rotation and elimination diet to confirm the results of his food sensitivity testing. The culprit turned out not to be based on his location after all. He was allergic to dairy and had a significant number of respiratory allergies, mostly to things in the Southwest and not the Midwest. I started him on sublingual immunotherapy (SLIT), which he took while both avoiding the foods to which he had an allergy and following my other recommendations, which included some general antioxidants, an omega-3 oil blend (see "The Role of Omega-3s in Treating Allergies"), and a good probiotic. A few months later, his mother called me from Minnesota to tell me that his allergic symptoms were much, much better. In fact, he was having no problems at all.

There are a few lessons to take away from this story. First, allergies can very much be based on where you live in the country, and a relocation can mean fewer allergy symptoms, more allergy symptoms, or a completely new set of allergy symptoms. The second is that, in most cases, allergy symptoms result from one of the most common allergens—pollen, pet dander, dust, dust mites, cockroaches, and certain foods.

There are thousands of substances that can cause allergies, which makes those of us who diagnose those allergies detectives, in a way. When we consider what may be causing a patient's symptoms, we must take into account diet, environment, and region of the country (see "Different Region, Different Allergy") because you never know what could be causing someone's allergic symptoms.

The Role of Omega-3s in Treating Allergies

When I treated the dairy-allergic boy from Minnesota, one thing that helped in controlling his food allergy was a supplement containing omega-3 fatty acids. Omega-3 fatty acids are polyunsaturated fatty acids your body needs but cannot make; you have to get them from foods or supplements. Food sources include flaxseed oil and oily fish (such as salmon, cod, and haddock) as well as flaxseeds and walnuts.

The reason omega-3 fatty acids can be so effective against allergies is that they contain eicosapentaenoic acid (EPA), which is a natural anti-inflammatory. And the lower the underlying levels of inflammation in your body, the lower your allergic potential.[1]

Different Region, Different Allergy

My young patient with the dairy allergy turned out not to be sensitive to his yearly change in region. However, his mother's thought that this annual migration might be a factor was a wise hypothesis. Different allergens are found in different environments; what causes seasonal allergies in upstate New York is completely different from what causes seasonal allergies in Phoenix—the two areas have nearly opposite climates and therefore grow very different plant species. So, naturally, people can undergo changes in their allergy symptoms when they travel from one area of the country to another. These new allergies can kick in immediately, or after a few months or years.[2]

COMMON SEASONAL ALLERGIES

The most common seasonal allergies include those to pollens from trees, pollens from weeds, and mold. Although mold is not a seasonal allergy in the classic sense, some molds have peak seasons in certain areas of the country. Here's an overview of these seasonal allergies and their symptoms.

Pollen Allergy

Pollen is a very fine powder given off by many different kinds of plants, from the grass in your backyard to the weeds and flowers in your garden. When a fertile plant begins to flower, it releases its pollen into the air. Pollen granules are the male cells of trees, grasses, and flowers, and they travel in search of a female plant to pollinate. Like matchmakers, in a sense, wind and—appropriately—birds and bees help the fertilization process, carrying pollen from one plant to another.[3]

Part of the reason pollen is so allergenic is that millions of particles can come from a single plant and travel up to 200 miles. As a quick glance at your yellow-coated windshield in May will tell you, when most pollination happens, in spring and fall, *tons* of pollen particles circulate through the air.[4]

Pollen allergy symptoms can range from mild to severe and may include sneezing, itchy throat, itching inside your ears, itchy eyes, swollen eyelids, runny or stuffy nose, coughing, wheezing, and trouble breathing.[5] Symptoms can also get better or worse based on the weather, with rainy days being less problematic for pollen allergy sufferers. (Precipitation literally rains on pollen's parade.)[6]

One of the most common allergic conditions caused by pollen is hay fever (also called allergic rhinitis), which involves itching in your nose, on the roof of your mouth, and in your throat and eyes; sneezing; runny nose; watery eyes; and dark circles under your eyes.[7]

Some people are allergic to only one kind of pollen, such as ragweed, while other unfortunate allergy sufferers react to multiple pollens from many different plants. Some of the other most common plants whose pollen can spark allergies include the following:[8]

TREES	WEEDS	GRASSES
Ash	Burningbush (also	Bermuda
Aspen	called summer	Johnson
Beech	cypress, Mexican	Kentucky bluegrass
Birch	fireweed, or kochia)	Orchard
Box elder	Cocklebur	Redtop
Cedar	Lambsquarters	Rye
Cottonwood	Mugwort	Sweet vernal
Elm	Pigweed	Timothy
Maple	Plantain	
Mulberry	Red (sheep) sorrel	
Oak	Russian thistle	
Willow	Sagebrush	
	Saltbush	
	Tumbleweeds	

Interestingly, in general, the less colorful the plant, the more likely it is to be allergenic. Pollen from the most colorful flowers and plants rarely causes symptoms because it is carried by insects and birds, which are attracted to the plants' vibrant hues. Duller plants and weeds, on the other hand, rely on wind to spread their seed.

Allergens and Their Seasons

By season, the offenders are:[9]

- **Spring (April and May).** Allergies most often result from pollen from trees, such as oak, ash, birch, western red cedar, hickory, maple, walnut, and sycamore.
- **Summer (late May through July).** Allergies most frequently result from pollen from grasses and weeds, such as timothy, redtop, Bermuda, orchard, sweet vernal, and bluegrass.
- **Fall (late August through the first frost).** Allergies most often result from pollen from ragweed, sagebrush, cocklebur, Russian thistle, tumbleweed, and pigweed.

In addition to following The Allergy Solution Plan (see page 231), you can try to control pollen allergies by paying attention to the pollen count in the air (which changes on a daily basis) and then adjusting your schedule so you don't have a lot of outside activities when the count is highest. Pollen count can largely affect whether or not you have a reaction. You can find out the pollen count by checking the weather section of your local newspaper or by entering your ZIP code on one of the popular weather information Web sites, such as The Weather Channel site at weather.com.

Mold Allergy

We've all heard of the scary black mold that can lurk behind bathroom walls and make you very sick. But there's also a somewhat less-threatening mold form that can cause allergy symptoms in your nose and throat.[10]

Molds are fungi that give off spores. These spores then float through the air and can get into your mouth, nose, and throat. Mold itself usually grows in dark, wet places, such as bathrooms, kitchens, and basements as well as outdoors on wet leaves and logs, but its spores can travel fast on dry, breezy days.

Mold allergy symptoms are generally similar to symptoms of pollen allergy and may include sneezing; congestion; itchy eyes, throat, or ears; swelling in your eyelids; coughing; trouble breathing; or wheezing. They can also range from mild annoyances to potentially severe anaphylactic reactions.[11] (See "Decoding Allergy Jargon" on page 59.)

Unlike pollens, which tend to be seasonal, molds can grow throughout the year if you live in a Southern or Western state. They do have peak seasons in other areas of the country, however; in warmer states, they peak in July, and in colder states, mold levels peak in October.[12]

COMMON ANIMAL ALLERGIES

The most common animal allergies are to household pets, but people can also develop allergies to outside pets like horses. Here's an overview of these animal allergies and their symptoms.

Pet Allergy

Ironically, one of the most common causes of allergies is man's best friend. Nearly two-thirds of American homes have a pet, and 161 million of these animals are cats and dogs. Some experts advise those with pet allergies to opt for a fish or turtle, instead, but millions of allergic pet lovers hold on to Kitty or Barkley anyway, for the love of their furry friends.[13]

Contrary to popular belief, fluffier pets are no more allergenic than their short-haired counterparts. Pet hair or fur can contribute to allergies by trapping other allergens, such as pollen or mold, but it's not the length of the dog or cat hair that matters—it's the dander, saliva, urine, and skin flakes that can spark allergic reactions or aggravate asthma in some people.

Also contrary to popular belief, there are no cats or dogs that are truly hypoallergenic. All pets have dander, saliva, and urine, and therefore, they can all cause allergies to some degree.

Another thing to keep in mind about pet allergies is that they can take a while to develop. Therefore, if you adopted a kitten last

Allergic Rhinitis versus Nonallergic Rhinitis: What's the Difference?

At least one out of three people with allergic rhinitis symptoms—runny nose, nasal congestion, sneezing—do not, in fact, have allergies. Instead, they have what is called nonallergic rhinitis, an allergic rhinitis imposter. These two conditions differ in that with allergic rhinitis, your immune system overreacts to an environmental substance such as pollen or mold, whereas with nonallergic rhinitis, your immune system does not get involved. Another important difference: Allergic rhinitis tends to come and go with the season, while nonallergic rhinitis hangs out year-round.[14,15]

week and everyone in your family is still symptom-free, you're not quite out of the woods yet. Pet allergies typically take between 4 and 6 months to fully kick in.[16]

For those with an established pet allergy, however, symptoms will show up shortly after exposure to a dog or cat—within minutes, in some cases. These symptoms may include itchy, watery eyes; sneezing; congestion; and runny nose. Less commonly, people with pet allergies may get itchy skin or hives.[17]

In addition to following The Allergy Solution Plan, starting on page 231, you can minimize pet allergies by limiting your snuggling time with your dog or cat, keeping your pet out of your bedroom, and brushing him or her outdoors. Using a high-efficiency particulate air (HEPA) filter in your vacuum cleaner or a HEPA air cleaner can also help.

Horse Allergy

A horse allergy is less common than an allergy to dogs and cats, but it can affect some people, especially those who live in states where horses may be a part of everyday life, such as Texas, Wyoming, and Arizona. People may be truly allergic to horses and their hair, or they may actually be reacting to the molds and spores given off by the hay horses sleep on and eat.[18]

Symptoms of horse allergy are usually mild and include allergic rhinitis, allergic conjunctivitis, itching, and hives. Horses may also spark asthma symptoms in some people or—in rare cases—can cause anaphylaxis, which may involve itching, hives, difficulty breathing, a drop in blood pressure, loss of consciousness, and potentially, death.[19]

If you think you may have a horse allergy, allergy testing can help you determine yea or "neigh."

COMMON HOUSEHOLD ALLERGIES

Americans spend most of their time indoors, so it's no surprise that some of the most common allergies are to household substances. Here's an overview of household allergies and their symptoms.

House Dust Allergy

House dust is like an allergen soup serving up a bunch of potentially allergy-aggravating ingredients. It can contain pet dander, fungi, dust mites, food remnants, fibers from drapes and carpeting, cockroach parts, and even dust from outside construction sites—anything you can think of that might be lurking in or around your home.[20]

Symptoms of a house dust allergy depend on the particular allergens that dust contains and may include sneezing; runny nose; itchy, watery eyes; and increased risk of asthma symptoms (such as wheezing, coughing, chest tightness, and difficulty breathing) in those who have asthma.[21]

Although an excessive amount of house dust may make allergy symptoms more likely to kick in, realize that in most cases, a dust allergy is not an indication that you're doing a bad job cleaning your home. Normal housecleaning simply isn't sufficient to remove dust—and a dust allergy—completely.[22] When it comes to house dust allergies, dust mites are the house dust component most likely to cause allergy symptoms. These little creatures belong to the arachnid family, which also includes chiggers, ticks, and spiders. Dust mites eat human and animal skin and dander, so they tend to hang out in places where they can find people and pets. They also love warm, humid spots—above 70°F with greater than 75 percent relative humidity. In fact, one of the best ways to kill dust mites is to drop the relative humidity below 55 percent; they cannot survive in conditions this dry.[23]

Decoding Allergy Jargon

Some of the most common allergic reactions are hiding behind some pretty technical-sounding names. Here's a quick overview of these reactions.

- **Allergic contact dermatitis.** This reaction occurs when your skin comes into direct contact with an allergen, such as poison ivy. It consists of red, swollen, itchy skin that may contain bumps or scales.[24]
- **Allergic conjunctivitis.** This condition occurs when the clear layer of tissue covering the whites of your eyes and your lids becomes swollen and inflamed as part of an allergic reaction to mold, pollen, pet dander, or another allergen.[25]
- **Anaphylaxis.** Also called anaphylactic shock, anaphylaxis is a severe, sometimes fatal reaction that begins within seconds to minutes after exposure and involves swelling of the lips, tongue, and throat; itchiness; a drop in blood pressure; difficulty breathing; and decreased blood flow to the brain, heart, and lungs.[26]
- **Angioedema.** Similar to hives, angioedema is swelling in the deep layers of the skin. Angioedema may occur with hives and often affects the skin of the eyelids, mouth, or genitals.[27] It can also affect the hands or feet, or the inside of the bowels or throat.[28]
- **Atopic dermatitis (eczema).** Eczema results from leakiness in the skin's barrier, which causes skin to become dry and therefore vulnerable to irritation and inflammation. Eczema typically shows up in the bends of elbows or knees, behind the ears, or on the hands and feet.[29]
- **Uticaria (hives).** When your immune system releases histamine in response to an allergen, small blood vessels leak, leading to swelling and redness on your skin. These hives may be itchy or painful, and they may appear as red and white raised bumps or welts.[30] They can show up anywhere on your body.

Dust mites are very small, so you can't see them with your naked eye. In fact, a single gram of house dust (about the weight of a paper clip) may contain as many as 19,000 dust mites. The mites live for about a month, during which time egg-laying females can produce 25 to 30 offspring. Each mite produces 10 to 20 waste particles per day. And in case you aren't grossed out enough yet, dust mites also eat their feces and coat those waste particles with even more allergenic proteins.[31]

Besides being thoroughly disgusting, the problem with dust mites is that the proteins in their bodies and feces cause allergy symptoms. These dust mite particles can float through the air, where you can breathe them in, or they can hide in pillows, mattresses, upholstered furniture, and carpeting, where they can be disturbed when someone vacuums the floor or changes the sheets. So to make a long and disgusting story short, dust mites multiply quickly and leave a lot of allergenic feces in their wake.[32]

To those who are allergic to them, dust mites and their waste can cause itchy, watery eyes; stuffy nose and ears; sneezing; eczema; respiratory problems; and in some cases, asthma.[33] To ease your willies a bit, you can rest assured that dust mites don't live on your body, they don't spread diseases, and they don't bite. If it weren't for allergies to them, we probably wouldn't even know they were there.[34] (Bedbugs, however, do bite and are becoming a problem for more and more people. While it remains to be seen what the allergic potential of bedbugs is, we do know that people develop IgE antibodies to these little critters.)[35]

Cockroach Allergy

When you hear the word cockroach, you may think of a dirty, infested, inner-city apartment. But actually, cockroaches have been around for an estimated 400 million years, so they've lived in the most rustic of country homes; their long history also proves that they are extremely resilient creatures.[36] Not only are cockroaches a stubborn nuisance but also they can cause allergy symptoms in some people.[37]

Cockroaches typically hang out in warm, dark, damp places

where they can find something to eat. They like to munch on human food, but they differ from us in that they also enjoy paint, newspaper, book-binding materials, and wallpaper paste. The bugs typically hide in grocery bags, in stacks of books, in wall and floor cracks, and under sinks. If you see a cockroach, there are probably many more: One roach can mean up to 800 more are lurking nearby.[38]

Although they may make your skin crawl, cockroaches are pretty harmless, except to those who are allergic to them. In allergic people, the bugs' waste can spark reactions like a persistent stuffy nose, skin rash, and asthma symptoms, such as coughing, wheezing, difficulty breathing, and chest tightness. Cockroach allergies are a particularly strong risk factor for asthma in children.

In addition to following The Allergy Solution Plan in Chapter 14, you can fight a cockroach allergy by doing what you can to get rid of the bugs: Don't leave food out in your kitchen; cover trash cans tightly with lids; avoid leaving bowls of pet food on the floor; mop your floors at least once a week; and fix leaky pipes, dripping faucets, and other moisture problems in your house.

COMMON FOOD ALLERGIES

Food allergies result when your immune system mistakes a food you've eaten for an invader. Instead of digesting the food and using it as nourishment, your body launches an attack (see page 39), which can lead to symptoms that range from mildly unpleasant to potentially fatal. In their most severe form, food allergies can cause life-threatening anaphylaxis.[39]

When we talk about food allergies, it's important to distinguish them from food intolerances or sensitivities. A true food allergy is a hypersensitivity of the immune system to a food component, usually a protein. With a food sensitivity, on the other hand, the immune system is not usually involved. For example, lactose intolerance is a food sensitivity. People with the condition lack the enzyme necessary to break down milk sugar (lactose), so when they eat dairy products, lactose intolerant people may experience gas, bloating, and diarrhea. Although they may be uncomfortable and embarrassed, these symptoms are not life-threatening, as some true food allergies can be.

Here's are the most common food allergies.

Peanut Allergy

One of the most common food allergies, peanut allergy is also one of the most potentially dangerous. Peanuts are among the foods most likely to cause anaphylaxis, and peanut allergies are on the rise. According to the Food Allergy Research and Education (FARE) study, peanut allergies more than tripled in the United States between 1997 and 2008.[40]

Unlike most other food allergies, which kids typically outgrow, peanut allergies are a lifelong condition—only about 20 percent of people with allergies to peanuts ever get rid of them. These allergies tend to run in families, with younger siblings of kids with peanut allergies at an increased risk of developing them, as well.[41]

Peanuts are a member of the legume family; other members include peas, lentils, and soy. Legumes differ from their cousins, the tree nuts (walnuts, cashews, and almonds), in that they grow in the ground. Although people with peanut allergies are no more likely to be allergic to other legumes, they *are* more likely to be allergic to tree nuts. Recent research shows that between 24 and 40 percent of people with peanut allergies also have tree nut allergies.[42]

Symptoms of a peanut allergy may include hives; eczema; stomach cramps; diarrhea; vomiting; runny nose; sneezing; itchy, watery eyes; and asthma symptoms, such as coughing, wheezing, and difficulty breathing. In its most severe form, peanut allergy can cause—within minutes—the sudden allergic reaction anaphylaxis.[43]

Another reason peanut allergies are such a concern is that just a tiny amount of a nut can trigger a big reaction in sensitive people. If someone with a peanut allergy touches a surface where a peanut or some peanut butter sat and then touches his or her eyes, for example, it can be enough to set off a serious allergic reaction.[44]

Because trace amounts of peanuts can spark a severe response, and because peanuts can lurk in many unsuspecting foods, people with a peanut allergy—or any true food allergy—simply can't be too careful. If you have a severe food allergy, you should carry an EpiPen at all times, and make sure you and those around you know how to administer it and are prepared to use it at any time.[45]

As a peanut allergy sufferer, you must also be vigilant about reading food labels. The Food Allergen Labeling and Consumer Protection Act (FALCPA) requires all foods containing peanuts that are sold in the United States to list the word "peanut" clearly on the label. However, keep in mind that the use of the phrase "may contain peanuts" is voluntary, so you still need to know what you're eating.

It's also important to be aware of foods and ingredients that may contain peanuts. These include the following:

- Artificial nuts
- Baked goods
- Candy
- Chili
- Egg rolls
- Glazes and marinades
- Mandelonas (peanuts soaked in almond flavoring)
- Marzipan
- Nougat
- Pancakes
- Pet food
- Specialty pizzas

Tree Nut Allergy

Tree nuts are, as their name suggests, nuts that grow on trees. They include almonds, walnuts, hazelnuts, pistachios, Brazil nuts, and cashews.[46]

Tree nut allergies are similar to peanut allergies in that they tend to cause severe reactions and usually last a lifetime. Even fewer kids with tree nut allergies than with peanut allergies ever outgrow them. Tree nut allergies also tend to run in families, with younger siblings of children with tree nut allergies at an increased risk of developing them, too.[47]

People with tree nut allergies are frequently allergic to more than one kind of tree nut, so they're advised to avoid all nuts and to check all ingredients. The FALCPA now requires food companies to list specific tree nuts on all labels of foods sold in the United States. Even so, those with allergies to tree nuts should be aware that these nuts can pop up in the most unusual places, such as barbecue sauces, flavored coffees, and alcoholic beverages. (Note that alcoholic beverages are *not* required by the FALCPA to list potential allergens on their labels.)[48]

If you have a severe tree nut allergy, you should also look out for the following substances:

- Gianduja (chocolate with hazelnut paste as an ingredient)
- Litchi
- Marzipan
- Pesto

Milk Allergy

Cow's milk is the most common allergy in infants and young kids. About 2.5 percent of children younger than age 3 are allergic to milk. Those with an allergy to cow's milk can also react to the milk of other animals, such as goats and sheep.[49]

Milk allergy symptoms are variable and can range from mild to severe. Some individuals react after ingesting only a tiny bit of milk, while others can drink a moderate amount and react only slightly. Mild reactions tend to take the form of hives, and severe reactions can include anaphylaxis.[50]

The good news is that most kids with milk allergies outgrow them. There are also a number of healthy dairy-free baby formulas available, so mothers of milk-allergic kids who choose not to breast-feed have other options. As you'll see in "Soy Allergy" on the opposite page, soy alternatives are not always a good choice because many people are also allergic to soy-based foods.

Luckily, the FALCPA now requires that all milk-containing products sold in the United States actually list the word "milk" on the label. Even so, it's helpful for parents of kids who are allergic to milk—and for the kids themselves—to be as educated as possible on hidden cow's milk sources. It's also important to realize that milk can show up in the most unexpected places, such as in deli meat (when meat slicers are used to cut both meat and cheese), meats that use casein as a binder, and medications that contain milk protein.

Here are some milk-containing ingredients to look out for:[51]

- Casein
- Caseinates
- Curd
- Diacetyl
- Ghee
- Lactalbumin
- Lactoferrin
- Lactose
- Lactulose
- Recaldent
- Rennet casein
- Tagatose
- Whey

Egg Allergy

Egg allergies are also common in kids, second only to milk. Luckily, most children outgrow their egg allergy by age 5. Those who are sensitive react to the proteins in the white of the egg. People with chicken egg allergies should also avoid eggs from ducks, geese, turkeys, and other birds, because they may contain some of the same allergenic proteins. Symptoms of an egg allergy range from mild skin reactions to severe anaphylaxis.[52]

Children who are most allergic to eggs can react after just smelling egg fumes or getting a tiny bit of egg white on their skin. Because eggs have the potential to cause anaphylaxis, those who are at risk should carry an EpiPen to use in the event of accidental exposure.[53]

The FALCPA requires all egg or egg product–containing packaged foods meant for distribution in the United States to say "contains eggs" on their labels. But eggs can still show up in unexpected places, such as in surimi, the foam toppings of coffee drinks and on pretzels. (They're in the egg wash used before the pretzels are dipped in salt.) Therefore, you can't be too educated about eggs' many whereabouts. Some of the less-obvious names for egg-containing ingredients include albumin (or albumen), meringue, and ovalbumin.[54]

Soy Allergy

Soy is another common food allergen, especially in infants and children. About 0.4 percent of children have a soy allergy. Some kids outgrow it by age 3, and the majority outgrow it by age 10.[55]

Soybeans are legumes (plants that have seeds in pods; other legumes include peas, lentils, and peanuts). Having a soy allergy does not make someone more likely to have an allergy to another legume, such as peanuts, however. And in most cases, soy allergies tend to be much milder than peanut allergies.

Symptoms of a soy allergy may include hives, itching, eczema, canker sores, abdominal pain, diarrhea, nausea, vomiting, or dizziness.[56] More severe anaphylactic reactions to soy can also occur, but these are rare. Those who are at risk for an anaphylactic reaction from soy should carry an EpiPen. (You can learn if you're at risk through specialized testing.)

The FALCPA requires all packaged foods that contain soy and that are sold in the United States to say "soy" on the label. However, it's still helpful to recognize foods and ingredients that may contain soy. These include the following:[57]

- Edamame
- Miso
- Natto
- Shoyu
- Soya
- Tamari
- Tempeh
- Textured vegetable protein (TVP)

Beyond the obvious soy milk and soy products like tofu, soy can also be found in unexpected foods, including canned meats and fish, cereal, crackers, energy bars, and infant formula.[58]

Fish and Shellfish Allergy

Like peanut allergies, fish and shellfish allergies often stick with people for their entire lives. In fact, seafood allergy is one of the top food allergies among adults. It also sends more people age 6 and older to the emergency room than any other food allergy because like nut allergies, an allergy to fish and shellfish can bring on a severe anaphylactic reaction.[59]

When it comes to seafood, those with fins are the most allergenic, with salmon, tuna, and halibut being the worst offenders. People who are allergic to one type of fish are frequently also allergic to another. However, fish and shellfish come from different families, so having an allergy to shellfish doesn't necessarily mean that you'll also be allergic to finned fish, or vice versa.[60]

In terms of shellfish, crustaceans within the shellfish family are most likely to cause allergic reactions. These include shrimp, lobsters, and crabs. Unfortunately, these are also some of the most popular shellfish for people to eat.[61]

If you are allergic to fish or shellfish and are at risk for anaphylaxis, you will want to avoid these foods at all costs. On a positive note, fish and shellfish hardly ever hide behind strange ingredient names or in surprising foods. And if a packaged food contains shellfish, the label must list it.[62]

However, it's important to keep in mind that deep fryers in restaurants are often used to fry multiple kinds of foods, so your plate of innocent French fries may have been dipped in the same oil as someone else's fried seafood sampler Hibachi restaurants are another danger zone for people with seafood allergies, because chefs use the same open grill to cook everyone's meals. If you have a shellfish allergy, your safest bet is to avoid seafood restaurants altogether, and *especially* any foods that have been deep-fried.[63]

In addition, because fish and shellfish allergies can cause anaphylaxis, carrying an EpiPen is a good idea for those who have these allergies.

Wheat Allergy

Wheat allergies most commonly show up in kids, who usually outgrow them by age 3. And just as a milk allergy should not be confused with lactose intolerance, a wheat allergy should not be confused with celiac disease or gluten intolerance, which is a sensitivity to the sticky protein (called gluten) that's found in wheat. Wheat allergies in their true form are reactions to the proteins in wheat and are mediated by the immune system; IgE antibodies are secreted within minutes to hours after a person eats a wheat-containing food.[64] Symptoms of a wheat allergy can range from mild hives, rash, digestion problems, itching, and swelling to severe, life-threatening anaphylactic reactions that involve wheezing, trouble breathing, and loss of consciousness.[65]

In someone with celiac disease or with wheat gluten *intolerance*, there is an abnormal immune system reaction to gluten (but not a hypersensitivity, which occurs with allergy). Left untreated, celiac disease can lead to malnutrition and serious damage to the intestines, so it's important for people who suffer from it to avoid wheat.[66]

Whether you have a wheat allergy or an intolerance, avoiding this ingredient can be challenging because wheat is America's most commonly used grain. It's also used as a filler in many foods that you wouldn't suspect, such as salad dressing, soy sauce, lunch meat, and ice cream. Good alternatives to wheat flour itself include corn, oats, quinoa, rice, barley, and amaranth. To best avoid wheat, you should also become educated on all of its imposters. These foods and ingredients contain wheat:

- Bulgur
- Couscous
- Cracker meal
- Durum
- Einkorn
- Emmer
- Farina
- Kamut
- Matzoh
- Seitan
- Semolina
- Spelt
- Triticale

Corn Allergy

The most profitable crop in the country, corn is used in almost everything these days, including as a filler in processed meats and as a sweetener in candies, cereals, and jams.[67] It's not yet considered a common food allergen in the United States, but based on the patients I've seen in my practice, I think corn is on its way to this list. In one study, 2 percent of people self-reported an allergy to corn.[68]

One reason I think corn allergies are underrecognized is because they can be so difficult to diagnose. When you use a standard skin or blood test, there can be cross-reactions between corn and other common allergens, such as grass pollens, grains, and seeds; therefore, a corn allergy can be difficult to tease out.[69]

When they do show up, corn allergies may cause symptoms such as hives, rash, runny nose, nausea, vomiting, cramps, diarrhea, headaches, sneezing, and asthma. Some people also experience severe anaphylactic reactions to corn and corn products, including the cornstarch used on surgical gloves. If you are severely allergic to corn, you should avoid both raw and cooked corn and carry an EpiPen in case of a reaction.

5

When Good Things Go Bad: Allergies and Inflammation

A FEW YEARS AGO, I saw a 34-year-old mother of two who had been having trouble losing weight after giving birth to her second child. This wasn't an unusual reason for an office visit in and of itself, but she also complained of constantly feeling gassy, bloated, and fatigued. She had previously gotten her hormone levels checked and was told that everything looked fine. She had also seen a gastroenterologist who had ordered a battery of tests that all came back normal. The last doctor she saw suggested she take an anti-gas agent and sent her on her way.

Frustrated because she wasn't getting any relief, this woman found her way to my office. We discussed her health history, including her diet and lifestyle habits. She wasn't aware of any food allergies, but she did say she had terrible springtime allergies that were not well controlled with over-the-counter antihistamines.

So I performed some testing and determined that she had a sensitivity to wheat. She admitted that breads and pastas were some of her favorite foods and that she had been enjoying them without restraint for her entire life. I encouraged her to try a wheat-free diet for a week. She was reluctant at first, believing that being "wheat-free" was a fad and thinking that eliminating wheat would be difficult. I assured her that having a sensitivity to wheat was a very

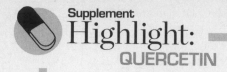

Supplement
Highlight:
QUERCETIN

In the story of my 34-year-old patient who was having trouble managing her weight and controlling her seasonal allergies, one of the remedies that worked well was a supplement called quercetin. Flavonoids like quercetin are antioxidants—molecules that neutralize harmful free radicals. (Through a process called oxidative stress, free radicals damage DNA, harm cell membranes, and increase your risk for many health problems, such as heart disease and cancer.)[1]

In terms of allergies, quercetin appears to fight symptoms like sneezing, runny nose, hives, and swelling because it acts as a natural antihistamine and anti-inflammatory. It stabilizes mast cells, the immune system cells that release histamine, which is the chemical that causes these allergic reactions.[2]

Quercetin comes in supplement form (pills or capsules), which is what my patient took to help ward off her spring allergies. Quercetin supplements sometimes also contain bromelain, an enzyme found in pineapple that acts as a natural anti-inflammatory.[3]

You can also get quercetin from fruits and vegetables such as apples, blackberries, blueberries, citrus fruits, dark cherries, onions, parsley, and sage. Or you can drink a dose, since it's also found in tea and red wine.[4]

real thing and that those who had it generally described symptoms similar to hers. We talked about how wheat contains substances that may cause her to gain weight and also inhibit weight loss. One substance found in wheat, gliadin, can actually stimulate appetite by binding to opioid receptors, which are specific receptors in the brain. I also talked to her about another component of wheat, amylopectin A, which is a highly digestible carbohydrate with the potential to cause a person's blood sugar to become markedly elevated. I further explained that she wouldn't have a tough time finding replacements for all her wheat-containing favorites. She decided to give it a try.

Within just one week of being on the wheat-free diet, this

woman noticed a big positive change in the way she felt. Her gas and bloating were gone, and she was beginning to believe that wheat might actually be part of her problem. Because her respiratory allergy testing had also revealed several allergies to grasses and pollens, I recommended starting sublingual immunotherapy (SLIT) for treatment of her seasonal allergies at that time. As the spring allergy season was right around the corner, I also recommended that she begin taking quercetin, a natural antihistamine found in onions and garlic, to help provide symptomatic relief for her allergies while the SLIT started to work (see "Supplement Highlight: Quercetin").

After a month or so of being wheat-free, my patient reported that her seasonal allergies had improved. Her body had been experiencing an increased degree of inflammation as a result of her diet, which had been worsening the severity of her seasonal allergy symptoms. In addition, her fatigue had improved and she had also lost a few pounds without increasing her exercise or limiting her diet in any other way. As a bonus, she was pleasantly surprised to find that being on a wheat-free diet improved her acne. We ended up using a combination herbal allergy formula along with the quercetin to alleviate her symptoms throughout the remainder of the spring allergy season. Today, she is continuing to lose weight, her allergy symptoms are dramatically improved, and she is working on continuing her full course of SLIT. (See page 48 for more information on SLIT.)

My patient's story illustrates the connection between allergies or sensitivities and other health issues that may, at first, seem completely unrelated. It is likely that the large amounts of wheat she was ingesting and her correspondingly large intake of amylopectin A were promoting her weight gain. They were also causing her to have elevated levels of inflammation. Amylopectin A causes extremely high levels of blood sugar, which causes higher-than-normal insulin secretion. Excessive insulin secretion promotes inflammation. Furthermore, her digestive symptoms were certainly a by-product of her wheat sensitivity. Her seasonal allergies were also likely worsened by the inflammation caused by her diet. When she adopted a less-inflammatory diet, her seasonal allergy symptoms improved.

Inflammation and allergies have a lot in common. They both

result from a number of biological, cellular, and immunological processes in your body, some of which they share.[5] In this chapter, we will explore the interdependent relationship between allergies and inflammation and how the two immune system responses contribute to overall health.

INFLAMMATION NATION

As scientists learn more about the physiology of disease, one common perpetrator continues to emerge at the top of the "most wanted" list—inflammation.[6] Inflammation is your immune system's response to injury, irritation, or infection. It involves increased white blood cells, redness, pain, swelling, and heat. Inflammation can affect any

The Power of Antioxidants

Quercetin, a natural antihistamine, is an example of antioxidants that can neutralize free radicals.[7] Free radicals can be so damaging because when they accumulate inside cells, they cause damage to cellular components, including DNA. This damage to the DNA can promote dysfunction that leads to the development of tumors. Because they fight free radicals, antioxidants help control this damage and prevent a number of diseases and conditions, including allergies.[8]

Some of the most powerful antioxidants are vitamin C (ascorbic acid), beta-carotene, and vitamin E. There are plenty of good sources of each of these antioxidants.[9]

Vitamin C	Beta-Carotene	Vitamin E
• Broccoli	• Carrots	• Almonds
• Green peppers	• Collards	• Bran cereal
• Red peppers	• Spinach	• Hazelnuts
• Oranges	• Squash	• Peanuts
• Papaya	• Sweet potatoes	• Sunflower oil
• Strawberries		• Sunflower seeds
		• Wheat germ

part of your body and is often described with "itis." For example, rhinitis is inflammation of the nose, arthritis is inflammation of the joints, and sinusitis is inflammation of the sinuses. (However, asthma means inflammation of the airways, so the "itis" rule doesn't always apply.)[10]

Many things in your environment can cause inflammation; the world we live in these days is very proinflammatory. Environmental toxins; high-fat, high-sugar processed foods; stressful lifestyles—they all cause your body to become hyperinflamed. These stressors also change the way your body functions and heals, acting on receptors, enzymes, mediators, and cells involved in both allergies and inflammation.[11]

The problem is, once your body switches into a proinflammatory state, it doesn't operate in an optimal fashion. It's in a state of high alert. There is something wrong, and your body knows it. It wants to eliminate the problem, but sometimes it has a hard time doing so. It could be that it is hard to avoid the problem (such as pollution, if you live in a city) or that your body doesn't have the resources to deal with the problem effectively (for example, due to a nutrient-deficient diet). As a result, your body becomes increasingly inflamed and thus becomes vulnerable to even *more* breakdown and disease, which ultimately causes more inflammation.

Allergies are one of the many conditions that can result from this vicious inflammatory cycle. An inflamed body is more sensitive to things in its environment, and is therefore more likely to overreact to food, pollen, animal dander, and other allergens. Other conditions—such as diabetes, heart disease, cancer, obesity, and chronic pain—can also result from uncontrolled inflammation.[12]

A Crash Course in Inflammation

To understand the connection between inflammation and allergies, you must first understand the physiology of inflammation. The term "inflammation" comes from the Latin word *inflammo*, which means, "to set alight or ignite." Similar to allergies, inflammation starts out as a well-intended immune response. Inflammation is often confused with infection, but the two are distinctly different. Infection

INFLAMMATION GLOSSARY:
The Biggest Players in the Inflammatory Process

Arachidonic acid (AA): AA is a proinflammatory omega-6 polyunsaturated fatty acid made from membrane phospholipids.

Cyclooxygenase (COX): COX is an enzyme required to convert arachidonic acid to prostaglandins.[13] There are two different forms of COX, COX-1 and COX-2. Both COX-1 and COX-2 work to induce pain by allowing prostaglandins to cause inflammation. These two enzymes are similar, but COX-1 promotes clotting, protects your stomach, and is involved in pain, while COX-2 is more involved in the pain that results from inflammation in your body.[14]

Cytokines: Among the most important players in inflammation, cytokines are proteins that help immune cells communicate and coordinate the inflammatory response. They also stimulate hematopoietic stem cells to multiply and turn into immune cells. Cytokines include IL-1, IL-6, and TNF-alpha.[15]

Dendritic cells (DCs): DCs are like the police out on patrol for criminals. They search for and pick out certain foreign antigens and they take them to local lymph nodes to activate T cells, natural killer cells (NKs), and B cells.

Histamine: When mast cells encounter an allergen, they release histamine, which starts the allergic reaction. Histamine increases blood flow and encourages fluid and protein to leak into tissues, causing swelling and redness.

results from invading bacteria, viruses, or fungi. Inflammation, on the other hand, is your body's response to these infections. It is part of a complex biological reaction to protect your body from potentially harmful invaders, be they viruses, bacteria, trauma, or allergens, such as pollen and mold. Without inflammation, wounds would never heal, tissue would become more damaged, and your body would eventually die from any wound it received.[21]

So in short bursts, inflammation can be a good thing. But when it goes on too long and becomes chronic, inflammation can turn bad and put you at risk for all kinds of diseases and health issues.

Interleukin-1 (IL-1): IL-1 is a cytokine. It is produced by platelets, macrophages, and monocytes. IL-1 stimulates a number of responses, including blood clotting, activating T cells during the immune response, decreasing blood pressure, and inducing fever.[16]

Interleukin-6 (IL-6): A protein that acts as both a proinflammatory and an anti-inflammatory cytokine. Macrophages and T cells secrete IL-6, usually in response to trauma, such as burns or tissue damage.[17]

Leukotrienes (LT): Inflammatory substances released by mast cells during an allergic reaction or an allergy attack.[18]

Natural killer cells (NKs): Part of the innate immune system, natural killer cells are white blood cells that reject tumors and viruses by attacking and "killing" the invaders.[19]

Prostaglandins: Prostaglandins are fatty acid derivatives of arachidonic acid involved in a number of bodily processes, including pain sensation.

Tumor necrosis factor-alpha (TNF-alpha): When mast cells are stimulated, they quickly release TNF-alpha. All cells involved in inflammation have TNF-alpha receptors, or TNF-alpha tells those cells to make more TNF-alpha on their own. As more TNF-alpha gets produced, the inflammatory response amplifies.[20]

The inflammatory process is complicated, and it involves quite a few chemicals. Here's one example of how inflammation occurs in the body: One of the big players in the inflammatory process is an enzyme called cyclooxygenase-2 (COX-2). COX-2 converts arachidonic acid (an omega-6 fatty acid and another big player in the inflammatory arena) into a protein called tumor necrosis factor-alpha (TNF-alpha) and the cytokines interleukin-1 (IL-1) and interleukin-6 (IL-6). Both TNF-alpha and IL-1 cause your body to release free radicals; these free radicals work to attack invaders, but they can also do major damage to your body by destroying cells and DNA.[22] This damage—which is the major problem when it comes to inflammation in your body and resultant disease—is called oxidative stress.[23]

To help my patients better grasp the concept of inflammation without having to introduce complicated physiology, I often use the example of the drug celecoxib (Celebrex), which is a COX-2 inhibitor. This prescription anti-inflammatory drug does exactly as advertised and reduces inflammation quickly. It also comes with some serious potential for side effects, including risk of death.

Celebrex works by blocking the action of COX-2—one of the most powerful enzymes for producing inflammation in your body. When you block COX-2, you literally stop pain in its tracks.[24] The opposite is also true: When you help facilitate COX-2, you make inflammation much more likely. I mentioned that COX-2 converts the omega-6 fatty acid arachidonic acid into inflammatory chemicals, which lead to free radicals and tissue damage. When you take in excessive omega-6 fatty acids (by eating lots of foods that contain refined vegetable oils such as snack foods, cookies, and crackers) without taking in an appropriate amount of anti-inflammatory omega-3 fatty acids (you should aim for a 2:1 ratio of omega-6 to omega-3 fatty acids), you give COX-2 that much more proinflammatory material to work with. Eating too many omega-6 fatty-acid–rich foods is like adding fuel to the inflammation fire.[25]

The Connection Between Allergies and Inflammation

There is a clear connection between allergies and inflammation; the two immune responses are linked in several ways. For one thing, inflammation is an important part of the allergic response. In hay fever, mucous membranes in your ears, nose, and throat become inflamed. In asthma, inflammation affects your airways. And during the life-threatening anaphylactic allergic reaction that can result from certain allergies, usually to foods, inflammation can affect your entire body.

In someone with allergies, the key chemical behind this allergic inflammation is histamine. During an acute allergic reaction, the immune system reacts to a substance that nonallergic people's immune systems would view as harmless. Allergens bind to IgE antibodies, which trigger mast cells to release histamine, which triggers allergy symptoms to set in. In the case of asthma, histamine causes the airways to become inflamed and to swell, which makes breathing more difficult.[26]

Allergies are prime examples of chronic inflammation in the body. Research has shown that people with allergies don't just experience inflammation during a flare; they actually have a higher baseline inflammation level all the time, particularly during the 2 months following allergy season. This minimal persistent inflammation, as it is called, then makes allergy sufferers more vulnerable to an allergy attack—and to having even more inflammation—when allergens do show up.[27]

On a deeper level, allergic inflammation involves an intricate communication between several proinflammatory cells, including mast cells, lymphocytes, eosinophils, basophils, dendritic cells, and at times, neutrophils.[28]

In terms of asthma, a few different inflammatory mediators, including T-helper cells, cytokines, prostaglandins, and leukotrienes, are involved in an asthma attack.[29] The mast cells, "allergy cells" in the body, are key players when it comes to initiating inflammation. Here is a general overview of what mast cells do.

- Mast cells' cytoplasm is loaded with granules that mediate the inflammatory process.
- These mediators recruit white blood cells, including:
  - *The monocytes that become macrophages when they leave the blood and enter the tissue.*[30]
  - *Neutrophils, which help fight off infections, especially those caused by fungi and bacteria.*[31]
  - *Eosinophils, proinflammatory cells that become active in response to certain invaders, including allergens and bacteria.*[32]
  - *Lymphocytes, including the B cells, T cells, and NK cells. B lymphocytes turn into cells that make antibodies, substances*

that attach to antigens and help the body destroy them. T lym-
phocytes directly attack antigens and release cytokines, chemicals
that control the immune response. Together, B and T cells help
create your immune system's memory, so it can easily attack
invaders it has seen before.[33]

In addition to recruiting these white blood cells, mast cells release their own inflammatory chemicals, one of which is histamine. Histamine brings on allergy symptoms like sneezing, runny nose, and hives, and it also causes inflammation by increasing blood flow and encouraging fluid and protein to leak into tissues.[34]

There are other elements of the allergy and inflammation connection that are more complicated and less well understood. Researchers are still learning more. In a 2011 review published in the journal *Immunological Reviews,* researchers said people with allergies may have defective anti-inflammatory mechanisms and molecules, including problems with lipids and cytokines. So over time, both allergies and inflammation get worse.[35]

THE ALLERGY AND OBESITY CONNECTION

The more scientists learn about allergy and obesity, the more the two seem to be related. Rates of both conditions are steadily climbing throughout the world, making researchers scratch their chins and consider a connection between the two. According to the World Health Organization, in 2008, more than 1.4 billion adults in the world were overweight and 500 million were obese, and these numbers are rising. At the same time, 235 million people had asthma, and those numbers are going up as well.[36] In addition to asthma, scientists have found connections between obesity and a variety of other allergic diseases, including allergic rhinitis, allergic conjunctivitis, and atopic dermatitis (eczema).[37]

In a review published in the September 2013 issue of *International Archives of Allergy and Immunology,* researchers examined the connection between obesity and allergies. The review showed that overweight children were more likely to have eczema, and the more overweight they were, the worse their skin conditions tended to be.[38]

They also found a clear connection between asthma and obesity. In one study, risk for wheezing went up steadily with increasing body mass index (BMI), showing that the heavier a person was, the worse his asthma. However, the question remains as to whether obesity *causes* asthma or the reverse is true. (It's the old "chicken or egg" puzzle.) Some think people with asthma are less likely to exercise for fear of suffering an attack, and therefore, they're more likely to gain weight. However, there are more studies to support the notion that the opposite is true—obesity worsens asthma.

One such study looked at 17,316 adults ages 18 to 65 and 10,700 children ages 5 to 17, all of whom had persistent asthma in 2008. The study members fit into one of three different categories based on their BMIs—normal, overweight, or obese. Researchers then looked at whether or not the participants had an asthma attack in the spring, summer, fall, or winter of 2009. The results: Both BMI and season exacerbated asthma symptoms. Higher BMI increased risk for asthma attacks in adults and kids with persistent asthma, especially in fall and winter.[39]

Another study published in the *British Journal of Sports Medicine* looked at 452 adult men and found that those with higher BMIs had increased white blood cell counts (markers of inflammation) compared to men of a normal weight. The researchers looked at the individual types of white blood cells (neutrophils, lymphocytes, monocytes, basophils, and eosinophils) and found that levels of *all* of these white blood cells were higher in overweight men.[40]

But perhaps the biggest link between obesity and allergies is in the arena of food allergies. We talked about the connection between food allergies and inflammation. Food allergies, being overweight, and excessive inflammation all seem to be interconnected as well. For one thing, overweight people seem to be more sensitive to food allergens.[41] I have seen patients steadily lose weight after they identify and cut out a food allergen, like the wheat-allergic mother of two. Interestingly, underweight people seem to be more sensitive to food allergens, too, but researchers aren't sure why.[42]

Types of Inflammation: The Good, the Bad, and the Ugly

When your immune system spots an invader, inflammation is one of the ways in which it prepares your defenses. Inflammation is an important first step in the fight against invading microorganisms or allergens, and it activates your body's healing processes.[43] There are two main types of inflammation—acute and chronic.

Acute inflammation happens quickly following an injury or illness, such as a sore throat, appendicitis, or a scratch or cut on the skin. It usually lasts for a few days but can go on for as long as a few weeks.[44]

During acute inflammation, your body goes through the following steps.

1. Your body senses an irritant, let's say a scratch on the skin of your elbow. The small branches of arteries that supply blood to your elbow skin dilate, leading to increased blood flow. The area around the scratch turns red.

2. Your capillaries change and become more permeable, so fluid and blood proteins can move through the spaces between cells (called interstitial spaces) and start the healing process.

As your body goes through these stages, there are five signs of acute inflammation: pain, redness, immobility, swelling, and heat.

Pain. Inflammation usually causes pain, which results from swelling

Food Allergies and Inflammation

Naturopathic physicians are taught to always think about the functioning of the liver and the gastrointestinal (GI) tract when assessing a person's health. If either the liver or the GI tract is not working well, then overcoming other health problems will certainly be more difficult.

As evidence of the influence that the GI tract may have on other organ systems, consider the GI-skin connection. People who have food allergies leading to increased GI aggravation and inflammation will frequently also have skin issues. In fact, when people are able to heal their GI tracts, their skin issues often resolve as well. In pushing on nerves. Pain can also result from chemicals released specifically to stimulate nerve endings. We all know pain is no fun, but it is an important warning sign that tells you something is harming your body.[45]

Redness. As blood vessels dilate and capillaries fill with more blood, an inflamed area turns red.

Immobility. Depending on the degree of inflammation, the affected area may not move or function as it normally would.

Swelling. Inflammation can cause a buildup of fluid, and therefore, swelling.

Heat. Excess fluid in the inflamed area can make it feel hot.[46]

Chronic inflammation. Inflammation that persists for several months and, in some cases, years. In contrast to acute inflammation, chronic inflammation is harmful to your body. When a disease or condition persists for too long—such as an autoimmune disease, like multiple sclerosis or rheumatoid arthritis; allergies; or asthma—the inflammatory response can backfire and become misdirected. Instead of healing tissue, they way acute inflammation does, chronic inflammation can actually lead to tissue destruction and cause many more problems than the initial invader that sparked it in the first place. This puts sufferers at risk for diseases and conditions that include hay fever, heart disease, and some cancers.[47,48,49]

Chapter 3, I talked about a college-age patient whose skin cleared up when she stopped eating foods to which she was allergic. I've repeatedly seen, in her case and in others, that when you heal the gut and functioning improves, the skin clears up as well.

The idea that the GI tract is significant in determining the health of an individual seems to be gaining support in the conventional medical world. The more scientists learn about the immune system and inflammation, the more they uncover the many inflammatory reactions that take place in the digestive tract and can cause cramping, nausea, vomiting, and bloating.

There's research to support this food allergy and inflammation connection. In a 2007 European study, researchers looked at two groups of kids—an overweight group and a normal-weight group. They then measured three indicators of inflammation: high-sensitivity C-reactive protein (CRP), a marker of inflammation in the body; plaque in the carotid arteries; and levels of immunoglobulin G (IgG). All three of these markers indicate delayed food allergies.[50]

They found that the overweight children had three times the CRP and 2½ times the IgG as the normal weight kids. The overweight kids also had thicker arteries and early signs of atherosclerosis. These results suggest that food allergies may actually cause inflammation and obesity, not vice versa.[51] Of course, it may be a vicious circle: The allergy causes the inflammation, which predisposes you to increased sensitivity.

One explanation for the study findings by the authors is something called leaky gut syndrome, which is exactly what it sounds like. Food allergies and leaky gut often coexist. For various possible reasons, including food allergies, a poor Standard American Diet, or microbial overgrowth, your GI tract can become irritated—so irritated that it actually breaks down and develops "cracks" in its lining. These cracks allow food particles to move out of your intestines and into your bloodstream. When these particles leave your gut, they are immediately recognized by your immune system as a foreign substance. In response, your immune system reacts by setting off a series of reactions aimed at eliminating this foreign substance, many of which are mediated by inflammation. These inflammatory processes can be very powerful, as there are large numbers of immune cells surrounding your GI system. The inflammation can be so powerful that it does not stay contained within your GI tract but rather can be felt throughout your entire body.[52]

Over time, the inflammation that results from a leaky gut can lead to conditions like nonalcoholic fatty liver disease and insulin resistance, which can cause obesity.[53] This leaky gut inflammation can also make people even more susceptible to food allergies, thus creating more inflammation.[54]

One way to help prevent leaky gut—and the inflammation, obesity, and other conditions that it can promote—is to create a healthy bacterial ecosystem in your GI tract. You don't realize it as you go through your daily life, but there are literally millions of bacteria living both on and within you at all times. Making sure they're the right types of bacteria can actually improve your health. Some of the bacteria have names that you might recognize, such as *Lactobacillus* or *Bifidobacterium*. Others have names that you might consider scary, like *E. coli*. When these bacteria live in the right proportions, they promote optimal GI system health. It's when the bacterial society within you gets disrupted that GI inflammation and illness may ensue.

The bacterial society within your gut regulates itself to a large extent. Each strain of microorganism is kept in check by the presence of the other strains also living within your system. The type of bacteria is also influenced by the types of foods that are regularly processed through your GI tract. A high-sugar diet, a high-protein diet, and a vegetarian diet all favor different strains of bacteria.

Some of the bacteria in your GI system have the potential to be pathogenic, if their population gets large enough. This can occur for reasons such as poor dietary habits or antibiotic use. Changes to the internal milieu (or environment) can also occur when the wrong type of bacteria is introduced into your system, as in the case of food poisoning. If the undesirable bacteria dominate the gastrointestinal society for extended periods of time, damage can occur to the lining of the intestines, allowing partially digested food to enter your bloodstream and stimulating your immune system. And that stimulated immune system can promote further inflammation throughout your body and increase your risk of obesity, heart disease, autoimmune disease . . . and allergies.[55]

To demonstrate the importance of good bacteria in the gut, researchers fed thin mice a high-fat diet to change their intestinal bacteria from good bacteria to the bad type. (High-fat diets feed toxin-promoting bacteria in the GI tract and kill good bacteria that fight off invaders.)[56]

Researchers found that the mice that ate the high-fat Standard American–like Diet favored a bacterial population that produced a toxin called lipopolysaccharide (LPS). This toxin was then able to seep into the bloodstream through the leaky gut that had also occurred due to the poor diet. In people, LPS is known to promote the production of proinflammatory molecules such as IL-1, IL-6, and TNF-alpha. The resulting inflammation, especially when it's chronic in nature, can cause insulin resistance, fatty liver, and obesity.[57]

Further research suggests that a less-than-ideal ratio of good to bad bacteria may also promote food allergies. Referring back to the hygiene hypothesis (see page 18), some scientists think that our lack of exposure to a range of bacteria early in life leaves our guts without the beneficial bacteria they need to stave off food allergies.[58]

A study published in *Proceedings of the National Academy of Sciences* supports this. Researchers compared the gut bacteria of 14 kids from a rural African village in Burkina Faso to the gut bacteria of 15 children in Florence, Italy. They found that the bacteria in these two groups of children were very different. The children in the African village live in a community that produces its own food, and they eat a mostly vegetarian diet similar to the one humans ate 10,000 years ago. The Italian kids, on the other hand, eat a diet close to the SAD—high in animal fat, sugar, and empty calories. The bacteria in their guts was less varied (or less biodiverse) than the bacteria in the guts of the African children. The study authors concluded that the difference in the bacterial flora in the two groups of kids was due to the extreme differences in their diets.[59]

Children who live in developing third-world countries have much lower rates of food allergies, and their protective gut bacteria may have something to do with it.[60] The moral of the story: Keeping your GI system and gut lining as healthy as possible is vital not just for digestive wellness, but also for overall health.[61]

Fighting Inflammation and Allergies: Going with Your Gut Instincts

We've established that allergies and inflammation are connected, not just because allergies cause inflammation but also because the two processes share some of the same proinflammatory chemical messengers. So the big question is, can you control inflammation in your body and start curing your allergies? The answer is yes, and The Allergy Solution Plan in this book (see page 231) will provide

Paving the Way to a New Diet with Probiotics

When I see patients who are making an effort to adopt a healthier vegetable-based diet, I often hear them complain of increased gas. One reason this occurs is that the bacterial populations in their digestive systems haven't had time to properly adapt to their new diets. I'll often prescribe a probiotic and a digestive enzyme to help them more easily transition to their new diets.

you with a comprehensive program for doing so. At this stage, I just want to introduce you to some of the important parts of the plan.

First, to stop the inflammatory process in its tracks, one of the most important things you can do is maintain an optimal weight. I believe that breaking out of the vicious cycle of obesity and inflammation is one of the best things a person can do to help control inflammation. This is not just my opinion, either; in one study, researchers found that postmenopausal overweight or obese women who lost at least 5 percent of their body weight had fewer inflammatory markers than they did before they dropped the pounds.[62]

Second, you can reduce your intake of proinflammatory omega-6 fatty acids (the ones that can be converted to TNF-alpha, IL-1, and IL-6) and *increase* your intake of the anti-inflammatory omega-3 fatty acids. Foods rich in omega-3 fatty acids have great potential to reduce inflammatory cytokines and thus lower systemic inflammation. The best omega-3 fatty acids are eicosapentaenoic acid (EPA) and docosahexaenoic acid (DHA); they can actually help your body make anti-inflammatory prostaglandins and reduce its own inflammation.[63] This means that you need to eat less vegetable oil and fewer processed foods (which contain omega-6s) and eat more cold-water fish, nuts, and flaxseed (which contain omega-3s). As I've mentioned, you should aim for an omega-6 fatty acid to omega-3 fatty acid ratio of 2:1, or better yet, a ratio of 1:1.[64]

And third, you can boost the number of beneficial bacteria living in your gut by taking probiotics. You can get probiotics from foods like yogurt or sauerkraut, or you can take them in supplement form. If you choose supplements, look for probiotics that contain *Lactobacillus* and *Bifidobacterium*.[65]

This again brings me to one of the main themes of this book: Treating the cause of disease. Too often people treat their allergies the same way they treat a lot of other health conditions—by only treating the symptoms and ignoring the cause. By looking at your body as a whole and addressing underlying risk factors, such as chronic inflammation, it is possible not only to improve and eliminate allergic symptoms but also to significantly reduce your risk of other diseases as well. Essentially, it's a two-for-one deal: Use a healthy lifestyle approach to treat your allergies, and make a drastic improvement to your overall health. After all, who doesn't want that?

6

Preventing Age-Associated Inflammation

ONE OF MY OLDEST PATIENTS, B. G., is in his late 80s; he's also one of my most inspirational patients. He's lived a very rich life and is also a colon cancer survivor. Since his cancer diagnosis, this gentleman has been very proactive about his health. He exercises every day, eats a healthy vegetable-based diet, and takes high-quality supplements specifically prescribed for him based on his needs.

One of those supplements is an omega-3 fatty acid supplement derived from molecularly distilled fish oil. As we've discussed previously, omega-3 fats are an essential component of a healthy lifestyle. Omega-3s decrease inflammation, improve cognitive function, and—important for this patient—can help to inhibit colon cancer growth.[1] I recently saw B. G. in my office for his yearly checkup, and at that time, I ordered an omega-3 analysis to assess his body's levels of these healthy fats. When his results came back, I was surprised by what I saw. This 80-plus-year-old guy had the best omega-3 fatty acid levels I had ever seen in a patient. His overall levels were in the high-normal range, and he had a nearly perfect ratio of omega-6 to omega-3 fats.

One of the things that I find so remarkable about this patient is his level of physical fitness. In one of my consultation rooms, I have a pair of funky-looking chairs that were made in the 1960s. They're great chairs, but they are truthfully a little low and hard to get in and out of, so they probably aren't the best patient chairs. Recently, B. G. was sitting in one of those low-slung chairs while we talked about his health. He was concerned that maybe he needed to be doing more to promote his health. He then proceeded to effortlessly stand up and get out of the chair he had been sitting in. At that point I told him, "You know, I have 40-year-old patients who have trouble getting out of those chairs, and here you are closing in on 90, and you get into and out of them without a problem. You're an example of what we should all strive for."

This patient is a shining example of the power of good lifestyle habits to keep us young. He is also an illustration of how much inflammation—or a lack thereof—contributes to overall health. As we age, we have an increased risk of developing a number or diseases and adverse health conditions, such as heart disease, arthritis, cancer, Alzheimer's, and yes, allergies. One reason for this is the accumulation of inflammation that typically accompanies the aging process. While some degree of inflammation is an inevitable part of aging, there are some things that you can do to set yourself up for less inflammation, both now and later in life.

B. G. is the perfect example. He does everything in his power to combat inflammation—he eats well, exercises, and takes a variety of herbs and supplements, including the powerful anti-inflammatory omega-3 fatty acids. He also makes time every day to do something to set his mind at ease and reduce stress. He tells me he has virtually no aches and pains. "My brother-in-law calls me a liar when I say nothing hurts, but it really doesn't," he says. He's also had no recurrence of the colon cancer that plagued him 15 years ago. And he is allergy-free.

When it comes to aging, I don't think any of us can ever completely escape the effects of time. We will never be able to completely fight all of the wrinkles and gray hair, nor will we be able to remove all of the inflammation from our bodies. However, if you take care of yourself and make an effort to reduce inflammation and promote health, you might be able to easily get in and out of some cool, low-slung, retro chairs when you reach your nineties. You will also be less likely to suffer from diseases associated with the aging process, including allergies.[2]

AN INTRODUCTION TO AGING AND INFLAMMATION

Scientists still have a lot to learn about the aging process and why some people age faster than others.[3] One established reason for the inevitable physical breakdown that comes with age is that our bodies become increasingly more inflamed as they get older. In general, elderly people have higher levels of inflammatory chemicals in their bodies, such as C-reactive protein (CRP), tumor necrosis factor-alpha (TNF-alpha), and interleukin 6 (IL-6). Once that inflammation sets in, research shows that it makes us age even faster.[4,5]

A number of studies support this link between increasing age and chronic inflammation.[6,7] In a 2013 study published in the *Canadian Medical Association Journal*, researchers looked at 3,044 middle-age adults who had no history of stroke, heart attack, or cancer and monitored them for 10 years. At the beginning of the decade-long study, they measured participants' levels of IL-6, an important marker of inflammation.[8] (IL-6 is a good marker of inflammation in the body because it helps control the release of other cytokines and inflammatory molecules that directly impact your muscles and brain.)[9]

After 10 years, 721 (23.7 percent) of the participants had aged successfully, based on the researchers' criteria. Of the remaining participants, 321 (10.6 percent) had heart disease, 147 (4.8 percent) had died, and 1,855 (60.9 percent) fit the criteria for normal aging.[10] The most important finding: The participants with the highest IL-6 levels were 47 percent less likely to age successfully when compared to those with normal IL-6 levels. Those with elevated IL-6 were also more likely to have suffered a heart attack or to have died from a condition not related to heart disease.[11]

Based on these results, researchers concluded that chronic inflammation reduces your likelihood of disease-free aging. In other words, the higher your inflammation levels, the "older" you are.[12]

Which Came First, the Candles or the Flame?

Scientists know for sure that most people become more inflamed as they get older. But it's not entirely clear whether inflammation levels increase and then consequently promote disease, or whether the diseases and conditions come first, causing people to become more inflamed.[13]

Some studies have shown that elderly people have inflammation regardless of whether or not they have any diseases, which would indicate that aging alone invites the swelling and tenderness in our tissues. One contributing factor may be that people tend to gain weight as they gain years. As we learned in Chapter 5, obesity certainly contributes to inflammation.[14] However, other studies have not shown increased inflammatory markers in older people *unless* they have an underlying condition or disease, which would indicate that the diseases come first, then the inflammation.[15]

It may also be a combination, where aging makes us more inflamed, while age-related inflammation then accelerates the aging process.[16] For instance, researchers at Albert Einstein College of Medicine in New York City have found that as a particular area of the brain called the hypothalamus becomes more inflamed with age, people are more likely to develop metabolic syndrome, a group of risk factors that includes a large waistline, high blood pressure, high blood sugar, and high cholesterol and triglycerides. Metabolic syndrome raises your risk of heart disease and other health problems.[17,18]

To further explore this connection, researchers activated a specific biochemical pathway, called the NF-kB pathway, within the hypothalamus. This study was performed on mice, and the activation of the NF-kB pathway led to decreased muscle strength and skin thickness in the mice tested. It also made it more difficult for those mice to learn, and it decreased their life spans. In short, when researchers stimulated the NF-kB pathway, the mice aged. Therefore, the hypothalamus and the NF-kB pathway appear to play an important role in the aging process.[19] Generally speaking, activation of this pathway appears to play a central role in inflammation, which, in turn, can accelerate the aging process.[20]

There are a number of additional theories on the aging and inflammation connection. One possible explanation is something called the free radical theory of aging. As we noted in Chapter 5, highly reactive atoms called free radicals can destroy cells and DNA in a process called oxidative stress.[21]

This free radical–induced damage can make a person more vulnerable to many age-related diseases and disorders, including diabetes, heart disease, and cancer.[22] (See "The Cancer Connection".) Oxidative stress is, in fact, one of the main causes of disease. And in general, as people age, they have more oxidative stress as well as less ability to use antioxidants (the molecules that can stop free radical damage) as protection against that stress.[23]

Another theory is that as people age, their bodies become less able to recover from periods of acute inflammation. To give you an example, imagine that a 70-year-old woman contracts pneumonia. To fight the infection, her body becomes acutely inflamed. But once the infection clears, the inflammation doesn't fully go away. Then,

The Cancer Connection

The link between age and increased cancer risk has been proven. With almost every cancer type, rates steadily increase with age. There are probably a few reasons why.

For one, immune function declines with age and puts older people at risk for cancer and autoimmune diseases. Put simply, like an old car, the aging immune system doesn't work as well as it once did. As a result, it can't put the brakes on a progressing tumor.[24] The biggest factor seems to be the decline in T cells, the immune system cells that look for fragments of antigens on the surfaces of cells that are infected or cancerous.[25]

For another, research has also linked cancer with allergies, claiming that people with allergies are more likely to develop certain types of cancer. Chronic inflammation is one of a few different explanations for this link. The thinking is that the ongoing inflammation caused by allergies causes oxidative stress, which damages tumor-suppressor genes. As a result, those genes can't inhibit cancer cell growth as effectively as they should. More research needs to be done, but the take-home message at this point is this: Do your best to keep yourself as inflammation-free as possible, and you will help prevent many diseases and conditions.[26] And if you also reduce the number of toxins to which you are exposed over your lifetime, you're sure to decrease inflammation.

when the next threat comes along—say a cold virus or an allergen—
her already-inflamed body overreacts and stays even more inflamed
once the cold or allergic reaction is gone. This vicious circle continues and the leftover inflammation mounts.[27]

Yet another study points to a group of genes to explain the connection between aging and inflammation. In a study that was
funded by the National Institutes of Health and published in the
journal *Molecular Cell*, researchers discussed what they found out
about a family of genes called AUF1. A family of four related genes,
AUF1 controls the inflammatory response in your body by turning
off inflammation to stop the onset of septic shock.[28] (Septic shock is
life-threateningly low blood pressure that sets in as a result of a serious infection.)[29] When researchers turned off AUF1, aging accelerated, which suggested that the genes actually helped slow the aging
process. AUF1 also appears to help protect chromosomes, thus preventing rapid aging and cancer.[30]

ALLERGIES AND AGING

We've established the connection between aging and inflammation,
but what does all of that have to do with allergies, you ask? Put simply, the chronic inflammation that increases with age puts people at
a higher risk of allergies.[31] And when it comes to allergies, let's face
it—the dark circles under your itchy, watery eyes and your constant
runny nose, not to mention the other unpleasant symptoms that go
along with allergies, don't make you feel healthy or young (see
"Anatomy and Allergies in the Elderly").[32]

Allergies are often thought of as childhood conditions, and
there's a good reason for that: Many children outgrow their allergies, especially food allergies to milk and eggs. In addition, a number of studies have shown that levels of immunoglobulin-E (IgE),
the antibody responsible for releasing histamine, decrease with age.
In one study of 326 people with allergies, IgE levels peaked in the
twenties and thirties and decreased from there on out. Other studies have shown that as allergic people get older, they have gradually
fewer allergen sensitivities.[33]

Anatomy and Allergies in the Elderly

In addition to battling the inflammation that often comes with age, older people undergo anatomical changes that can make allergy symptoms worse. According to an article published in the journal *Allergy, Asthma, and Clinical Immunology*, as you get older, the tip of your nose droops, resulting in decreased airflow through your nostrils and worsened hay fever symptoms. In addition, nasal hairs are less active in postmenopausal women, so allergens are more likely to build up in the nose and throat and cause symptoms in these individuals.[34]

But—and this is a big but—there are also a number of allergic conditions that persist into adulthood and the senior years as well as some allergies that make their initial appearance later in life.[35] Allergies and asthma can show up for the first time at any age, even as late as 70 or 80 years old.[36]

Additionally, as allergy rates are increasing in the general population, they are also rising in the elderly. Doctors report seeing more older patients for allergy symptoms than ever before.[37] In one study, the rate of allergies in people over age 60 was estimated to be 4 percent.[38] Other studies put the number at 5 to 10 percent. Considering the fact that people 65 years old and older are the fastest-growing segment of the population in developed countries, the number of elderly people with allergies will be an increasingly important part of the overall allergy picture.[39]

When it comes to asthma, according to the Centers for Disease Control and Prevention, about 10 percent of the 14.5 million asthma sufferers are age 65 or older.[40] Considering the way that things are trending, the number of elderly people suffering from asthma will double over the next 20 years. Furthermore, experts think the numbers of older people with allergies and asthma are underreported, so the actual number of elderly with allergies is probably much higher. Unfortunately, there are fewer studies done on older people with allergies, and therefore, fewer statistics on rates in this group.[41]

In addition, symptoms of other conditions of older age, such as shortness of breath, wheezing, and chest tightness may mimic symptoms of allergies and asthma; as a result, allergies and asthma are tough for doctors to pinpoint. Older people are also more likely to take medications with side-effects similar to allergy and asthma symptoms. For example, ACE inhibitors, which are popular drugs for treating diabetes, high blood pressure, and heart disease, can cause a dry cough. And the beta-blockers used to treat high blood pressure and glaucoma can constrict the airways and lead to difficulty breathing.[42]

But allergies and asthma in older adults are nothing to sneeze at. When they do show up later in life, these conditions tend to be more severe. Older adults with asthma are more likely to suffer respiratory failure and are less likely to go into remission than younger people with the disease.[43]

Why do allergies sometimes wait decades before rearing their ugly heads? There are a few possible reasons. For one thing, it can take years of exposure to an allergen before your body makes IgE antibodies and finally reacts to that allergen.[44] In addition, as people age, they seem to be more sensitive to IgE than they were earlier in life, making them more likely to react to allergens like cockroaches, dust, and mold, even if these substances had never bothered them before. Not only do allergy symptoms persist in elderly people whose IgE levels remain relatively high, but they are also more likely to lead to asthma.[45]

Second, some scientists think that the same hygiene hypothesis that may explain why people of all ages are experiencing more allergies may also explain why older people are more vulnerable to first-time allergy symptoms. Because of smaller family size, increased sanitation, and less exposure to viruses and bacteria, people are suffering fewer infections; as a result, their relatively inactive immune systems are more likely to react to everyday things like dust, pollen, and mold. Increasing air pollution in our developing world may also play a role.[46]

In terms of asthma, older people are also more likely to suffer asthma attacks in response to nonallergen irritants, such as cold air, potent perfumes and other smells, and respiratory infections. (And

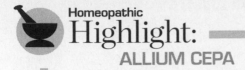

Highlight:
ALLIUM CEPA

Latin for "onion," *Allium cepa* is a homeopathic remedy that treats allergy symptoms mimicking those you would experience from cutting the pungent vegetable. People who benefit most from *Allium cepa* are those who suffer allergy symptoms such as watery discharge from the eyes, burning eyes, and burning acrid discharge from the nose.

when those respiratory infections hit in older asthmatics, they are more likely to be severe.) And older people with asthma are likely to suffer more severe declines in lung function than their nonasthmatic friends of the same age.[47]

In addition, having allergies earlier in life seems to put people at increased risk for asthma later on. In the Normative Aging Study, researchers followed a large group of people ages 21 to 80 and found that those who were allergic to cats were more likely to develop asthma in old age.[48]

It works both ways: Researchers have also found that older adults with asthma are more likely to have allergies. In a 2013 study published in the *Annals of Allergy, Asthma, and Immunology*, researchers looked at 2,573 people who took part in the National Health and Nutrition Examination Survey (NHANES) 2005–2006 and compared allergic sensitization of two groups—adults ages 20 to 40 and adults age 55 years old and older. In the younger group, 6.7 percent had asthma, and in the older group, 4.5 percent had asthma. Of the asthmatics, researchers found that 65.2 percent of the older group also had at least one allergy, making them nearly three times more likely to have an allergy than the participants who didn't have asthma. The most common allergies in the older people with asthma were dust mites and rye grass. As an interesting side note, allergies were most common in women, especially those who were overweight or obese.[49,50]

Which brings me back to one of the main themes of this book: By virtue of being more inflamed than they were in their twenties, older people become more vulnerable to all sorts of conditions, allergies included. The inflamed body is more sensitive, and therefore has more potential to overreact to dust mites, pollen, and other allergens.[51]

DON'T TAKE INFLAMMATION LYING DOWN

As my patient B. G. demonstrated, you shouldn't shrug your shoulders, put your feet up, and accept inflammation and increased risk of disease as an inevitable part of getting older. There are a number of things you can do to keep yourself healthy and nimble.

We will delve into this more in The Allergy Solution Plan, but exercise is one of the most effective ways people can fight inflammation as they get older.[52] In the short term, it is true that exercise can increase inflammation, especially if that exercise is intense and prolonged. If you've ever worked out particularly hard one day and then dreaded climbing stairs the next, you've experienced this kind of inflammation.

However, once your body adapts, regular aerobic exercise seems to be one of the best ways to *reduce* inflammation, especially as you age. At least nine studies have shown that the more physical activity older people (average age over 60) report, the fewer inflammatory markers they have.[53]

In a study published in the *Journal of the American Geriatrics Society,* researchers put half of 424 sedentary, overweight 70- to 89-year-olds on a moderate-intensity walking program and put the other half in a health education program that didn't include exercise. They then measured levels of two inflammatory markers—CRP and IL-6. After 12 months on their respective programs, levels of both inflammatory markers went down more in the exercise group than they did in the nonexercise group, especially levels of IL-6. Similar studies have shown the same results—regular aerobic exercise lowers inflammation in people age 60 and older.[54,55]

In addition to exercise, eating fewer calories may also help reduce age-related inflammation. Since the 1930s, studies done on mice have found that restricting calories helps decrease inflammation and

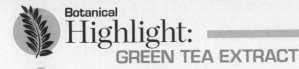

Botanical
Highlight:
GREEN TEA EXTRACT

Green tea has superpowers when it comes to fighting all kinds of age-related conditions and ailments, allergies included. The list of conditions green tea can help combat includes numerous forms of cancer, including breast, ovarian, prostate, pancreatic, and stomach; diabetes; liver disease; and inflammatory bowel disease. There's also evidence that green tea can help keep you trim.[56]

Researchers think green tea is such an effective medicine because it contains chemicals called polyphenols, which act as antioxidants. As we've discussed, antioxidants are molecules that neutralize the free radicals that can cause damaging oxidative stress.[57]

In terms of allergies, in a study published in *Scandinavian Journal of Immunology,* researchers at the State University of New York (SUNY) Downstate Medical Center in Brooklyn looked at a component of green tea extract called epigallocatechin gallate (EGCG) and its power to suppress immunoglobulin E (IgE). (To refresh your memory, IgE antibodies are proteins the body makes when exposed to allergens. IgE antibodies lead to inflammation.) They found that the EGCG in green tea extract indeed helps suppress IgE in human allergic reactions.[58]

You can take green tea in standardized extract form, as dried tea leaves made into tea, or in capsules. I tell my patients to look for a decaffeinated green tea extract standardized to contain 90 percent of the green tea polyphenols, which are the antiallergic portion of the leaves. The supplements I recommend are also standardized to contain at least 40 percent of EGCG—the most active part of the green tea plant that suppressed IgE in the SUNY study. I recommend that most people aim for 500 to 1,500 milligrams of green tea extract per day, depending on how well it works.

As a side note, whenever you buy supplements, keep in mind that they aren't regulated by the FDA, so you have to do your homework to find out what you are really getting. Look for supplements that are as pure as possible, with no unnecessary or extraneous ingredients. Also, beware of terms like "proprietary formula," which could mean 30 ingredients but no efficacious doses of any beneficial supplements or herbs.

slow the aging process. When rodents are fed a diet that has 30 percent fewer calories than usual, they live up to 40 percent longer than they normally would. Researchers at the National Institutes of Health are currently looking into whether the same is true in monkeys and other nonhuman primates. They have also started preliminary studies to look at the effects of calorie restriction in humans.[59,60,61]

As we discussed in Chapter 5, people who are overweight or obese tend to have more inflammation in their bodies because fat tissue, especially abdominal fat, produces cytokines that stimulate inflammation. And the more you exercise and the fewer calories you eat, the less fat tissue you will have.[62]

Overall, we know that exercise and healthy eating are cornerstones of any strong lifestyle routine. It's not just the changes in muscles and breathing that exercise brings on but also the positive mental changes, the improved body mass index, and the decreased inflammation that help combat both the physical breakdown accompanying aging and the increased allergy risk that can result.

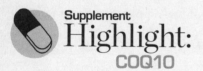

Supplement
Highlight:
COQ10

Coenzyme Q10 (CoQ10) is a substance found in your body that helps with cell growth and maintenance. It also functions as an antioxidant, fighting the free radicals that can cause oxidative stress. CoQ10 levels tend to decrease with age and in people with certain conditions, including cancer, diabetes, heart disease, and allergies.[63]

CoQ10 is a good allergy remedy because it acts as an antihistamine; it quickly works to combat allergy symptoms like sneezing, hives, and runny nose.[64] To boost levels of this natural antihistamine, you can take CoQ10 in supplement form. Personally, I like the chewable CoQ10 supplements because they taste like chocolate and are a lot better for you than a candy bar or a brownie. To help prevent allergy symptoms, I recommend taking about 300 milligrams of CoQ10 a day.

Peg's Story

Many people develop allergies in childhood, but for Peg, 52, they first kicked in when she reached middle age.

"In my 40s, I developed sneezing, rhinitis, and watery eyes that would last for months out of every year," says the nurse. "I tried several over-the-counter medications with no success."

On top of her allergies, Peg struggled with high blood pressure, which she was also unable to control with conventional drugs. "I visited many doctors and tried a number of medications, but nothing worked," she says. With high blood pressure combined with a high stress job, she was a ticking time bomb.

So at the recommendation of a friend, Peg went to see Dr. Psenka, who prescribed supplements—fish oil, curcumin, and vitamin D—as well as sublingual immunotherapy (SLIT). He also encouraged Peg to exercise regularly.

Peg found Dr. Psenka's plan easy to follow, and she saw results right away. "My blood pressure improved immediately," she says. "With the allergies, it took a couple of weeks, but my symptoms are definitely better." She also began sleeping more soundly under Dr. Psenka's care.

For Peg, Dr. Psenka's natural remedies for treating her allergies and high blood pressure worked. "I would tell anyone suffering from seasonal allergies to try naturopathic medicine and SLIT," she says.

7 Tipping the Scale: The Additive Effects of Inflammation

I RECALL TREATING A PARTICULAR 50-YEAR-OLD professional guy a few years ago. To say that this gentleman was not a picture of health would be an understatement. This guy was overweight, unhappy, and fatigued. He claimed that in the past, around 30 years ago, he had been a heavy exerciser, but like many middle-age men, he had fallen into a sedentary lifestyle. He was eating an unhealthy Standard American Diet (SAD). His blood pressure, blood sugar, and cholesterol were all elevated, and he had problems with impotency and insomnia as well. On top of all that, he complained about having tremendous gastrointestinal (GI) issues—gas, bloating, and diarrhea were the rule, rather than the exception, for him.

This patient had seen another doctor, who had offered him prescription medications to treat his hypertension and elevated blood sugar and cholesterol levels. But the potential side-effects of these medications scared him, so he sought out naturopathic care, looking for a more natural approach to addressing his health issues.

When this man came to me, we started slowly. I ordered some baseline laboratory tests, including food allergy testing, and I also instructed him on how to begin eating a healthier diet. It turned out that he had a wheat intolerance. When he removed wheat from his diet, he reported that his GI issues diminished dramatically, and he also felt more energetic than he had in a long while. We talked about the importance of regular exercise, and I persuaded him to get back into a regular exercise routine. Once he implemented this, he noted that his sleep improved and his fatigue went away.

By the time about a year had passed, my patient had dropped close to 80 pounds; his GI issues were resolved; his blood pressure, cholesterol, and blood sugar all normalized; and his other symptoms were all greatly improved. His health had completely turned around—and he never took one prescription medication.

This man's experience reinforces my theory about the downward spiral that can result from unhealthy habits. As a person succumbs more and more to a state of *dis*-ease and begins developing a number of lifestyle-related diseases and conditions, as my patient did, his or her levels of inflammation also rise dramatically. This rise in inflammation is additive and systemic. As your levels of inflammation increase, your body becomes more and more vulnerable to additional health problems.

So many of the conditions and diseases that are making people sick in today's world—obesity, heart disease, diabetes, cancer—are largely diseases of lifestyle, meaning that they arise or become worse due to poor dietary, exercise, and stress-management habits.[1] Most of the aforementioned diseases have substantial inflammatory components. When people have chronically unhealthy habits, they stimulate their bodies to produce increasingly higher levels of systemic inflammation, which further increases their risk of developing these diseases.

As we discussed in Chapter 5, allergic diseases are also promoted through an inflammatory cycle. So as you become more and more inflamed, you become even more likely to overreact, with allergic symptoms such as sneezes and hives, to substances in your body. In short, you become more allergic.[2]

The Inflammation Cup Spills Over

When talking to patients, I often make an analogy between allergic symptoms and an overflowing glass. You can only fill a glass with so much fluid before it gets filled to the top and begins spilling over.

The same concept holds true for inflammation: Your body can only adequately control so much before the levels get too high, symptoms are felt, and disease risk is elevated. When it comes to allergies, if your body is already feeling inflamed when allergy season arrives, the first speck of pollen is more likely to leave you suffering swollen, itchy eyes and a runny nose than it is for someone with lower levels of inflammation.

Back to the glass analogy: Let's say you have an empty glass in front of you and you have four known allergens—dog, cat, rye grass, and oak tree. Each one of those allergies causes the glass to fill up by a quarter. With exposure to all four allergens, your glass is 100 percent full, right to the brim.

Now let's say you also have a wheat intolerance—not an allergy to wheat or celiac disease, but an intolerance that makes your stomach hurt with gas and bloating whenever you indulge in a wheat-containing food. You go out for pizza with your friends and you eat three slices—crust and all. It is delicious, but the next morning you pay dearly with terrible gas and bloating. Your glass has spilled over.

This is a common scenario. Many of us are at the brim of our glass or, like my 50-year-old patient with the wheat intolerance, already have liquid pouring over the top. One reason so many of us are overflowing

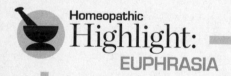

Homeopathic
Highlight:
EUPHRASIA

Also called eyebright because of its benefits to the eyes, *Euphrasia* is a purple-flowered plant. As a homeopathic remedy, *Euphrasia* seems to work best for eye-related allergy symptoms, including burning, stinging, or watery eyes as well as nasal discharge that gets worse when you lie down.[3] I generally recommend a 30c dose a couple of times per day for acute eye allergy symptoms. (Note: Homeopathic remedies are measured on the centesimal, or "c," scale, which represents the dilution.)

with inflammation is that there are proinflammatory substances all around us. The preservatives in your morning cereal, the chemicals that cause the "new car smell" in your brand new SUV, the fumes coming out of the factories you pass on the road, and the anxiety you feel once you open your full e-mail inbox—these things all add to your inflammation glass and take away from your health.

The CRP Connection

The nature of the relationship between inflammation and disease is something scientists continue to investigate. Some studies support the notion that inflammation builds, leading to increased risk for body dysfunction and disease. One marker of this inflammatory buildup is a protein called C-reactive protein (CRP), or HS-CRP for high sensitivity CRP.[4]

Like inflammation itself, CRP does have some beneficial actions in your body. It triggers many immune system responses that help fight off fungi, viruses, and bacteria. Short-term bouts of increased CRP are fine; it's when those CRP levels stay elevated due to chronic inflammation that they can do harm and cause tissue destruction.[5] Some doctors now perform blood tests to measure HS-CRP levels as a means of evaluating a patient's risk of developing a sudden heart problem, including a heart attack.[6]

Some scientists think CRP levels slowly build in the body as people experience diseases and infections. So the more illnesses a person has fought in his or her lifetime, the higher the potential inflammation and resultant CRP levels, and therefore the greater the risk of an untimely death. In the United States, people are much less likely to die at an early age today than they were 200 years ago. One thought is that people who lived hundreds of years ago died at a young age because they experienced many more infections and as a result, they had higher CRP levels.[7]

One 2008 study published in the *Journals of Gerontology, Series A: Biological Sciences* and *Medical Sciences* explored this theory. Researchers couldn't re-create the unsanitary conditions of hundreds of years ago, but they could take a good look at a population that lives under similar circumstances today. Because of limited access to modern medicine, the Tsimane people of Bolivia have high rates of infection and a low life expectancy. In fact, their current mortality rate is the same as that of people who lived in 19th-century Europe.[8] To paint a more practical picture, at the time of the study, more than two-thirds of the Tsimane participants were actively infected with at least one species of intestinal parasite.[9]

What the researchers found was interesting: As a result of years of infections, the Tsimane had higher levels of the inflammatory marker CRP throughout their lives. By age 35, the average Tsimane had spent more years with high CRP than the average American has at age 55. The CRP levels of young Tsimane people were higher than those in Americans age 65 and older. The life expectancy of the Tsimane was about half of the life expectancy in the United States, which at the time of the study was 77.2 years.[10]

So what do these findings really mean? We know that inflammation contributes to many age-related diseases, including metabolic syndrome, diabetes, heart disease, and cancer. But the results of this study show that inflammation can also result from infection and disease and can build up in your body over time; therefore, the more your body goes through in terms of infection and illness, the more inflamed it may become. In a sense, if your body fights off too many bacteria, viruses, and parasites, it can prematurely age. The take-home message is this: The more you can do to protect yourself from illness and infection, the less inflamed you will be. (One interesting footnote is that a number of recent studies have demonstrated that a range of environmental toxins can lead to increased risk for a number of diseases—including cardiovascular disease—by promoting inflammation.[11])

Diseases That Increase Inflammation

With the Tsimane in mind, one important thing you can do to prevent excess inflammation—and therefore, allergy symptoms—in your body is to work to stay healthy. There is only so much you can do to avoid bacteria and viruses, but there are steps you can take to help prevent some common promoters of inflammation. Many lifestyle-related diseases not only may arise in the face of chronic inflammation but also they actually increase inflammation once they have developed. These include obesity, diabetes, heart disease, some digestive disorders, and cancer. In the next few chapters, I will teach you some simple steps to help prevent and potentially reverse these health problems. First though, let's explore the relationship between chronic inflammation and the diseases of lifestyle.

OBESITY

One of the most important conditions to avoid is obesity, because the development of other lifestyle diseases can be hastened by carrying excess weight.[12] Obesity is the biggest health problem in the United States, with almost 155 million adult Americans now overweight or obese, according to 2013 figures from the American Heart Association.[13,14] Scientists are constantly learning more about obesity and what—other than simply eating too much—causes it. They do know it is a disorder of metabolism caused by numerous factors, including inflammation and oxidative stress.[15]

There is some debate among researchers about which comes first—the inflammation or the obesity.[16] (It's the ever-present chicken-or-egg conundrum.) There's actually research to support both sides of the debate. Those who believe that the inflammation precedes the obesity describe a series of steps like this: When you eat a food to which you are allergic or sensitive, your body becomes inflamed. That inflammation then causes your adrenal glands to secrete adrenal hormones that destabilize your blood sugar and insulin levels, causing them to become elevated. High insulin levels affect the activity of two enzymes, lipoprotein lipase and triglyceride lipase, which tell your body to store fat rather than to burn it for energy.[17] The high insulin levels also promote inflammation.

As a result, over time, you gain weight. Then, to make matters worse, having a high-body-fat percentage makes your body even more inflamed. People assume that fat tissue is just fat tissue and that other than making your jeans tighter, it doesn't do anything. However, fat is, in fact, very metabolically active and plays lots of different roles, both good and bad, in your body. One of the bad: It causes other tissues to behave differently and to become more inflamed—and more inflammation means even more sensitivity to allergens.[18]

Let's look at this in more detail. Contrary to popular belief, when you gain weight, you do not gain more fat cells. You are actually born with a set number of fat cells, and you keep that fat cell total for your entire life. When you gain weight, these cells become larger and fill with more fat; when you lose weight, they shrink. As you gain weight and your fat cells swell, they can become stretched to the point where they develop holes and they leak. To clean up the messy fat that seeps out, your immune system sends out a type of cell known as a macrophage. As they clean, the macrophages release inflammatory chemicals. The inflammation that results from this cleanup process may be the mechanism behind a lot of the negative health effects of obesity.[19]

There's more still: To counteract this inflammation, your body produces anti-inflammatory chemicals. Fighting inflammation is a good thing, but it comes at a hefty price. Some anti-inflammatory chemicals appear to interfere with leptin—the hormone responsible for keeping your body at a healthy weight. (Leptin is the reason some people can eat whatever they want and not gain weight; if these people overeat, leptin kicks in to boost metabolism and decrease appetite.) Inflammation can cause a condition called leptin resistance, where leptin doesn't work properly to control appetite and metabolism. As a result, people struggle to maintain a healthy weight.[20]

The process I just described is one of the ways people develop the condition called metabolic syndrome. Metabolic syndrome is a group of five factors that raise your risk for a number of diseases, including heart disease, diabetes, and stroke. The five risk factors are high blood pressure, high blood sugar, high triglycerides, abdominal fat, and a low level of good (HDL) cholesterol.[21] People with metabolic syndrome usually have high levels of the inflammatory marker CRP, too.[22]

Most people with metabolic syndrome go on to develop insulin resistance, which changes the way the body processes sugar and fat. As such, insulin resistance is a precursor to diabetes and nonalcoholic fatty liver disease—a condition that limits the liver's ability to perform its functions. Once people develop nonalcoholic fatty liver disease, also known as nonalcoholic steatohepatitis (NASH), they get very high cholesterol and triglyceride levels, as well as elevated blood sugar, and liver enzymes, potentially leading to severe liver dysfunction. So the more you can do to prevent inflammation, the better.

HEART DISEASE

In terms of specific disease states, the one with probably the closest connection to inflammation is heart disease. These days, fewer people are dying from heart disease in this country, but more and more people are being diagnosed with the condition. In fact, more than one in four American adults has some form of heart disease.[23]

Although no one has proven that inflammation directly causes heart disease, study after study on cardiovascular disease points to inflammation as a major contributing factor, especially to atherosclerosis.[24] Atherosclerosis is a condition in which fatty deposits called plaque build up inside the arteries. Atherosclerosis can lead to serious health problems, including heart attack and stroke.[25]

It works like this: Just like a knife can injure the tip of your finger with a cut, smoking, high-fat foods, and high blood pressure can damage your cardiovascular system. As a response to these irritants, plaque is deposited in your arteries, narrowing the lining of the vessels and potentially causing a blockage.[26]

In addition, your body sees plaque in your arteries as a foreign invader and tries to protect itself by separating that plaque from your bloodstream. One result of this attempted separation: blood clots, which are one of the biggest causes of heart attack and stroke.[27]

Researchers have also discovered that there may be a direct link between heart disease and allergies. Scientists at the Einstein Medical Center in Philadelphia looked at health information on more than 8,600 adults who participated in the National Health and Nutrition Examination Survey (NHANES). They found that people with heart disease often had allergies. They also discovered that people with wheezing had two times the risk of heart disease, and people with stuffy nose and itchy, watery eyes (rhinoconjunctivitis) were 40 percent more likely to have heart disease than people without these allergic conditions. The researchers think allergies and the inflammation that goes along with them may lead to thickening of artery walls and, eventually, to heart disease.[28]

More recently, researchers have connected allergic episodes to acute coronary syndromes. In a Turkish study published in *Inflammation and Allergy-Drug Targets,* researchers linked the inflammatory mediators released during an allergy attack—namely, histamine—to coronary artery spasms and plaque erosion or rupture.[29]

DIABETES

Diabetes, especially type 2, which is directly tied to poor lifestyle choices, is one of the fastest-growing diseases in the world. In the United States, the number of people with diabetes went from 1.5 million in 1958 to close to 19 million in 2010. This rise is mainly due to poor lifestyle habits, such as lack of exercise and eating the Standard American Diet (SAD).[30] These bad habits lead to obesity, which is a primary risk factor for diabetes. Both bad habits and extra fat tissue lead to more inflammation in the body, which researchers have also tied to diabetes risk.

New research from Denmark looked specifically at the inflammatory nature of type 2 diabetes. In one 2014 study, researchers looked at how type 2 diabetes unfolds in mice. They found that during the early stages of the disease, macrophages invade the pancreas and, in the process, release proinflammatory cytokines. Those cytokines then destroy the beta cells that produce insulin, leading to insulin resistance and diabetes.[31]

DEPRESSION

It seems that inflammation is not only associated with physical conditions but also can arise as a consequence of a person's mental health. For example, in a study at the University of Miami researchers found that depressed patients taking selective serotonin reuptake inhibitors (SSRIs) were less likely to see beneficial results from the drugs if they'd experienced a negative event (or emotional trauma) early in life. Patients who hadn't experienced such an event were more likely to respond to the drugs. Inflammation caused by the early life stressor appears to have inhibited the drugs' effects.[32]

There's also a pretty clear link between depression, asthma, allergies, and inflammation. On the surface, dealing with a chronic condition such as asthma or allergies can, in and of itself, be depressing.

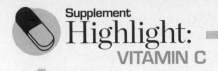

Supplement
Highlight:
VITAMIN C

American chemist Linus Pauling thought vitamin C was nature's best medicine. When it comes to fighting inflammation and allergies, he may have been on to something.

Vitamin C is a water-soluble vitamin found naturally in citrus fruits, tomatoes, and broccoli. It's important for growth and repair of tissues, especially skin, ligaments, tendons, and blood vessels. Vitamin C is also important for bone and tooth health as well as for wound healing.

The healing power of vitamin C stems from the fact that it is an antioxidant, and therefore it combats some of the damage caused by free radicals. Because of these properties, vitamin C can help treat allergy symptoms such as hay fever, asthma, and eczema.[33] When you're treating allergies, typical doses of vitamin C range from 1 to several grams per day, usually in divided doses.

A study published in *Psychosomatic Medicine* showed that people with hay fever had higher rates of depression and decreased feelings of pleasure during the early fall ragweed season. This is the opposite of the general population, which tends to get the blues during the winter months.[34] But the relationship seems to go deeper than that, to cytokines—the chemicals secreted by immune system cells to start or stop inflammation. Both conditions are connected to increased levels of these proinflammatory types of cytokines.[35]

IRRITABLE BOWEL SYNDROME

For a long time, scientists didn't think there was any connection between irritable bowel syndrome (IBS)—a chronic bowel disorder characterized by abdominal pain and intermittent diarrhea and constipation—and inflammation. But they've changed their tune. There seems to be some low-grade inflammation in the digestive tracts of some people with IBS.[36]

Some people may develop IBS as a result of gastroenteritis, often referred to as a stomach bug.[37] Most of us have suffered the acute inflammation of a stomach bug: As soon as you got infected, mast cells and cytokines were quickly recruited into action to fight against the infection. The release of these substances caused abdominal pain, cramping, vomiting, or diarrhea. Then, after a day or two of feeling poorly, chances are you started to feel better.[38]

Research points to the possibility that, in some people with IBS, the inflammatory process persisted long after the stomach infection resolved. In fact, up to 30 percent of people with IBS claim their symptoms started after a stomach infection or food poisoning. In these people, the mast cells continue to stay mildly activated, causing ongoing cramps and diarrhea.

Since mast cells are involved, this research also helps support a connection between IBS and allergies to foods and other substances. Many people with IBS report that certain foods make their symptoms worse. Plus, many people with IBS who go on food elimination diets tend to feel better, which suggests that food allergies or sensitivities may be at play.[39]

Besides food, research has shown a link between IBS and respiratory and skin allergies as well. A 2008 study found that people with hay fever and eczema were much more likely to have IBS than people without these allergies. On the flip side, IBS sufferers are more prone to eczema and hay fever than people without IBS.[40]

CANCER

Scientists have long recognized the link between cancer and inflammation, but they have yet to understand the exact reasons for the relationship.[41]

In a 2007 study published in the journal *Cell*, researchers at The University of California, San Diego, found a specific protein called p100, which is common to both inflammation and cancer. Simply put, p100 helps regulate the balance of inflammation and cellular development in your body. Someone with chronic inflammation may have too much p100, which leads to the development of more cells, including cancer cells.[42]

In a more recent review published in *Clinical and Experimental Allergy*, researchers took the relationship between inflammation and cancer a bit further and looked at how allergies fit in as well. Among other theories, they examined the *chronic inflammation hypothesis,* which says that the inflammation connected to allergies may increase cancer risk by causing oxidative stress. This oxidative stress damages tumor suppressor genes, thereby making cancer more likely to grow.[43]

I want to stress that the world we live in is very proinflammatory. We're constantly being bombarded with substances that increase our inflammation, and bad habits like choosing the couch instead of a workout and supersizing our meals certainly aren't helping. Remember the glass of inflammation analogy: It can only get so full before it starts running over the rim and causing symptoms or increasing disease risk. If you want to improve your health, not just with respect to curing your allergies but also relating to your mental and physical fitness, read on. The Allergy Solution Plan in Chapter 14 will provide tips to help you do just that.

8

Firing Yourself Up: Anxiety and Inflammation

A FEW YEARS AGO, I consulted with a very nice woman who had recently been diagnosed with metastatic breast cancer. She had been struggling with chronic anxiety even before her cancer diagnosis, and facing the condition understandably made her all that much more anxious. As with all of the patients I see, I asked this lady how she perceived her anxiety levels. On a scale of 1 to 10, with 1 being the lowest anxiety level and 10 being the highest, most people rate their average anxiety levels at about a 7 or an 8. She wasn't any different, stating that she was normally about an 8, but since her diagnosis she had been a 10-plus.

The next question I asked was more important: What did she do on a daily basis to compensate for the 10-plus stress level she was experiencing? Her answer was the same as that of many of the people I see. She didn't do anything, though she had been using Ativan to help her deal with her daily stress and to help her fall asleep at night. I asked her what she did for fun. She didn't have an answer. I asked her if she practiced any sort of religion or engaged in any artistic outlets. She did not.

I suggested that this patient find something she could do to help offset her anxiety. We discussed many different options, such as meditation, guided imagery, religion, exercise, and art. At one point,

I suggested gardening. She said she had a yard, but it was mainly just dirt with a few scraggly plants on the sides. She had never given much thought to gardening, but because she was sick of being constantly anxious, she decided to give it a try.

As time passed, this woman slowly but surely became less anxious, even during her cancer treatments. Along the way, I would ask her how the gardening was going; she would always smile and say, "Oh, it's coming along."

A few years later, the same woman who had come into my office with no hobbies and a chronic anxiety issue told me she was planning to host her parents' 50th wedding anniversary in the garden she had created in her backyard. Once she had incorporated a little stress-relieving gardening time into her day, she became gradually less dependent on the antianxiety medication and was eventually able to stop taking it altogether. I'm happy to share that she also overcame the metastatic breast cancer.

This particular patient did not suffer from allergies, but she is a good example of the power anxiety and stress have to take over your life as well as the importance of including enjoyable, stress-relieving activities in your daily routine. Her story also illustrates the toll mental problems can take on your physical health. Anxiety is more than just a feeling; it has a very tangible effect on your body. Most notably, anxiety causes surges in the adrenal hormones cortisol (the "stress hormone"), epinephrine, and norepinephrine, and chronically elevated levels of these hormones set up your body for inflammation.

As we've discussed, inflammation puts a person at greater risk not just for allergies but also for a whole host of other disorders and conditions, including heart disease, diabetes, obesity, and cancer.[1] There is no way to determine whether my patient's chronically elevated anxiety level contributed to her cancer, but it certainly didn't help. Over the years that I have been in practice, I have visited with many women diagnosed with breast cancer, and the vast majority of them reported having significantly elevated stress levels just prior to their diagnoses. I'm very happy that my breast cancer patient, and many others like her, found an activity to help compensate for and treat their anxiety. Reducing anxiety levels can only improve your health, no matter what your health challenges may be.

What Are Anxiety and Depression?

Anxiety disorders are among the most common mental disorders in the United States.[2] In fact, about one in five Americans suffers from anxiety in some form.[3]

Anxiety is complex and can be difficult to understand, even for experts. In simple terms, it is an abnormal level of apprehension about the future, especially concerning challenging tasks. There are a number of categories of anxiety disorders, including generalized anxiety disorder, social anxiety disorder, phobia, post-traumatic stress disorder (PTSD), and obsessive compulsive disorder (OCD).[4] Each disorder has its own unique symptoms, but they all share two common elements: irrational fears and feelings of dread. Anxiety disorders often accompany other mental or physical illnesses; substance abuse and depression are two of the biggies.[5] And while anxiety is worrying about the future, depression can be defined as overthinking the past.[6]

Similar to anxiety, there are a number of different depressive disorders, each of which has its own unique symptoms. But in general, symptoms of depression can include sadness, irritability, crying spells, changes in sleeping and eating habits, difficulty making decisions, short temper, overeating, problems concentrating, pain, avoidance of people, and decreased interest in activities you used to enjoy. In the most severe cases, depression can include thoughts of suicide.[7] Nearly as many Americans suffer from depression as from anxiety.[8]

During my years in practice, I have come to believe that anxiety is one of the biggest health problems affecting our society. Nearly all of the patients I see in my practice report having elevated anxiety. Often, it's unchecked, meaning that these patients have anxiety but no method for relieving it. I make it a point to educate all of my patients on how to incorporate relaxing, stress-relieving activities into their everyday routines. Doing so promotes living a healthier, less-stressed lifestyle and reduces inflammation, and therefore improves overall health, including allergy symptoms. With The Allergy Solution Plan in Chapter 14, I will help you do the same.

WHAT IS STRESS?

In order to have anxiety, you must first have or anticipate having stress. Stress is any factor in your life that requires you to adapt and react, either physically or mentally. It can be emotional (losing a loved one), physical (an injury), social (pressure to attend parties you'd rather skip), technological (your constantly beeping and ringing cell phone), or economic (a layoff). In some cases, these stresses are real. In others, they are exaggerated in our own minds.[9]

Stress can act as a motivator, so it can be a good thing in small doses. (This positive stress is sometimes referred to as eustress.) After all, in the absence of any stress, we'd all still be in our pajamas at noon, flipping through the channels instead of halfway through a productive day. It's when the stress starts and becomes chronic and unrelenting, eventually taking over our lives, that it becomes problematic.[10] Unfortunately, stress seems to be a major problem for most people in this country. According to the American Psychological Association, most Americans believe they are moderately or severely stressed.[11]

The trouble stems from a mismatch between the way the human stress response was originally designed to operate and our current stress-riddled lifestyles. In times past, our stress response, the fight-or-flight response, kicked into gear when we were in danger. The fight-or-flight response is orchestrated by our adrenal glands and the hormones that they produce, namely epinephrine and norepinephrine. These hormones change our bodies physiologically to prepare us to do one of two things, fight or run. Defending oneself or being able to escape from danger served our ancestors well when we were still living in the wild.

I often use an example taken from some of our closest animal relatives, the chimpanzees, to help people more fully understand this concept. Everyone is familiar with chimps; they are social apes that live in tightly knit groups in Africa. Most of a chimp's day is spent foraging for food and reinforcing the strong social bonds that tie their families together and keep things calm. One way that chimps reassure each other and promote a lowered stress level is though grooming, and they have been observed doing this behavior for much of the day. It is only every now and then that a jaguar springs out of the bushes and sends the chimps into a frenzy, triggering their fight-or-flight responses. The chimps operate in this state until the danger has passed, likely 10 to 15 minutes, and then they go right back to grooming each other.

While having the fight-or-flight response is helpful in dangerous situations (such as escaping from a hunting jaguar), having a chronically stimulated fight-or-flight response can lead to problems. Today, most of us live very busy lives with not nearly enough relaxation time, and that puts our bodies in a near-constant state of fight-or-flight. As a result, our bodies, acting under the direction of the adrenal glands and the fight-or-flight response, are chronically preparing to either fight or run. In this state, there are very few bodily resources devoted to essential health-promoting functions such as digestion, repairing, and rebuilding. Digestion is impaired, leading to problems with nutrient absorption and gastrointestinal function, which often lead to symptoms such as stomach cramps and diarrhea. Immune function is also lowered, making you more susceptible to illness. Researchers have also found clear connections between chronic stress and chronic depression.[12] Excessive anger and irritability are linked with chronic stress states as well. In some people who are chronically stressed, the reproductive system may even stop working as it should. Based on this, it's clear that the stress and anxiety levels experienced by most people today are contributing to

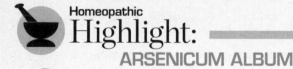

Homeopathic
Highlight:
ARSENICUM ALBUM

Made from white arsenic that will cause severe gastroenteritis if taken at a high dose, *Arsenicum album* taken in homeopathic doses can help with gastrointestinal symptoms as well as anxiety and depression. I recommend this treatment to my patients with food intolerances or mood disorder symptoms. I generally recommend a 30c dose to start.

the development of disease, and what we should be doing is spending more time picking the fleas off our friends—figuratively speaking, of course.

The Connection Between Anxiety and Inflammation

Researchers know that there's a definitive connection between anxiety and inflammation in your body, and they are constantly learning more about the reasons why. Unlike other organs, your brain has no pain nerves. So instead of pain, inflammation in your brain manifests as mental conditions like anxiety, depression, or fatigue.[13] And chronic brain inflammation can be dangerous. When it goes on too long, this inflammation can cause decreased communication between brain cells and fewer signals between nerves.[14]

A recent study done by researchers at Ohio State University has found that chronic stress may actually change the way genes in immune cells behave before they enter the blood. By comparing mice and humans in stressful situations, the research found that the two experience similar changes in their bone marrow when they're under stress.[15]

To create stress in the mice, researchers forced a group of male mice to live together in close quarters for enough time to create a hierarchy. They then introduced an aggressive male mouse to the group for 2 hours at a time. (The mouse equivalent of social defeat, which put them in chronic fight-or-flight mode.) The human participants in the study had poor socioeconomic status, which is a strong predictor of chronic stress.[16]

To give you some context, each day, your bone marrow releases billions of red blood cells and many different types of white blood cells. If your immune system senses a threat, your bone marrow produces special energized white blood cells that are primed for an immediate and powerful defensive response even when there is no actual infection or trauma present. These immune cells can then cause unwanted and excessive inflammation, even if the signal for the cellular activation was a faulty one.[17]

When the researchers examined the immune cells taken from

the blood of the stressed mice, they found four times the number of immune cells compared to mice that weren't stressed.[18] The stressed humans had more proinflammatory cells as well, and some of the changes in the humans' gene expression were similar to the changes seen in the mice. These results indicate clear links between mind and body, and in particular, between stress and inflammation.[19] To put the findings in practical terms, if you have prolonged periods of stress, you can actually change the gene expression in your immune system to create more inflammation in your body.[20]

Another study done at Carnegie Mellon University in Pittsburgh showed a similar connection between psychological stress and the inflammatory response. This study found that people with chronic stress can develop problems regulating inflammation, leading to an increased risk of disease.[21] The study was built off of previous research concluding that people who experienced stress were more likely to come down with a cold when exposed to a cold virus.[22]

In this follow-up study, researchers assessed 79 healthy people for their ability to control the inflammatory response. They then exposed those people to a cold virus and monitored their production of cytokines, the chemical messengers that trigger inflammation. The researchers found that those who were worst at regulating inflammation were more likely to come down with the cold.[23]

The researchers' conclusion was that the immune system's ability to regulate inflammation helps explain how stress can promote disease. Inflammation is in part regulated by the stress hormone cortisol, and when cortisol doesn't function like it should, inflammation can go haywire.[24] It works like this: Prolonged stress alters cortisol's ability to regulate the inflammatory response because it makes tissues less sensitive to the hormone. Because cortisol also helps regulate the inflammatory response, decreased sensitivity to cortisol can cause your body to become more inflamed, and this uncontrolled inflammation promotes the development of a number of diseases.[25,26]

Personality can also play a role in how people deal with stress, and therefore whether or not their bodies become inflamed in the presence of adversity. People who dwell on negative events in their lives seem to be more vulnerable to inflammation, according

Gender and Age Differences in Anxiety and Depression and Inflammation

In general, more women than men suffer from anxiety and depression.[27] But there are some interesting differences in the way that men and women respond to chronic stress and anxiety. For one, men with anxiety disorders tend to have low-grade inflammation in their bodies, and therefore they have higher levels of C-reactive protein (CRP).[28]

In a study published in *Psychosomatic Medicine*, researchers looked at data from 6,149 people who took part in the third National Health and Nutrition Examination Survey (NHANES). They found that men who had a history of major depression had elevated CRP, but that the same results were not found in women.[29]

In a more recent study published in the *Journal of Occupational Health Psychology*, researchers looked at 933 men and 630 women and found that once again, depressed men had higher levels of CRP as well as elevated fibrinogen, another inflammatory marker for heart disease. They also uncovered something new: Women suffering from burnout (defined as fatigue, emotional exhaustion, and cognitive weariness) were more likely to have elevated CRP than men with burnout. Scientists think that these gender differences may have something to do with sex hormones. Another theory is that men answer interview questions and self-disclosure questionnaires about depression differently than women do.[30]

Aside from gender, age also seems to play a role in the different relationships between mood disorders and inflammation. The highest CRP levels occur in both men and women who developed their anxiety disorder at an older age, particularly after age 50. One possible explanation is that psychological and physical stress build over time, eventually causing immune system changes that lead to anxiety and depression.[31]

to a study done at Ohio State University. When study participants were asked to ruminate about a stressful incident, their levels of C-reactive protein rose.[32] (To give you a refresher, C-reactive protein, or CRP, is an important marker of inflammation in the body. It is produced by the liver and rises as part of the immune system's initial inflammatory response to trauma, infection, or injury. Elevated CRP has been linked to heart disease and a number of other chronic diseases and conditions).[33]

To get to their findings, researchers asked 34 healthy young women to give a speech about their potential job candidacy to stone-faced interviewers in white lab coats. Then half of the participants were asked to think about their performance during the interview, and the other half were asked to think about nonstressful, neutral activities, like a trip to the grocery store or sailing on a boat. Researchers measured CRP levels before the women completed the interview and then again after they were asked to think the stressful or neutral thoughts. An hour later, CRP levels continued to rise in the women who thought about the interview. In those who thought about neutral things, CRP levels returned to normal.[34]

Also linked to inflammation is anxiety's cousin, depression. In a study published in the journal *FuturePundit*, researchers looked at 28 men, half of whom were diagnosed with major depression, and exposed them to mildly stressful situations for 20 minutes. Researchers took the men's blood every 15 minutes, starting right before the stressful situation and for the 1½ hours following. In these blood samples, they measured the inflammatory cytokines interleukin-6 and a proinflammatory signaling molecule in white blood cells called nuclear factor-kB. The results: Both the depressed and nondepressed men showed an inflammatory response to the stressful task, but the depressed patients had the greatest increases in inflammation.[35]

In a related 2003 study, men with depressive symptoms were found to be more likely to have heart disease and increased mortality than men without depression. And among people with cardiovascular disease, the study showed that those who were depressed had twice the risk of death compared to people without depression.[36]

ANXIETY AND ALLERGIES

So what's the connection with allergies, you ask? It all goes back to the allergy and inflammation connection.[37] As we've discussed,

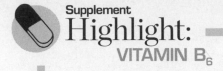

Supplement
Highlight:
VITAMIN B₆

Vitamin B₆, or pyridoxine, is one of the eight water-soluble B vitamins that help your body convert food into energy. The B vitamins assist with metabolism and also support healthy skin, hair, eyes, and liver. They also support your nervous system and brain function, helping to prevent mental disorders like anxiety and depression. More specifically, vitamin B₆ helps your body make the feel-good hormone serotonin.[38]

Significant B₆ deficiencies are rare, but some people can be mildly deficient, especially kids and older people. Symptoms of a deficiency may include nervousness, depression, problems concentrating, and memory loss.[39]

In terms of stress and anxiety, vitamin B₆ can help assist in the tryptophan-serotonin pathway; low levels of vitamin B₆ can lower serotonin and therefore increase a person's risk for anxiety and depression. In a 2004 study published in *Psychotherapy and Psychosomatics,* researchers looked at the association between depression and blood levels of vitamin B₆ in 140 people. They found a significant link between low plasma levels of B₆ and symptoms of depression. I recommend that you take vitamin B₆ as part of a B-complex vitamin, which can provide significant help for stress and anxiety. It can also help to control PMS, some neurological problems, and acne.[40]

short-term anxiety is likely not a major issue; it's when that anxiety persists and becomes chronic that it causes problems, namely through inflammation. Because anxiety and depression are pro-inflammatory, they make people more vulnerable to allergic reactions.[41] Stress not only worsens asthma and some allergies but also it can stimulate mast cells in your coronary system (called coronary mast cells), which can lead to inflammation in your coronary arteries and contribute to heart disease.[42] Conversely, allergies seem to worsen anxiety and depression by triggering the release of pro-inflammatory cytokines into the blood.[43]

A 2011 research review published in *Innovations in Clinical*

Neuroscience took a good look at the relationship between allergies and mood disorders and found that the majority of studies showed associations between the conditions. The review proposed a few possible explanations for the connection.[44]

- Allergies may affect people's ability to think clearly and therefore worsen mood disorders like depression and anxiety.

- Allergies may cause insomnia by making it more difficult for sufferers to breathe, and the resulting lack of sleep then makes mental disorders like anxiety and depression more pronounced.

- Some people may have genetic factors that put them at increased risk for both anxiety or mood disorders and allergies.

Studies have also been done to directly examine the relationship between allergies and mood disorders. In a study of more than 85,000 people, researchers found that people with allergies had rates of depression that were 1.7 times higher than those of people without allergies.[45] A similar, more recent study of 12,000 people found that people with nonfood allergies were more likely to suffer from major depression than individuals who were not allergic.[46]

Additionally, having a severe allergy or asthma can in and of itself be stressful, causing anxiety. A 2013 study published in the journal *Annals of Allergy, Asthma, and Immunology* found that patients with asthma were 43.5 percent more likely to suffer from anxiety than patients without asthma. The researchers concluded that all patients with asthma should be screened for anxiety.[47]

THE FATTY ACID FIGHT

In addition to anxiety and depression, another contributing factor when it comes to inflammation in the brain is the omega-6 fatty acid arachidonic acid (AA). This fatty acid produces inflammatory hormones called eicosanoids.[48]

The best way to counteract AA is with its antithesis fatty acids—the omega-3s. There are two omega-3 fatty acids in your brain:

docosahexaenoic acid (DHA) and eicosapentaenoic acid (EPA). Together, these two fatty acids help decrease inflammation. When their levels drop too low, brain cells become inflamed, disrupting communication between cells and nerves.[49]

Several studies back the theory of the anxiety-fighting power of omega-3s. In a 2008 study that was published in the journal *Progress in Neuro-Psychopharmacology and Biological Psychiatry,* alcoholics and substance abusers who took high doses of EPA (more than 2 grams per day) had less anxiety than those who took a placebo. (Anxiety is one of the main reasons alcoholics and substance abusers tend to relapse.) In addition, the substance abusers with the best ratio of AA to EPA in their blood had the greatest reductions in anxiety. In other studies, taking EPA seemed to make people happier and better able to roll with stress. So it seems to help with depression as well.[50]

In another study done at the University of Montreal, researchers looked at the effectiveness of omega-3 fatty acids in treating major depression. Researchers gave 432 patients with major depression without anxiety either an omega-3 supplement containing high concentrations of EPA or a placebo for 8 weeks. The researchers found that the omega-3 supplements worked as well as conventional antidepressant treatments for depression in these patients.[51]

In a 2009 review published in the journal *CNS Neuroscience and Therapeutics,* researchers looked at three studies on the treatment of depression and found that omega-3 fatty acids were more effective than a placebo for treating depression in both adults and kids.[52]

Another study done at Ohio State University found that omega-3s reduced anxiety and inflammation in young, healthy people. The research, published in the journal *Brain, Behavior, and Immunity,* looked at a group of medical students to see if omega-3 supplements would decrease their production of proinflammatory cytokines. The study followed earlier research from the same scientists showing that stress from exams affected the medical students' immunity.[53]

This time, the researchers took 68 first- and second-year medical students and divided them into six groups. Multiple times throughout the study, the students took surveys to gauge their levels of stress, anxiety, and depression and gave blood samples that measured their

Anxiety and Sleep

One of the most common and potentially serious side effects of anxiety is sleep deprivation. I see patients with insomnia all the time in my practice. Most insomniacs do not have an organic disorder that prevents them from sleeping; they can't sleep because they lie down at night, put their heads on their pillows, and the wheels start turning. They can't stop thinking about the meeting they had with their boss, the things they have to do tomorrow, or how they'll make that car payment. Then they wake up in the morning and get themselves back into the same bad routine that contributed to the insomnia in the first place: They eat junk food, avoid exercise because they are tired, and maybe have a few extra cups of coffee to help them stay alert.

Meanwhile, the body is doing whatever it can to stay awake, too. When stress becomes chronic, the adrenal glands can actually lose the ability to produce enough stress hormones to meet the demands of the body. As a result, the body turns to other places for energy, one of which may be the brain. In response, your brain pumps out excitatory neurotransmitters; these chemicals will give you energy during

levels of inflammation. Half of the students got omega-3 fatty acid supplements containing four or five times the amount of fish oil in one serving of salmon, and the other half got a placebo.[54]

Due to a change in curriculum, the students didn't have the level of stress the researchers had originally anticipated; however, researchers were still able to measure the students' anxiety. What they found was interesting: The students who took the omega-3 fatty acid supplements reported 20 percent less anxiety than the students who took the placebo. And when they measured levels of three markers of two important proinflammatory cytokines—interleukin-6 and tumor necrosis factor-alpha—there was a 14 percent reduction in these cytokines in the students taking the omega-3s. The bottom line: The omega-3 fatty acids reduced both inflammation and anxiety in these students.[55]

To make a long fatty acid story short, one of the best things you the day, but unfortunately, they also keep you up at night. This is a common phenomenon. According to the American Psychological Association, 42 percent of people who report having stress say they frequently lie awake at night.[56]

There's also a connection between allergies—specifically food allergies—and insomnia. People who have this condition, called food allergy insomnia, have trouble falling asleep and staying asleep after eating certain foods. The insomnia usually happens after eating a new food or drink, for example, cow's milk (a common culprit in adults who don't typically consume dairy products).[57]

No matter the reason for insomnia, it is extremely detrimental to your health. If it goes on for a long time, sleep loss can lead to increased risk of high blood pressure, obesity, diabetes, depression, heart attack, and stroke.[58] So needless to say, for the sake of staving off allergies and protecting your general health, it's very important to get your Z's.[59]

can do to combat anxiety is to consume less omega-6 fatty acids and more of the omega-3 fatty acids EPA and DHA. In terms of food, that means eating less vegetable oil, processed foods, and refined carbohydrates. It also means eating more cold-water fatty fish, like salmon and mackerel. I do think that eating more omega-3 foods is good, but most people will benefit from taking a supplement as well. The dosages studied are higher than what could be achieved by adding fish to your diet once or twice per week. Again, I recommend a 2:1, or better yet, a 1:1 ratio of omega-6 to omega-3 fatty acids.

THE ANXIETY SOLUTION

So with all of this information on the relationship between anxiety and inflammation, what's a stressed-out, potentially allergic person to do? In mainstream medicine, doctors usually put people with anxiety or depression on antidepressant or antianxiety prescription medications. In some cases, these drugs are a good choice, and they give people a marked improvement in their quality of life. In other cases, these medications provide only temporary relief or put patients in a permanent fog.[60] No matter how a patient responds, these prescription medications may not address the underlying causes fueling the mental conditions they are designed to treat.

The Allergy Solution Plan will provide more information (see page 231), but in the meantime, here are some of the things I advise my anxious patients to do to ease their stress and help decrease inflammation.

Don't ignore symptoms. Far too often, people with stress, anxiety, and depression chalk up their symptoms to normal reactions to the inevitable frustrations and challenges of life. Or, they may simply be in denial. My gardening patient is a prime example. She ignored her anxiety symptoms for far too long. Only after she faced her symptoms could she start to incorporate the changes that helped her go back to enjoying life.

If you feel stressed, anxious, and depressed most of the time, you are probably doing significant harm to your health; you need to talk to your health-care professional or a counselor and address your symptoms as soon as possible.

Find an outlet. There's a simple reason why so many people in this country are stressed-out: We don't handle stress well. According to the American Psychological Association's Stress in America Survey, 36 percent of people report eating unhealthy foods and 27 percent say they skip meals due to stress.[61] Other unhealthy stress relievers include smoking, using drugs, and drinking too much. These bad habits are all proinflammatory and increase disease risk; therefore, by using these coping mechanisms, you are adding fuel to the inflammation and anxiety fire.[62]

Instead, one of the best ways to deal with stress is to spend time doing things you enjoy, especially activities that make you feel like you're making a difference in the world. This doesn't mean forcing yourself to participate in a stress-relieving technique you don't enjoy; that won't work. Make sure you do things that truly give you pleasure. Take a long bike ride on a Saturday morning. Volunteer at a local homeless shelter. Or, like my patient, create a masterful garden. Do something you enjoy every single day. You'll be amazed at how much better you will feel.

Change your perspective. In our fast-paced, competitive society, a lot of our stress is self-imposed. We feel pressure to say yes to every social engagement and request we get, we try to be too many things to too many people, and we spend too much time sweating the small stuff. Give yourself a break now and then. Take time to think about all you have to be thankful for, and step back to assess what's really important. These simple switches in your thinking can do wonders for your stress level and overall health.

Exercise. We will dive much deeper into this in Chapter 13, but we know that exercise is a cornerstone of any healthy lifestyle routine. And it's not just the benefits in cardiovascular conditioning, muscle tone, and weight loss that exercise brings, but the positive *mental* changes physical activity provides that make such an enormous difference. I don't suggest that people with allergies or asthma exercise vigorously. In fact, the best approach is slow and steady. The best forms of exercise are mind-body practices such as yoga and tai chi. In addition to calming your mind, these time-tested exercise forms do wonders for staving off allergies and supporting good physical health.

Balance your omegas. To get the amount of EPA shown to reduce anxiety in the medical student study, you would need to consume about 2 pounds of salmon per day. The Japanese are able to eat this much, but they are the largest fish consumers in the world. For you and me, that's a difficult goal—not to mention the risk of mercury exposure associated with eating this quantity of fish. So I tell my patients to eat more omega-3s as part of an anti-inflammatory diet (see Chapter 10 to learn exactly how) and to take purified fish oil supplements daily.[63]

Kyle's Story

"Your body can heal! Find someone who understands this, and let that person help you help."

Such is the advice from Kyle Cass's mother, who has watched her 12-year-old son's allergy and asthma symptoms get better thanks to Dr. Psenka's all-natural plan. "I wish all doctors would use the body's natural ability to heal instead of pills, and when intervention is necessary, use the most natural way possible," she says.

Before they went to see Dr. Psenka, not wanting to put their son on steroids, Kyle's parents watched their son's allergies and asthma get gradually worse. "We used his primary care doctor and limped along with just an inhaler," Kyle's mom says. As a result, Kyle had to rest during recess or sports and use his rescue inhaler on a regular basis. He would also occasionally wake up breathless in the middle of the night and need to reach for his inhaler to get his breathing under control.

Because Kyle's parents believe in prevention instead of treatment, they took him to Dr. Psenka.

The plan was an easy assimilation for Kyle, who had already started making some nutritional changes. "We were on the right track before we came to Dr. Psenka, but we have seen much better results under his guidance," Kyle's mother says.

With the dietary changes, Kyle saw changes in his allergy and asthma symptoms within a month. He also started sublingual immunotherapy (SLIT), which lead to noticeable improvements after six to nine months.

As a bonus, the whole family has changed their eating habits along with Kyle. "Before we saw Dr. Psenka, we were eating 50/50 good and bad foods. Now we crave the good foods and are at about 80/20 healthful to unhealthful foods. Our bodies are doing great," Kyle's mother says.

Today, Kyle is much more active, both on and off the sports field. He is no longer waking up at night to use his inhaler, and he has much more energy during the day. "And we are hoping to trash the inhaler altogether soon!" his mother says. To parents of other children with seasonal allergy and asthma symptoms, she says, "Get guidance with natural treatments. Even the smallest changes can make a huge difference."

9 When Foods Don't Agree with You: Diet and Inflammation

WHEN I THINK OF THE ADVERSE EFFECTS OF FOOD, I think of a 10-year-old patient I saw who was having trouble paying attention.

"She can't sit still," her parents said. The girl's hyperactivity, combined with the occasional outburst, was leading to problems in school. Her parents told me that their daughter had always been restless, and they were concerned that her behavior would end up being a disadvantage to her if they didn't do something about it.

While reviewing this girl's history, I discovered that her diet was probably at least partially responsible for her behavior. Both parents worked, and because of their busy schedules, time for meal preparation was minimal. Quick-and-easy foods were commonplace in their home, and processed foods and "juice drinks" were the main staples of the girl's diet.

We sat down and discussed some food preservatives known to have overstimulating effects and that have also been linked to attention deficit disorder (ADD). We also talked about how processed foods and refined sugars can cause kids to be hyperactive. I felt that getting this kid on a healthy diet plan was paramount. I presented a strategy to her parents and gave them some samples of healthy meals as well as a few cookbook recommendations.

When I saw the family back in my office a few months later, the parents were very happy with the results they were seeing in their daughter. She was having fewer problems at school, and her teacher had remarked about the improvements she saw.

This 10-year-old's case is far from unusual. There is often a relationship between a person's symptoms—in this case, behavior—and lifestyle factors such as diet. I find that many patients and parents of patients either don't know what really constitutes a healthy diet or they find themselves too crunched for time to prepare healthful food.

My hope, in my practice and in this book, is that by educating both children and adults, I will teach them healthy habits that they can use for a lifetime. It's never too late to start eating better, both for the sake of your allergies and your overall health.

CHANGING OUR DIETS FROM SAD TO HAPPY

The food you put in your body is so important. In the days before medications, doctors used foods as medicine, and some of us still do. Many foods have strong healing powers, but what you eat can also trigger inflammation. Repeatedly eating the wrong foods can cause a chronic inflammatory state within your cells, tissues, and organs. Your immune system treats these junk foods like invaders and goes into attack mode, and with no virus or bacteria to zap, this causes inflammation.[1]

As we've discussed, the diet most Americans eat—the Standard American Diet (SAD)—is sad in every sense of the word. It's way too high in processed foods and excessive sugars, and it's deficient in fruits, vegetables, and healthy protein sources.

It's important to keep in mind that if you have a sensitivity or intolerance to a food and you choose to splurge and eat that food, it will lead to inflammation. So while walnuts may be completely anti-inflammatory in a nonallergic person, they may cause *lots* of inflammation in someone with a walnut allergy or sensitivity.

The excessive levels of inflammation that can result from eating the wrong foods can contribute to all kinds of problems in your

The Power of Prenatal Diets

All medical experts agree: Pregnant women should eat a healthful, nutrient-filled, toxin-free diet to ensure the best possible outcomes for their babies. And of course, I wholeheartedly agree with this advice. As soon as a woman conceives, she is literally eating for two.

But when it comes to allergy risk, the guidelines for pregnant moms have been anything but clear. Women have been told to avoid potential allergens to help prevent food allergies in their babies, and they've also been told to eat these foods without restraint.

The latest research tells pregnant women to eat up. A 2014 study published in the *Journal of Allergy and Clinical Immunology* looked at 1,277 mother-child pairs. Researchers used food frequency questionnaires to assess the mothers' diets during their first and second trimesters, specifically their intakes of common food allergens. They then assessed their kids for food allergies, allergic rhinitis, and asthma by using questionnaires and measuring IgE levels when the kids reached an average age of 7.9. The results: The moms who ate lots of peanuts during their first trimester were 47 percent less likely to have a child with a peanut allergy. The moms who drank lots of milk during their first trimester were less likely to have kids with asthma and allergic rhinitis. And the moms who ate lots of wheat during their second trimester were less likely to have a child with eczema.[2]

A related study published in the *British Journal of Nutrition* looked at pregnant moms' intakes of fatty acids and the risk of eczema, wheezing, and allergic rhinitis in their children once they reached age 5. Results suggest that a higher ratio of omega-6 to omega-3 fatty acids may be linked to increased risk of allergic rhinitis, and eating larger amounts of omega-3 fatty acids may decrease the risk of allergic rhinitis in kids.[3]

The advice to eat lots of different foods seems to continue after birth. New research also shows that encouraging kids to eat a variety of foods during their first year of life may help prevent them from developing food allergies, asthma, and food sensitivities years later.[4]

body, even putting you at risk for diseases like heart disease, diabetes, and cancer. Not surprisingly, eating the SAD can also lead to weight gain. Inflammation causes your adrenal glands to secrete hormones that can cause a dysregulation of your blood sugar and insulin levels. Chronically elevated insulin levels not only make your body hold on to fat but also they lead to inflammation. If that weren't bad enough, increased body fat also leads to—you guessed it—even more inflammation.[5]

As we discussed, high insulin levels and inflammation can also lead to a potentially serious condition called nonalcoholic steatohepatitis (NASH), which leads to fat, inflammation, and damage to your liver.[6] Therefore, in terms of both allergy and inflammation, it is imperative that you do whatever you can to incorporate a healthy diet into your life and to avoid the foods to which you are sensitive or allergic.

In this chapter, we will discuss the best and worst foods to eat when it comes to preventing inflammation and, as a result, allergies. Keep in mind as you read that the central goal is to improve your *entire* diet plan, not necessarily to maximize your intake of or avoid one particular food. It's what you do most of the time that has the greatest impact.

THE GOOD GUYS: ANTI-INFLAMMATORY FOODS AND NUTRIENTS

There are a number of foods and nutrients that can help decrease inflammation. Here are the most noteworthy.

Omega-3 Fatty Acids

As we've discussed, there is a lot of research to support the benefits of omega-3 fatty acids, especially when it comes to inflammation. In a review of studies on omega-3 fatty acids published in *American Family Physician,* researchers found that when given in doses of at least 3 grams a day, omega-3 fatty acids helped reduce inflammation, stiffness, and pain in people with rheumatoid arthritis.[7]

Some of the foods highest in omega-3s are oily fish like mackerel, tuna, salmon, and sardines. Look for salmon (wild king has the most omega-3s), wild or canned sockeye, sardines that are packed in

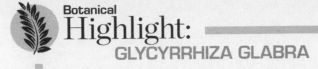

Botanical
Highlight:
GLYCYRRHIZA GLABRA

For thousands of years, healers in both Eastern and Western medicine have used *Glycyrrhiza glabra* (licorice) to treat a number of diseases and conditions, including the common cold, liver disease, asthma, and some allergies.[8] For eczema, a 1 to 2 percent topical licorice gel can help relieve itching, swelling, and redness.[9,10]

water or olive oil, herring, or black cod. Keep in mind that fish can be high in mercury, so keep your number of weekly servings to three or fewer.[11]

Not a fish eater? Fish oil supplements also get the job done, without the potential for mercury exposure. Look for a supplement that contains both eicosapentaenoic acid (EPA) and docosahexaenoic acid (DHA) in daily dosages of 2 to 3 grams.[12]

Other good sources of omega-3 fatty acids include omega-3 fortified organic milk and eggs, flaxseeds (freshly ground flaxseeds are the best), and hemp seeds.[13] Note that flax only contains alpha-linolenic acid (ALA) and no EPA or DHA, so it shouldn't be considered a good omega-3 supplement all by itself.

As a side note, diet alone is often insufficient to raise a person's omega-3s to a healthy level, and a supplement may also be needed. I use some specialized testing to get a clear picture of what a person's omega-3 levels are (broken down into EPA, DHA, and ALA). The testing also tells me a patient's omega-6 levels, so that helps determine how much omega-3 they should have. I run this testing on many allergic patients and also use it as part of a comprehensive health assessment panel I run on patients. For more on omega-3 fatty acid supplements, see Chapter 11.

Colorful Fruits and Veggies

A good rule of thumb: In general, the brighter the color of a fruit or vegetable, the richer it is in anti-inflammatory antioxidants. In-season fresh fruits and vegetables are best when it comes

Supplements or Foods: What's the Best Way to Get the Nutrients Your Body Needs?

The foods versus supplements debate is a hotly contended one. Most research shows that supplements are helpful for people who are deficient in a specific nutrient, but for people who have a good baseline, it's preferable to get nutrients from whole foods.[14]

After all, when you get nutrients from foods, not only are you living your life the way nature intended but also you can create fantastic combinations, both in terms of nutrients and taste.[15]

To get more bang for your nutrient buck, you can combine certain healthful foods. When you eat broccoli and tomatoes at the same time, for example, the sulforaphane in the broccoli and the lycopene in the tomatoes have stronger tumor-preventing powers than they do when eaten alone. And your body will absorb beta-carotene best when you eat it with a fat, so combine carrots with avocadoes or olive oil. Other good combinations include apples with blueberries and spinach with strawberries.[16]

to retaining nutrients. But frozen fruits and veggies are a good alternative because they are frozen at the peak of freshness, which means most of their nutrients are retained.[17] Within the bright-colored vegetables and fruits, there are some shining stars.

BERRIES

Whether they're blue, boysen, cran, black, or rasp, berries are great anti-inflammatory foods. Research done at Tufts University in Medford Massachusetts, shows that berries help prevent age-related inflammation by turning off proinflammatory signals sent by cytokines and the proinflammatory enzyme COX-2. Researchers think berries are so powerful because of their anthocyanins, the antioxidants that give them their rich red, blue, or purple color.[18]

DARK, LEAFY GREENS

When it comes to fighting inflammation, the rule is, the darker the greens, the better. Dark green veggies such as spinach, kale, collard greens, and broccoli contain vitamin E, which has been shown to help protect the body against proinflammatory cytokines. As a bonus, these greens serve up a bunch of healthful vitamins and minerals, including calcium, iron, and anti-inflammatory phytochemicals.[19] They're also very rich in antioxidants.

To measure the level of antioxidants in fruits, vegetables, and spices, the National Institute on Aging developed the oxygen radical absorbance capacity (ORAC) test. ORAC assigns a score to a long list of foods. The highest-scoring foods include brightly colored fruits and vegetables, such as blueberries, raspberries, apples, beans, and, you guessed it: leafy greens.[20]

TART CHERRIES

At a 2012 American College of Sports Medicine (ACSM) conference in San Francisco, researchers at Oregon Health & Science University proclaimed that cherries have "the highest anti-inflammatory content of any food." That's a bold statement. To come to this conclusion, the researchers studied women ages 40 to 70 who had inflammatory osteoarthritis. They found that women who drank tart cherry juice two times a day for 3 weeks had decreases in important inflammatory

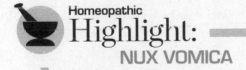

Homeopathic
Highlight:
NUX VOMICA

Nux vomica is a homeopathic remedy derived from seeds of the strychnine tree, which is native to India. It is traditionally used to treat digestive upset from food intolerances such as heartburn and stomach discomfort as well as nausea. *Nux vomica* can also help with other allergy symptoms.[21]

A few years ago, *nux vomica* was recognized in the medical journal the *Lancet* as one of 12 homeopathic remedies that can help fight hay fever symptoms.[22] I occasionally use *nux vomica* for patients with allergies, and when I do, I generally start with a 30c dosage.

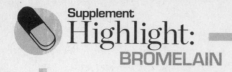

Supplement
Highlight:
BROMELAIN

An enzyme found in the fruit and stem of pineapple, bromelain is a natural anti-inflammatory that's often used to treat injured or damaged tissues and arthritis pain. Bromelain is also used to help control allergy symptoms, such as nasal and sinus swelling and thick mucus.[23]

In my experience, the efficacy of bromelain seems to be dose-dependent. Some people benefit from 150 milligrams per day, while others may need to take upwards of 1,000 milligrams daily. I usually recommend that my patients take 150 milligrams of bromelain three or four times per day.

An important side note: Some people are allergic to bromelain, and in these people, it can cause respiratory symptoms similar to those of a respiratory allergy. Because bromelain comes from pineapple, people who are allergic to tropical fruits should use caution when taking it.

You should always take bromelain on an empty stomach to maximize absorption.

markers. The women who had the greatest inflammation at the beginning of the study had the largest decreases in inflammation as a result of drinking the cherry juice. The researchers also found that you need to pucker to prevent pain—sweet cherries don't pack the anti-inflammatory punch of their tart relatives.[24]

TOMATOES

If the rule of thumb with greens is, "the greener, the better," the rule with tomatoes is, "the redder and juicier, the better." Tomatoes contain a chemical called lycopene, which reduces inflammation in the lungs and throughout the body. In a 2013 Iranian study published in the *British Journal of Nutrition,* obese and overweight women who drank tomato juice had significantly lower levels of inflammatory markers in their blood than overweight and obese women who drank water.[25]

Nuts

Nuts are a big part of the Mediterranean diet, which has been shown to help reduce inflammation in a matter of weeks (page 149). Almonds and walnuts are particularly packed with anti-inflammatory fats. Other good nuts for fighting inflammation include pecans and Brazil nuts. In fact, a 2008 study published in the *Asia Pacific Journal of Clinical Nutrition* found that people who frequently ate nuts had decreased concentrations of C-reactive protein (CRP), an important marker of inflammation in the body. They also had lower levels of another inflammatory marker, interleukin-6, in their blood.

Nuts also contain antioxidants, which can help protect your body from damage caused by inflammation.[26] Raw nuts—not roasted—provide the most benefits. An important note: Avoid eating nuts if you are allergic to them.

Olive Oil

When it comes to fighting inflammation, olive oil is one of the most powerful foods; it acts as an anti-inflammatory elixir of sorts. Studies have shown that a compound in olive oil, called oleocanthal, works similarly to nonsteroidal anti-inflammatory drugs (NSAIDS) in that it blocks cyclooxygenase-2 (COX-2), the enzyme that helps stimulate proinflammatory prostaglandins. By doing this, olive oil stops inflammation in its tracks. The stronger the olive oil's bitter bite, the higher its oleocanthal levels and the more anti-inflammatory it is. Olive oils from Tuscany or other regions that use the same variety of olives have the strongest bite and therefore the highest oleocanthal levels.[27]

In one study, researchers found that 50 milliliters of olive oil, or about 3½ tablespoons, is equal to a 200-milligram tablet of ibuprofen in terms of reducing pain and inflammation. This amount of olive oil serves up about 400 calories, so to avoid weight gain, use olive oil in place of other fats in your diet, such as butter or margarine.[28,29]

Garlic

Known for its immune-boosting properties, garlic is also anti-inflammatory. And it seems that in order to get the greatest reductions in inflammation, you will have to put up with a little garlic breath. A 2013 study published in *Food and Chemical Toxicology* found that fresh raw garlic contains higher levels of allicin, a compound that gives garlic its anti-inflammatory powers by reducing levels of proinflammatory cytokines. Garlic that has been heated contains less odiferous sulfur, but also less allicin, and is therefore not as strong of an anti-inflammatory as garlic in its raw form.[30]

Other Good Spices

Some spices aren't just good for adding zest and flavor; they can lower inflammation as well. Ginger, a popular antinausea remedy, can reduce inflammation in your intestines when taken in supplement form. Like olive oil, ginger inhibits COX-2 and therefore blocks proinflammatory prostaglandins that are important for pain sensation.[31]

A relative of ginger, turmeric (the spice that gives curry its yellow color), fights inflammation by helping to turn off NF-B, a protein that helps regulate the inflammatory response in your immune system.[32] Numerous studies have shown that cinnamon can also help reduce inflammation. In an Iranian study published in the *International Journal of Preventive Medicine*, researchers gave 60 healthy female tae kwon do athletes either cinnamon, ginger, or a placebo daily for 6 weeks. At the end of the study, the athletes taking the cinnamon and ginger had less muscle soreness than the athletes taking the placebo.[33]

The Bad Guys: Proinflammatory Foods and Nutrients

There are a number of foods and nutrients in the SAD that may be proinflammatory. Here are some of the worst offenders.

OMEGA-6 FATTY ACIDS

Through a fairly complex chain of events, many of the omega-6 fatty acids are proinflammatory. Simply put, omega-6 fatty acids activate the COX-2 enzymes that cause inflammation. Eating a diet high in omega-6 fatty acids (found in vegetable oil) and low in omega-3 fatty acids is associated with elevated levels of cytokines, proteins in cells that trigger inflammation, according to a 2007 study published in *Psychosomatic Medicine*.[34]

Foods rich in omega-6 fatty acids include corn, sunflower, safflower, soybean, and cottonseed oils; processed snack foods; margarine; fried foods; egg yolks; and meats. These foods tend to be the ones people overindulge in, leading to weight gain. Remember that it's very important to balance your intake of omega-6 fatty acids with a healthy intake of omega-3s.[35]

SUGAR

One of the worst parts of the SAD is an overabundance of sugar. We eat an excessive amount of sugar in this country, and it's no wonder; the sweet stuff seems to be in everything, from ketchup to soda to junk-food-in-health-food's-clothing, like energy bars and sports drinks. To give you an idea, the average American eats approximately 100 grams of sugar a day. But your body can only tolerate about 50 grams, so the excess sugar triggers irritable bowel symptoms like gas and bloating as well as inflammation.[36]

There are basically three different forms of sugar—fructose, sucrose, and high-fructose corn syrup (HFCS). Fructose is a natural form of sugar found in honey and many fruits. Sucrose is a naturally occurring form of sugar made of fructose and glucose. It is found in many plants but is usually extracted from sugarcane and sugar beets to make table sugar. Sucrose (table sugar) is 50 percent glucose and 50 percent fructose.[37]

High-fructose corn syrup is corn syrup with added enzymes that change some of the glucose to fructose. This process makes HFCS sweeter than regular corn syrup. It can range from 42 to 55 percent fructose.[38] It is a cost-effective sweetener used in many products, including cereal, bread, yogurt, ketchup, and fruit juice.[39] In the 40 years since HFCS was introduced in this country, obesity rates have skyrocketed from 15 percent of the population in 1970 to nearly one in three Americans today.[40]

The results of a study done at Princeton University and published in *Pharmacology Biochemistry and Behavior* are alarming.

Researchers conducted two experiments to test whether or not HFCS leads to weight gain. In the first experiment, they fed male rats water sweetened with high-fructose corn syrup or water sweetened with table sugar (sucrose) in addition to a standard rat-chow diet. The concentration of sweeteners in the two drinks was the same, but the rats that drank the HFCS solution gained significantly more weight than the rats that drank the sucrose solution.[41]

In the second experiment, researchers looked at weight gain, body fat, and triglyceride levels in rats that consumed HFCS for 6 months. Compared to rats on a standard diet, the HFCS rats developed a metabolic syndrome similar to the condition found in humans, complete with weight gain (they gained 48 percent more weight than the rats on the standard diet), increased triglycerides, and an abnormal degree of belly fat.[42]

Fructose isn't a much better option. While every cell in your body uses glucose for energy, fructose is only metabolized by your liver. Therefore, eating too much fructose can damage your liver just like alcohol and other toxins do. And like alcohol, fructose gets metabolized into fat instead of energy. It gets stored in your fat cells, which can lead to mitochondrial damage and, as a result, inflammation.[43]

SODA

I can't talk about sugar without bringing up one of its biggest customers: soda manufacturers. There is absolutely *nothing* good about soda (also called soft drinks). As if the piles of sugar it contains weren't bad enough, soda is also proinflammatory. In a Swiss study published in the *American Journal of Clinical Nutrition,* young men who drank about two cans of cola per day had CRP levels that rose by nearly 110 percent in only 3 weeks.[44]

REFINED CARBOHYDRATES

When you eat white bread, pasta, and rice, you might as well be eating sugar. The effects of these refined carbs are similar to sugar, and they increase your levels of proinflammatory cytokines.[45]

As evidence, in a 2010 study published in the *American Journal of Clinical Nutrition,* researchers looked at the carbohydrate intake of

1,490 postmenopausal women and 1,245 men who were 49 years old. They found that the women with the highest intakes of refined carbohydrates had nearly three times the risk of death from inflammatory disease compared to the women who ate the fewest number of refined carbohydrates.[46]

Processed Foods

Many processed foods are loaded with all kinds of flavor-boosting, freshness-preserving chemicals with long, scary-sounding names. And we *should* be frightened of these ingredients because many of them are potentially toxic and inflammatory.

One such chemical is monosodium glutamate (MSG), a flavor enhancer and preservative used in many processed foods, and traditionally used in Chinese food. In a 2008 study published in the *Journal of Autoimmunity*, researchers injected MSG into mice and found that it led to significant liver inflammation. The mice also developed obesity and type 2 diabetes. By the time they reached 6 and 12 months of age, all of the mice given MSG had developed liver inflammation, and some had developed lesions.[47] Another preservative commonly used in processed foods, butylated hydroxytoluene (BHT), has been shown to cause lung injury and inflammation in mice as well.[40]

Red Meat

Organic, grass-fed red meat eaten in moderation is an acceptable protein (and iron) source.[49] Unfortunately, overconsumption of unhealthy types of red meat is a serious problem and promotes unnecessary and unhealthy inflammation in the United States.

The fact is that red meat in the form of steaks and burgers is loaded with saturated fatty acids, which can lead to the formation of arachidonic acid. Plus, red meat—especially when charred—may contain toxic substances like heterocyclic amines, which have been linked to the development of cancer.[50]

Case in point: Asian men have much lower rates of prostate cancer than American men, and they are much less prone to inflammation in general. In Asia, the diet consists of lots of fish and very little red meat. Interestingly, the longer Asian men live in the United States, the higher their risk for prostate cancer. Asian men who live in the United States for 25 years or more have half the rate of prostate cancer of Caucasians. If their sons are born in America, their prostate cancer risk rises to the same as that for Caucasian American men.[51]

Why this difference between Asians and Americans? For one, Asians eat a lot more fish and a lot less red meat and poultry than Americans do. There may also be something to the way we prepare our meats in the United States. We know that when meats are cooked a certain way, they can produce those nasty carcinogens, heterocyclic amines. It seems that the more charred a meat, and the more times it gets flipped during cooking, the higher its level of these dangerous amines. The worst of these heterocyclic amines is called Ph1P. When laboratory animals ate large doses of this chemical, the males developed colon and prostate cancer and the females developed breast cancer.[52]

Some researchers think the level of carcinogens consumed by meat-eating Americans comes close to the equivalent of smoking half a pack of cigarettes a day. The best thing you can do is eat red meat only occasionally, in moderation. If and when you do eat them, stick to lean cuts.[53]

Allergenic Foods

In addition to foods that spark allergy symptoms by worsening inflammation, there are also foods that, in and of themselves, cause allergies. Going back to Chapter 4, there are a number of allergenic foods. The most common are wheat, peanuts, tree nuts, milk, eggs, soy, fish, and shellfish. Some food allergies fade with time and others, like nut allergies, tend to persist. The ones that hang on are usually those that carry the risk of anaphylactic shock. I recommend that people with these serious food allergies avoid the offending foods altogether. It's simply not worth the risk or the resultant inflammation in your body.

Beyond classic food allergies, there are also a number of foods that can worsen other allergy symptoms. For example, some people who are allergic to ragweed will experience itchiness and swelling in their mouths when they eat bananas, watermelon, or cantaloupe. People who are allergic to pollen may find that cherries, peaches, potatoes, carrots, or apples may make their symptoms worse. If honey contains some allergenic pollen, it can cause a reaction as well. People with these cross-reactions usually get symptoms all year long, but their symptoms often get worse at the height of hay fever season.[54]

Aside from avoiding the fruits and vegetables that cause you to sniffle and sneeze, there's only one thing you can do to deal with a cross-reaction: Cook the foods that give you symptoms. Of course this works better for some produce, such as potatoes and carrots, than for others, such as watermelon.[55]

Fruits and veggies aside, some people with hay fever also find that red wine causes their allergy symptoms to kick in. A 2011 study found that along with a buzz, some red wine serves up histamine, the chemical that causes allergic reactions such as a runny nose and sneezing.[56] If you already have hay fever, indulging in a glass or two can cause constriction in your bronchial tubes and difficulty breathing.[57]

SOME HELPFUL TIPS ON INCORPORATING ANTI-INFLAMMATORY FOODS

Now that you know about the benefits of anti-inflammatory foods, here's how to work them into your eating routine.

Plan your meals. Schedule all of your week's meals ahead of time so you can buy the ingredients you need in one trip to the market. Consider preparing all of your meals on Sunday and keeping them in the freezer or fridge until you need them later in the week.

Be wary of ridiculous health claims. As a general rule, if a product makes a special point of saying it contains something like a vitamin or mineral, be a skeptical consumer. For example, I recently saw a frozen drink that said, "Contains vitamin C!" in big, eye-catching letters on the label. Pure and simple, it was a Slurpee, and there are zero health benefits to drinking Slurpees. The 10 milligrams or so of vitamin C that come along with the bucket of sugar are negligible at best.

Another one of my pet peeves is the notion that sports drinks are good for you. Unless you are an elite athlete or labor in the heat all day, you probably don't need to consume sports drinks. They are loaded with sugar and they are not juice in any way, shape, or form.

Overall, it's important to keep in mind that not only does eating a diet full of healthy, anti-inflammatory foods help prevent allergies and other conditions but it also helps control your weight. As discussed, obesity is one of the biggest contributors to inflammation.

Each of the anti-inflammatory foods listed in this chapter is healthful in its own right, but these foods are most effective when eaten as part of an *entirely* anti-inflammatory diet. That having been said, giving in to a hamburger craving every now and then isn't going to make you inflamed. Read on, and I'll tell you more about how an anti-inflammatory diet can improve your health and reduce allergies.

10

Eating for Your Allergies

IT IS MY GOAL AS A NATUROPATHIC DOCTOR and as the author of this book to educate people about how to make healthy lifestyle choices. In fact, one of my favorite things to do as a doctor is educate people about their health. I believe that this should be an important part of what every physician does with his or her patients, and this concept of the doctor acting as a teacher is one of the guiding principles of naturopathic medicine. The doctor's role includes educating and encouraging the patient to take responsibility for his or her own health. The doctor should also empower and motivate the patient to make a healthful change, as it is the patient who ultimately creates the healing. I hope that you will use the information in this chapter as a guide for how to change your diet and daily lifestyle habits to be happier, healthier, and allergy-free.

Whether or not they have allergies, I always encourage those patients who may benefit from weight loss to do so by adopting a healthy eating and exercise plan. Nearly everyone who has ever tried to lose weight using anything else has experienced temporary results at best. You simply can't change your eating and exercise habits for a few months, drop some weight, and then expect to go back to your old habits and keep those pounds off. No matter what any 30-day diet claims, it *never* works that way.

That said, changing habits isn't always an easy thing to do. They're called habits for a reason: They're regular tendencies that are hard to give up. The best way to rewire your brain and change your habits is to replace them with new ones. The goal of making healthy lifestyle changes is all about creating new habits to achieve a state of sustained wellness.

For most Americans who are overweight, there are a number of different factors contributing to their condition. The unhealthy Standard American Diet (SAD), which is full of sugar and processed foods and is severely lacking in vitamins, minerals, and antioxidants, certainly plays a role. Undeniably, a lack of adequate physical activity also predisposes you to carrying extra weight. Stress and anxiety are also common reasons people gain and maintain an unhealthy weight, as there is a strong emotional attachment to food; many find it brings comfort during stressful or anxious times. If any of this sounds familiar, then get ready to make some changes. You'll be glad you did!

THE HEAVY HEALTH BURDEN OF OBESITY

Obesity is an epidemic in this country. A majority of adults—nearly 7 in 10—are carrying enough extra weight to put them at increased risk of health problems.[1]

Overweight and obesity are risk factors for all kinds of diseases, including heart disease, stroke, arthritis, type 2 diabetes, and some cancers.[2] As we learned in Chapter 5, extra weight also increases your risk for allergies. Therefore, keeping yourself at a healthy weight is extremely important, not just for your self-image but also for your physical health.

Obesity doesn't happen overnight; usually, the weight slowly accumulates over months or years as you tip the balance by taking in more calories than you burn. No matter what fad diets claim about the ratio of fat to carbohydrates you should be eating, pure and simple, if you want to lose weight, you have to burn more calories than you take in from food.[3] If you want to maintain your weight, you need to balance the calories you eat with the calories you burn through physical activity.

The correct balance between calories in and calories out differs from person to person. Different people have different basal metabolic rates (BMRs). Your BMR is the energy your body requires to maintain bodily functions, or just to "keep the lights on." Some people have fast metabolisms and others have slower ones. Those with slower BMRs may need to work harder to keep their weight in the healthy range.[4]

Losing weight can seem like an overwhelming task, especially if you have lots of extra weight or have failed at diets in the past. But you will find that getting the weight off is well worth the effort—losing just 5 to 10 percent of your body weight can make a big difference in your allergy symptoms and your overall health.[5] Remember, achieving a healthy weight seldom happens overnight. Losing 1 to 3 pounds per week is a good goal; slow and steady is the recipe for success.

The Starting Block: Understanding Your BMI

Aside from your social security number, one of the most important numbers for you to know is your body mass index (BMI). Body fat can be measured in a number of ways, from underwater weighing to calipers that measure folds of fat. The easiest and least-expensive way to measure your body fat is to determine your BMI. Although this doesn't directly measure your body fat percentage, in most cases, your BMI correlates closely and is a good screening tool to determine whether you are overweight or obese and need to lose some weight.[6]

In terms of BMI and allergy risk, a number of studies have demonstrated a connection. A 2011 study published in the *Journal of Asthma* examined 5,351 Taiwanese children ages 4 to 18 and looked at their BMIs, immunoglobulin E (IgE) levels, and history of allergies and asthma. They found that the kids with elevated BMIs were more likely to suffer from wheezing and eczema than children of a normal weight.[7] Another study published in 2013 in the *Journal of Allergy and Clinical Immunology: In Practice* found that both asthmatic children and adults with BMIs that classified them as overweight or obese were more likely to suffer an asthma attack, especially during the spring and fall allergy seasons.[8]

As we discussed in Chapter 5, the strongest link between obesity and allergies seems to be connected with food allergies. I have seen patients lose weight after determining which foods they are allergic to. Eliminating these foods from the diet can make losing stubborn weight much easier for some people.[9]

There is a mathematic calculation for determining your BMI: Take your weight in pounds and divide it by your height in inches squared, then multiply that number by 703. The resulting number is your BMI. If math is not your strong point, don't be alarmed—there are many BMI calculators to be found online, and all you need to know is your height and weight. You can try the one from the Centers for Disease Control and Prevention: by visiting my Web site: seasonalallergysolution.com.[10]

Alternatively, many physicians are starting to run their patients' BMIs in the office as part of routine visits. There are several machines available that can do this quickly and efficiently. It might be worth your time to ask your doctor if she can do this for you.

Once you know your BMI, you can determine whether you are classified as underweight, normal weight, overweight, or obese. To be at your healthiest weight, you want to aim for the normal range.

BMI	WEIGHT STATUS
Below 18.5	Underweight
18.5–24.9	Normal
25.0–29.9	Overweight
30.0 and over	Obese

As I mentioned, BMI correlates pretty strongly to your amount of body fat, but there are some exceptions. For example, highly trained athletes may weigh more due to increased muscularity. Their

BMIs may read as overweight when actually their ratio of fat to muscle is low. Conversely, women tend to have more body fat than men do at the same BMI. In addition, older people usually have more body fat at the same BMI than their younger counterparts.[11]

Once you know your BMI, you can determine whether you need to lose weight, and if so, about how much. If your BMI is 26, for example, you're just over the normal weight category and probably won't need to lose more than 5 or 10 pounds. If your BMI is 30 or above, you have significant weight to lose. Either way, you can do it, and my plan will show you how.

To determine approximately how many calories you will need to cut from your diet or burn with exercise in order to reach your weight-loss goal, you must first determine the number of calories you use each day—your basal metabolic rate, plus any calories you burn with everyday activities. To access an online calculator, visit seasonalallergysolution.com.

If you have a specific weight-loss goal in mind, you can pretty easily crunch the numbers and determine how many calories you should be eating and burning each day. Again, you can find an online calculator at seasonalallergysolution.com to help you verify that your goal weight is healthy and achievable.

EFFECTIVE EATING: THE MODIFIED MEDITERRANEAN DIET

Countless diet plans have gone in and out of the limelight, some touting health benefits and all claiming to help people lose weight. Many of these diets have been proven to be not only ineffective, but in some cases, also potentially dangerous.

However, one diet has stood the test of time and research, both in terms of health benefits and weight control: The modified Mediterranean diet. Based on the diet eaten for centuries by people in Mediterranean Spain and Italy, this diet is rich in plant-based foods and healthful, monounsaturated fats. It differs from the standard Mediterranean diet in that it calls for reduced servings of meat, wine, and starches.

The main elements of the diet are:[12]

- Plenty of fish and other seafood
- Very little red meat and chicken
- Use of anti-inflammatory olive oil as the main source of fat to flavor and cook foods
- Lots of vegetables and a moderate amount of fruit
- Minimal use of sauces and gravies
- Whole grains that naturally contain a high amount of fiber
- Very few sweets or sugary foods or drinks
- Very little butter and eggs

In addition to its heart-healthy benefits, the Mediterranean diet seems to help protect against allergies. In a 2007 British study, researchers assessed the respiratory symptoms and dietary habits of nearly 700 children who lived in Crete, Greece. They found that 80 percent of the children ate fresh fruit and two-thirds ate fresh vegetables at least twice a day. These produce-eating kids were less likely to develop airborne allergies, skin allergies, and asthma symptoms than kids who didn't eat fruits and vegetables in these amounts.[13] Conversely, kids who ate margarine had increased levels of allergic rhinitis and asthma. According to the study, the Mediterranean diet eaten by these Greek kids, which includes antioxidant-rich grapes and tomatoes, had something to do with their lower rates of asthma and allergies. As we learned, antioxidants help fight disease by neutralizing dangerous free radicals.[14]

The children in this study also consumed a lot of nuts that are rich in magnesium, which seems to help protect the lungs and, as a result, prevent asthma. Children with a high intake of nuts had lower rates of asthma.[15] Another study published in the journal *Allergy and Asthma Proceedings* found that both kids from urban Athens and rural areas of Greece who ate a Mediterranean diet had lower rates of asthma than kids who did not eat a Mediterranean diet.[16]

A more recent study published in the *Journal of Asthma* looked at the effects of a Mediterranean diet on 38 adults with asthma. Researchers put the participants into three groups—a high-intervention group, a low-intervention group, and a control group. The first two groups were encouraged to adopt a Mediterranean diet. They also received consultation sessions from a nutritionist, vouchers for purchasing appropriate foods, and written advice. To measure asthma symptoms, the researchers used asthma control questionnaires, food frequency questionnaires, asthma-related quality-of-life questionnaires, and spirometry (a common office test used to diagnose asthma and other breathing conditions). At the end of 12 weeks, those in the intervention groups had small but significant improvements in their spirometry and quality of life, indicating that the Mediterranean diet may be a feasible treatment for adult asthma.[17]

Additionally, research shows that expectant women who eat a Mediterranean diet during pregnancy are less likely to give birth to a child who later develops asthma or allergies than are pregnant women who do not eat a Mediterranean diet.[18] A 2008 study published in the British journal *Thorax* followed 460 Greek mother and child pairs from pregnancy until their children reached the age of 6. Sixty-four percent of the pregnant women ate a Mediterranean diet rich in fruits, vegetables, and omega-3 fats from fish and nuts, and the remaining 36 percent did not eat a Mediterranean diet. Researchers found that pregnant women who did not eat a Mediterranean diet were more likely to have children who later developed asthma and allergies.[19]

Modifying the Mediterranean Diet for You

I recommend the modified Mediterranean diet for more than just its potential as an antiallergy diet. Aside from its antiallergy powers—which are great—I recommend this diet to my patients because it is a varied, vegetable-rich plan; it has a low glycemic load, so it doesn't cause rapid elevations in blood sugar; and it provides adequate protein and fiber. Perhaps most important, the modified Mediterranean diet is not restrictive—it provides lots of food choices. With a lot of other diets, you're limited to eating certain foods for a defined period of time, but the modified Mediterranean diet is an eating plan you can stay on—and enjoy—indefinitely.

As an important side note, if you have an allergy or sensitivity

The Most Powerful Antiallergy Foods

There are a number of foods that can help curb allergy symptoms. Here's a quick look at a few of the most potent.

Onions and garlic. They might not be the best for your breath, but onions and garlic are great for allergy control. Both flavorful root vegetables contain quercetin, a natural mast cell stabilizer (antihistamine). Because of these antihistamine properties, quercetin helps fight the inflammation that accompanies the allergic response. Other foods that contain quercetin include apples and tea.[20]

Citrus fruits. Similar to quercetin, the vitamin C in oranges, tangerines, and other citrus fruits has antihistamine effects that can help fight allergy symptoms. Other good sources of vitamin C include strawberries, peppers, and tomatoes.[21,22]

Pineapple. The tart tropical fruit contains an enzyme called bromelain, which is a powerful anti-inflammatory. Research shows that it can ease sore throats and irritated sinuses.[23] And a 2012 study published in *Alternative Therapies in Health and Medicine* found that bromelain helped ease airway inflammation in mice, which is evidence that it may help with allergic asthma.[24] Plus, pineapple is a great source of the allergy-fighting antioxidant vitamin C. To get the most from pineapple, eat the fresh fruit.[25]

Broccoli sprouts. Recent research published in the journal *Food and Function* shows that broccoli sprout extract (BSE) may actually be able to protect against the allergy- and asthma-promoting effects of diesel exhaust particles (DEPs), which are pollutants that, for various reasons, actually have the power to exacerbate allergic reactions (see page 16). Researchers exposed 29 people to DEPs and then

to one of the foods in the modified Mediterranean diet, you will want to find appropriate substitutes for that food. Luckily, this eating plan is very flexible and offers lots of healthful alternatives.

To make the modified Mediterranean diet even more palatable, both in the true sense of the word and in terms of your lifestyle, here are some tips to try.

Boost your omega-3s. The most important element of the modified Mediterranean diet in terms of allergies, inflammation, and measured their inflammatory responses in terms of increases in white blood cell counts. Test subjects then got a dose of BSE in mango juice every day for 4 days. When participants took the BSE, their white blood cell response to the DEPs was 54 percent lower than when they didn't drink the BSE. The researchers concluded that eating broccoli and broccoli sprouts may help lessen the impact of particulate pollution on people with asthma and allergies.[26]

Red grapes, blueberries, and red wine. These deep purple treats have one important ingredient in common: a polyphenolic compound called resveratrol. In a 2013 study published in the *Journal of Nutrition*, researchers found that resveratrol helped suppress the IgE-mediated allergic responses in mice.[27]

Watermelon and tomatoes. Both of these summertime fruits are high in lycopene, which has been shown to decrease the allergic response and the accumulation of symptom-producing cell types in the lungs (specifically, the white blood cells eosinophils).[28] In a 2007 study published in the *Journal of Asthma*, asthmatics were found to have lower levels of lycopene in their blood than participants without asthma.[29]

Chocolate (cocoa). If you have a sweet tooth, I've saved the best antiallergy food for last. Cocoa has been found to have some antiallergy properties via reduction in IgE synthesis. In a 2012 study published in the journal *Pharmacoligical Research*, laboratory animals fed a cocoa-enriched diet for 4 weeks had lower levels of IgE than rats fed a standard diet.[30]

overall health is omega-3 fatty acids. As discussed, both omega-3 fatty acids and omega-6 fatty acids are essential, meaning your body doesn't make them; instead, you have to get them from food or supplements. Some omega-6 fatty acids, like those found in vegetable oil and many processed foods, are proinflammatory unless you balance them with the appropriate amount of omega-3 fatty acids. Most experts recommend aiming for an omega-6 to omega-3 ratio of 1:1 or 2:1.

Not only do omega-3 fatty acids help keep inflammation at bay by counteracting omega-6s, but omega-3 fatty acids may also help fight allergies.[31] One of the best sources of omega-3 fatty acids is oily fish, but there's a limit to how much fish you can eat. According to the Environmental Protection Agency, all fish and shellfish contain some mercury. To be safe, I recommend that you limit yourself to no more than two servings of seafood per week. This is especially important for children and women of childbearing age.[32]

Besides oily fish, there are a number of other food sources of omega-3 fatty acids. These include flaxseed, chia, and spirulina (a blue-green freshwater algae). Recently, food manufacturers have been making an effort to advertise their products as being fortified with omega-3s. Products like cereal, milk, and eggs are often labeled as good sources. Those with allergies or sensitivities to wheat, dairy, or eggs will obviously want to avoid these foods. Furthermore, how much beneficial omega-3 fatty acids these products really contain is sometimes suspect, so I certainly wouldn't rely on these foods to fulfill your omega-3 quota.

One of the best nonfish ways to get some omega-3 fatty acids is to consume flaxseeds. Flaxseeds are rich in alpha-linolenic acid (ALA), a type of omega-3 fatty acid that has been found to be protective against the symptoms of asthma.[33] You can buy flaxseed in bulk in most health food grocery stores. In order to get the most out of flaxseed, you should grind it into a meal before ingesting it. (The seeds are too small to be effectively broken down by your digestive tract and absorbed.) I generally recommend that people use whole flax, rather than a preground product, as the healthy fats contained in the seed can rapidly oxidize when exposed to air, losing some of their healthiness. A simple solution is to grind a couple of heaping tablespoons of whole flaxseeds in a small coffee bean grinder just prior to using them. Freshly ground flax makes a great addition to oatmeal or cereal; it adds a pleasant, nutty flavor to salads; and it is a good addition to a smoothie. A quick word of caution: If you add ground flax to a smoothie, make sure you add a little more liquid than usual, as the fiber contained in the seeds can make your drink pretty thick. It's important to note that flaxseeds do not contain the other omega-3 fatty acids, DHA and EPA, so they are not a complete source of omegas. There is evidence, however, that the ALA found in flax can be converted to DHA and EPA.

As previously mentioned, most people are deficient in omega-3s and, in addition to dietary measures, will benefit from taking a supplement to bring their levels up to optimal. A quality fish oil supplement or spirulina product is a good way to correct this deficit. The current recommendations for omega-3 fatty acids are 500 milligrams per day of EPA and DHA for healthy adults.[34]

I think that these levels are a little low to realistically achieve a healthy ratio of omega-6 to omega-3 fatty acids unless you also drastically reduce your omega-6 intake and increase your omega-3 intake from food. In Japan, it has been documented that people have eaten in excess of 1,200 milligrams of combined DHA and EPA for decades without adverse effects. While I tend to use higher doses of omega-3s, I recommend that people consult with a physician educated about such things prior to using supplements to boost their omega-3s. Personally, I feel the liquid is the best form. You may have to take up to eight capsules of some brands to get the 2,000 milligrams I recommend, but you can get this amount in just 1 teaspoon of the liquid.

Use olive oil whenever you can. The fat in olive oil is a monounsaturated fat, which has been shown to reduce inflammation, lower cholesterol, and help prevent blood clots. Olive oil is also rich in antioxidants, which can reduce inflammation and help prevent a number of inflammation-related diseases.[35] To reap all of these benefits, follow the guidelines of the modified Mediterranean diet and use olive oil as your main fat. Drizzle olive oil on your salad instead of topping it with ranch dressing, and use olive oil to cook your vegetables instead of other fats and oils.[36]

Keep in mind that olive oil has a very low smoke point (defined as the temperature something can reach before it starts to burn, smoke, and eventually catch fire), so you should only use it to cook at a lower heat—less than 325° to 400°F. Not only could high-temperature cooking with olive oil cause a fire, but when it reaches its smoke point, the oil starts to break down. It loses its antioxidants and can actually release toxic chemicals in its smoke, serving you carcinogenic free radicals—the very free radicals it helps fight in its cooler form. So avoid using olive oil to sear fish, meat, or chicken; to roast vegetables in an oven hotter than 400°F; when you are cooking in a wok or stir-frying in a pan; or when you are deep-frying anything. When cooking in these higher-heat instances, use refined coconut oil instead.[37]

Get four or five servings of veggies and two or three servings of fruit per day. As discussed in Chapter 9, fruits and vegetables— especially brightly colored varieties—are great sources of anti-inflammatory antioxidants.[38] But if you're not a natural fruits and veggies eater, don't panic. You don't have to munch on carrots and celery all day. Aim for four to five ½-cup servings of vegetables and two or three ½-cup servings of fruit per day.[39] Add strawberries (see "The Importance of Springing for Organic Strawberries") and blueberries to your oatmeal or flax cereal in the morning, have a spinach salad with tomatoes and avocado for lunch, and eat a serving of steamed asparagus with your dinner, and you've more than met your daily goal.

Eat your grains whole. Whole-grain breads, cereals, and rice are good for you because they contain dietary fiber. The soluble fiber in whole grains forms a sticky gel that protects the inside of your digestive tract from harmful substances in the foods you eat.[40] Plus, a 2014 study shows that dietary fiber may help protect against allergic asthma. Swiss researchers fed mice two different diets—one with

The Importance of Springing for Organic Strawberries

Strawberries are one of the most delicious, nutritious fruits you can eat, but unfortunately, they are also one of the most heavily contaminated foods. Along with grapes, apples, and peaches, strawberries are guilty of being on the "Dirty Dozen" list (see page 159). And strawberries are on this list for a good reason: They may contain up to 371 different pesticides approved by the Environmental Protection Agency, including methyl bromide; chloropicrin; captan; malathion; Dibrom; Kelthane; and avermectin. These chemicals can cause a number of health problems, including nerve damage, respiratory problems, and cancer.

Because nonorganic strawberries are potentially toxic, it's worth it to invest in organic strawberries if you can.[41]

4 percent fiber and one with 0.3 percent fiber. When they exposed both sets of mice to dust mite extract, the mice eating the lower-fiber diet had twice the number of immune cells associated with allergic inflammation in their airways compared with the mice eating the high-fiber diet.[42]

If you have an allergy or sensitivity, or just a general desire to avoid grain products, you can get soluble fiber from other foods, too. In addition to whole grains, nature provides a number of alternative sources of soluble fiber, including lentils, apples, beans, blueberries, carrots, celery, cucumbers, dried peas, nuts, oranges, pears, and strawberries.[43]

Don't rely on red meat and chicken as your primary protein sources. Red meat and chicken both contain proinflammatory arachidonic acid. That doesn't mean you have to cut them out completely, but they shouldn't be at the center of your diet.

To help minimize your dependence on these meats, consider trying some of the really good meat substitutes available. Textured vegetable protein (TVP) is a defatted soy flour product that has a similar protein content as meat. (There's a restaurant down the street from my house that serves meatless chicken wings made from textured vegetable protein, and you literally cannot tell the difference.) You can also use quinoa as a ground meat substitute in things like meatballs and vegetarian stuffed peppers. Veggie burgers and portobello mushroom burgers are also tasty alternatives to beef. Other good alternative protein sources include beans, lentils, nuts, and seeds.

I also want to highlight the importance of getting *complete proteins*—proteins that contain all nine of the essential amino acids necessary for human dietary needs—in the correct proportions. Most animal proteins, such as eggs, dairy products, meat, and fish, are complete proteins. If you are cutting one or more of these animal products from your diet, add quinoa; it's also a good complete protein source.[44]

Part of changing your eating habits to reduce your meat consumption involves giving your palate some time to adjust. Substitutes for meat, chicken, and other fattening and inflammation-promoting foods take some getting used to. As you start to adopt a less-meat-dependent diet, not only will you find that you feel better but

Genetically Modified Foods and Allergies

As discussed in Chapter 2, there are a number of theories to explain the rise in allergies in developed countries—particularly food allergies—ranging from our sterile society to the increase in pollution. One additional potential explanation for this increase is genetically modified (GM) foods. Genetically modified foods (also called genetically engineered foods) are foods that contain genes from other animals or plants in their genetic codes. Just like dog breeders have worked to create breeds that are more docile and domesticated, scientists have tried to create the "perfect food" in appearance and taste by moving desired genes from one plant or one animal to another.[45]

Genetically engineered foods do have some benefits. They may be more nutritious, require fewer pesticides, grow faster, have a longer shelf life, or have increased medicinal properties that allow them to be used in vaccines and drugs.[46] These benefits come with some significant risks, however, including unexpected genetic changes that may be harmful. For example, a food can contain a gene from another allergenic food, which could cause people allergic to Brazil nuts to react to soybeans, because the Brazil nut protein was transferred to the soybean as part of the genetic engineering process. In addition, genetically modified foods may interbreed with natural organisms and create hybrids, potentially leading to the genetic extinction of the original animal or food.[47]

According to the American Academy of Environmental Medicine (AAEM), genetically modified foods pose a serious threat to human health. The AAEM believes that introducing genetically modified

also your taste buds will change and you will crave those foods less and less.

DIETARY CHANGES AND YOUR DIGESTIVE SYSTEM

This brings me to my next point: Any time you are making significant changes to your dietary habits, your digestive tract will likely need foods into the food supply has correlated with rises in diseases and allergies, particularly allergies to foods.[48] The main reason genetically modified foods are contributing to food allergies is that, as a result of being manufactured, genetically modified foods may contain more foods than the food they were meant to become, as is the case of the Brazil nut and soybean just explained.[49]

My advice to people with allergies is to avoid genetically modified foods as much as they can. The best way to avoid genetically modified foods is to eat organic whenever possible. That means vegetables, fruits, fish, and—if you eat them—poultry, meat, and dairy. Eating an all-organic diet can be cost-prohibitive. I often tell people to visit their local farmer's market, as organic foods are often less expensive when you buy them straight from the farmer. I personally try to eat only organic animal products. As for produce, I use my dollars to buy only those foods that are not on the Environmental Working Group's "Dirty Dozen" list.[50] These are the foods that are most likely to contain potentially harmful chemicals.

The "Dirty Dozen" includes the following 12 fruits and vegetables:

1. Apples
2. Grapes
3. Strawberries
4. Spinach
5. Peaches
6. Cherry tomatoes
7. Imported snap peas
8. Sweet bell peppers
9. Cucumbers
10. Celery
11. Imported nectarines
12. Potatoes

some time to adapt. To digest high-fiber fruits, vegetables, and nuts, you will require different enzymes than you did while eating a meat-based diet. As a result, when you're suddenly eating more produce, you may experience an increased amount of bloating and gas. A good digestive enzyme supplement can help you through this transition.

Digestive enzymes are produced by your pancreas and secreted into your small intestine to help you break down the foods you eat. These enzymes are very important, as they work to digest food into a state in which it can be easily absorbed by your body. Quite often, patients with gastrointestinal symptoms will remark that their symptoms dramatically improved once they started taking a digestive enzyme. There are many good digestive enzyme supplements available, and for those people moving toward a more vegetable-heavy diet, an enzyme formulation containing alpha-galactosidase may help reduce the symptoms of gas and bloating. Digestive enzymes are generally taken right before meals.

All-Powerful Probiotics

I think just about everyone should try to incorporate probiotics into their daily plan. Regardless of whether you are making a significant dietary change, fighting allergies, or trying to improve gastrointestinal health, probiotics will likely be of benefit.

Probiotics, the health-promoting symbiotic bacteria that live on and in us, can help maintain a healthy balance of good to bad microorganisms. To illustrate the benefits of probiotics, consider this example: Most women have experienced a urinary tract infection (UTI) at one time or another in their lives. Generally speaking, the usual treatment for a UTI is an antibiotic. The antibiotic will eliminate the offending bacteria from the urinary system, but it often predisposes the woman to a subsequent yeast infection. This is because while the antibiotic destroys the bacteria responsible for the infection, it also damages the population of healthy, protective, good bacteria, called beneficial flora, in the urinary tract. With these good bacteria diminished, it creates an opportunity for yeast overgrowth, as yeasts are not affected by antibiotics. Taking a probiotic during a course of antibiotics, and especially immediately afterward, can nearly always prevent the yeast overgrowth.

In terms of allergies, research has shown that the right balance of beneficial to bad bacteria can help prevent your immune system from overreacting and can therefore prevent allergic reactions.[51] As mentioned in Chapter 2, kids who are exposed to a wider variety of bacteria early in life tend to have fewer allergies than kids who are more protected from germs.[52] Plus, because of our widespread use of antibiotics, we're unintentionally destroying some of the good, protective bacteria along with the bad ones, and that loss of good bacteria inhibits our immune systems from functioning properly.[53]

There's research to support the potentially protective effects of probiotics in people with allergy symptoms. In a 2013 review published in the journal *Current Opinion in Allergy and Clinical Immunology*, researchers found that probiotics may help prevent eczema as well as respiratory allergies.[54]

Here are some guidelines on taking probiotics.

- **Don't fall for the probiotic marketing hype.** Make sure to look for products that contain multiple strains of probiotics. Lactobacillus and acidophilus are common strains found in foods like yogurt.

- **Find the right probiotic supplement.** Most probiotic supplements should be refrigerated. Because they are living things, probiotics are sensitive and can lose efficacy if exposed to temperature extremes. There are a few probiotic supplements that don't need to be refrigerated (look for them in health food stores), but they are few and far between. Also look for supplements that have the following:

  - **A good range of bacteria, not just one kind.** *Your supplement should contain acidophilus, bifidobacterium, and lactobacillus.*

  - **Enough bacteria.** *Probiotics are measured in colony forming units (CFUs). Look for a supplement that has at least 5 billion CFUs.*

  - **Some variety.** *I think it's a good idea to switch your probiotic supplement every so often, because they all contain slightly different strains of bacteria. You don't want the same bacteria over and over. Instead, mix it up to add some fresh genetics to the gene pool, so to speak.*

Additionally, there are some foods that are naturally good sources of probiotics, such as miso soup, sauerkraut, yogurt with "live, active cultures," and kefir (a cross between milk and yogurt).

THE IMPORTANCE OF HYDRATION

Drinking water is one of the best things you can do for yourself. After all, more than half of your body is made of water—it makes up your interstitial fluids, intracellular liquid, and cerebrospinal fluid as well as other important liquids. Blood, for instance, is 83 percent water.[55]

Just as you have to change the oil in your car, for good health, it is a good idea to continuously flush your system with fresh water in order to promote health. You are constantly losing water through urine, sweat, breath, and stool, so you need to replenish your supplies constantly.[56] Unfortunately, many of us are walking around semi- or completely dehydrated. Most of us are busy, and drinking water doesn't make it onto our to-do lists. We confuse sensations of thirst with hunger and reach for a snack, rather than for the water we really need.[57]

Making sure you get enough water is imperative. Without enough water, your blood can't deliver oxygen, nutrients, and other important substances to your tissues.[58] Dehydration can lead to all kinds of problems, including digestive upset, especially acid reflux and constipation, as well as depression and irritability. Anyone who

Drinking and Drugging?

If you drink municipal water, you may be getting more than you bargained for. A number of studies have found high levels of pharmaceutical drugs in drinking water. In fact, according to an Associated Press study of 24 major US cities, 41 million Americans may be getting drugs in their drinking water. These medications include drugs for pain, asthma, mental illness, high cholesterol, and infections.

To help protect yourself and your family from these unwanted drug treatments, consider a home water-purification system or water filter. Also, make sure to engage in lifestyle activities that promote good health, such as healthful eating and exercise, which will help flush things through your system and prevent accumulation of these drugs as well as unwanted toxicity.[59]

has ever had a hangover knows the mental fog that dehydration can bring. In fact, when dehydration persists, blood volume can get so low that it can temporarily reduce blood flow to the brain and impair clear thinking.[60]

In terms of allergies, dehydration can cause an immune system imbalance and increased histamine levels. Therefore, if you do encounter an allergen, such as from a mold or a cat, when you are thirsty, your allergic reaction could be exaggerated.[61] Hydration, on the other hand, can also protect against allergy symptoms by thinning mucus and helping your sinuses drain. Since congestion also leads to a dry mouth and lessens the protective properties of saliva, drinking lots of water can help boost your immunity.[62]

To stay hydrated, I recommend you drink *water.* My general recommendation is half of your body weight in ounces of water each day. For me, a 200-pound guy, this equates to about 100 ounces per day. Activities that cause you to sweat will obviously increase your water needs. To stay hydrated:

- **Drink water throughout the day.** Don't wait until 6:00 p.m. to drink your daily requirement; nobody likes to be up all night going to the bathroom.
- **Keep water with you at all times.** One of the biggest obstacles to drinking water is not having access to it. If you have a water bottle on your desk or in your car, you will drink from it. Get a good water bottle and take it with you wherever you go. Look for a container that is free of harmful chemicals such as bisphenol A (BPA).
- **Make sure you have good water in your home.** Consider installing a quality drinking water filter (see "Drinking and Drugging?"). It's not a bad idea to install chlorine filters on your showerheads, too. Both of these types of filters are readily available from a variety of sources.
- **Forgo bottled water.** The FDA doesn't require water-bottling companies to undergo water-quality tests. In the past few years, some bottled water has been recalled due to contamination with bacteria, mold, arsenic, and even some cleaning compounds.[63]

- **Make sure your water isn't too pure.** Reverse osmosis is a water-purification process that converts saltwater into fresh drinking water. It is such a powerful cleansing tool that it strips all of the minerals out of the water, too, so you're left with pure H_2O. With nothing to buffer it, water purified through reverse osmosis can be quite acidic, and drinking it can actually remove some of the minerals from your body. To buffer the acidity, I recommend that people who drink this water head to the health food store and purchase liquid minerals. Add a few drops to your water bottle to buffer the acidity, and you're good to go.

SLOW AND STEADY WINS THE RACE

Changing your lifestyle to lose weight—or just to become healthier and less allergic—is a big commitment. In order to succeed, you have to be kind to yourself and take things slowly.

Be flexible. One of the great things about the modified Mediterranean diet is that there are so many foods you can eat as part of it, which means you can eliminate foods you can't eat or don't like. If you dislike eggplant or avocados, for example, you can substitute in other healthful vegetables and nuts, such as squash and chickpeas. If you don't like seafood or are allergic to fish or shellfish, you can still enjoy a healthful, anti-inflammatory eating plan. Some suggestions for shellfish substitutes in recipes include green leafy vegetables, like spinach; walnuts, Brazil nuts, hazelnuts, and pecans; flaxseed oil; canola oil; eggs; sesame butter (tahini); soybeans and soybean oil; soy milk; and tofu.[64]

Be accountable. To stick to healthy lifestyle changes, it can help to be accountable to someone or something, be it a trainer at your gym, an exercise buddy, or an online journal—whatever works best for you. When it's just you, it's really easy to talk yourself into or out of something. Walking through the grocery store, you could be doing great, pushing a cartful of organic greens and fish. Then, for whatever reason, you head down the frozen food aisle and there is your favorite macadamia nut crunch ice cream. It feels good to eat ice cream, so you reach out, grab it, and throw it into your cart without really thinking. If it is in your freezer, you have a higher probability of eating it. Now, if you made a point of bringing a friend with you to the grocery store, or you just promised yourself you would tell a friend all of the things you bought, you would be a lot less likely to give in and toss the ice cream into your otherwise healthful array of purchases.

Another example: Many of my patients complain about having to fit exercise into their busy schedules. It usually requires a change in routine—getting up earlier in the morning or going to the gym later at night. So you tell yourself you are going to get up at 6:00 a.m. to run. But when that alarm goes off, you smack it, roll over, and go right back to sleep. If you have a friend waiting on the corner to run with you, it will be a whole different story. Not only will you feel guilty for letting yourself down if you skip the run but also you will have to live with knowing you let your friend down, too. So the point is, whether it's for exercise or weight loss or any major lifestyle and habit change, accountability is very important.

I also like the idea of keeping a food journal. Writing down what you eat and when you eat it not only provides positive feedback about how great you're doing, but it can also help identify foods that might be causing GI upset. I think it's smart to keep a food journal for about the first 2 weeks of any new diet plan.

Make it a family affair. I see this a lot: One member of a family decides to lose weight or just start to make healthier eating choices (usually the wife), and the other family members (usually the husband and the children) choose to continue to eat their regular diets. Typically, the wife is the cook in the family, so now she has to cook two meals, not to mention dealing with the temptation of continuing to have unhealthy foods around the house. So I think it is really important for people undergoing a lifestyle change to make sure they have a real, honest discussion with their family members about their plans *before* they get started. Spell out how you plan to improve your health, and encourage your family members to adopt the same habits—not only to give you support but for the sake of their own health as well. That's one of the beautiful things about this plan: It's not just for allergies, it's for good health in general!

Spencer's Story

Ever since he was a kid, Spencer suffered from severe allergy symptoms—eye watering, puffy, itchy eyes he could barely keep open, sneezing, running nose, and food allergies that interfered with his quality of life. "As a kid, I missed a lot of school due to my allergies," he says.

Later, as an adult, he missed work and activities he enjoyed. "Working or riding motocross are the only two places you'll find me. Both were impossible when I couldn't see and felt miserable," says the 22-year-old.

In addition, Spencer suffered stomach unrest gastroenterologists couldn't fix. After trying numerous anti-anxiety medications to help with serotonin levels, as well as a range of antibiotics, Spencer did not feel any relief. "The GI doctors didn't support the idea of bacterial overgrowth or leaky intestinal lining. They weren't willing to consider it as an actual condition," Spencer says.

Fed up, he decided to visit someone who would take his symptoms seriously: Dr. Psenka.

"I was never a believer in 'natural treatments.' I felt there was a pill for everything," says Spencer, a personal trainer at Orange Theory Fitness. For the old Spencer, energy drinks, stress, and binge drinking were a regular occurrence. He also ate whatever he wanted. "Somehow, those habits coupled with a bacterial infection is how the whole mess started. I wish I would have always been eating healthfully like I do now."

Don't go cold turkey. Just like trying to quit smoking, most people have to wean themselves off of their old diets and ease into a their new ones. Switching to a new eating plan overnight is a recipe for failure. My advice: Take a week or so and mentally ease into the idea of your new eating plan. Consider doing some research and finding some recipes for the modified Mediterranean diet. Look for some cookbooks with ideas for healthy meals (I like Asian, and specifically Thai, cookbooks myself), because these recipes are typically in line with Mediterranean diet food choices.

This 'eating healthfully' means following the Specific Carbohydrate Diet (SCD), which eliminates carbohydrates that are difficult to digest and cause inflammation in the gut—primarily grains, starches, sugars and dairy.

In addition, Spencer is now using sublingual immunotherapy (SLIT) to fight his seasonal nasal and ocular allergies. Within the first two weeks on SLIT, he started feeling better. "Since I started using the SLIT, I haven't had one bad day like I used to have," he says. "My life is now allergy- and worry-free."

The SCD is working well, too. "It took about two months for the diet to eradicate the bacterial overgrowth, but I now feel I am on the path to healing my intestinal lining," he says. "When my stomach feels good, I am a far happier and more outgoing person, and I feel less stressed."

Spencer has also lost weight. "I dropped from a 34 waist size to a 30 to 32, and I went from 200 to 185 pounds," he says. And his weight dropped from 200 pounds to 185.

All this thanks to Dr. Psenka's plan, which Spencer says was easy to follow and well laid out.

For all these reasons, today, the once natural remedies skeptic is now a first believer. "I have learned keeping your body healthy can fix a lot more problems than one medicine can," he says. "I will now see Dr. Psenka first for whatever problems I am having."

Set small goals. The safest way to lose weight and keep it off is to do it slowly, losing no more than 2 to 3 pounds in a single week. Monitor your weight loss closely, weighing yourself a few times throughout the week to make sure you are losing at a good pace. Also, keep a record so you can see your progress over time. This is great positive feedback that will help keep you enthusiastic and on track.

11

Treating Allergies the Natural Way: Supplements and Herbs

DURING THE 12 YEARS THAT I HAVE BEEN PRACTICING as a licensed naturopathic physician, I have used dietary supplements to help a great number of people. When used correctly, supplements can help improve a person's health in a variety of ways. For example, people who are just beginning to eat a healthy diet can use supplements to give their bodies a boost of a particular substance, like omega-3 fatty acids, and quickly correct any nutritional deficiencies that may exist. Once these deficiencies have been corrected, then diet alone can be used to maintain healthy levels.

It's important to note that physicians will often suggest using supplements along with conventional medications in hopes that this synergistic approach will deliver better results than either treatment could alone. Special attention should be paid in these cases, because not all supplements and medications work well together. Sometimes supplements can be used by themselves to address specific symptoms in much the same way that prescription medications are. If a natural supplement can alleviate symptoms just as well as a medication, but without the potential for adverse effects, then my recommendation is to use the natural supplement.

It's also a good idea to use food to improve your health whenever possible. I would much rather see people eating wholesome foods than taking a handful of supplements. Food as medicine is always the ideal, but as you'll discover in this chapter, it's sometimes helpful to use supplements to aid healing and find relief from allergies.

Now, I am not recommending that you immediately discontinue prescription medications for allergies or asthma, but rather I'm hoping to encourage you to learn how you can safely integrate medications and supplements. But—and this is a big but—keep in mind that just because something is natural doesn't mean it is safe. Poison ivy, for example, is natural, but we all know it isn't safe to touch. It's also important to remember that herbs and supplements are not regulated by the FDA the way other medications are, so they don't have to undergo the same type of testing before they hit the shelves.

It's a good idea to consult with a physician experienced in using natural supplements before taking anything new. This is especially true if you have health issues, are pregnant, or are taking any pharmaceutical medications. Consulting with a doctor can not only help you avoid any unpleasant adverse effects that may arise but also it can help ensure that your dosage is correct and that the product you are taking is of high quality.

In addition, some supplements may actually aggravate allergy symptoms. Echinacea, for example, belongs to the same family as ragweed, so it can make hay fever worse. The same goes for chamomile.[1]

Supplements and herbs may also cross-react with some prescription or over-the-counter medications.[2] For all of these reasons, it's important to follow dosage recommendations and directions whenever you take any herb, supplement, or medication. And *always* talk to your health-care provider and pharmacist before you start taking any new substance.

SUPPLEMENTS AND HERBS FOR ALLERGIES AND ASTHMA

With all of the above information in mind, here are some of my favorite supplements and herbs for treating allergies, asthma, and the inflammation that can exacerbate these and other conditions.

SNEEZE-STIFLING SUPPLEMENTS

Bromelain

Bromelain, which was first produced in Hawaii and Japan, is a protein-digesting enzyme (aka a proteolytic enzyme) that can significantly reduce inflammation. As an anti-inflammatory, bromelain has the potential to help many conditions, such as strains, sprains, arthritis, back pain, and of course, allergies.[3]

HOW IT FIGHTS ALLERGY OR ASTHMA SYMPTOMS

Bromelain has been shown to decrease inflammation in the respiratory tract, and therefore it can help reduce allergy symptoms, such as nasal and sinus swelling.[4,5] Bromelain can also thin mucus, easing nasal congestion. There's also some evidence that it can boost your immune system.

In a 2005 study published in the journal *In Vivo*, researchers found that children under age 11 who were diagnosed with acute sinusitis responded well to bromelain. The participants got one of three different treatments—bromelain (200 milligram tablet), bromelain combined with a standard treatment, or the standard treatment by itself. The group treated with the bromelain alone had the fastest recovery—6.66 days, compared to 9.06 days for the kids treated only with the standard therapy.[6] It is also important to point out that none of the children in the study experienced any serious adverse reactions to bromelain. However, one child did have an allergic reaction, and it was later determined that this child had a pineapple allergy.

HOW TO GET IT

While you can get bromelain from eating fresh pineapple, most of the enzyme is found within the pineapple stem, which isn't a good part of the pineapple to eat. The best way to use bromelain is to take it as a supplement.[7]

Bromelain is usually measured in gelatin dissolving units (GDUs), milk clotting units (MCUs), International Pharmaceutical Federation units (FIP), or milligrams (mg). (To convert milligrams to FIPs, simply multiply them by 2.5.) It's a good idea to look for a bromelain supplement that is enteric coated, which protects the bromelain from becoming active in your stomach. When bromelain becomes active in your stomach, the enzyme works to digest any food that is in there. Therefore, it is best to take bromelain supplements on an empty stomach.

The German Commission E monograph for bromelain suggests a dosage of 80 to 320 milligrams. The effectiveness of bromelain seems to be dose-dependent and, for many, dosages up to 1,000 milligrams per day have been used. It is best to take bromelain three or four times per day, rather than as a single dose. I usually recommend that my patients take 150 milligrams three or four times a day.

CONTRAINDICATIONS AND THINGS TO CONSIDER

Bromelain has a good safety profile and is well-tolerated by most people. That said, it does have the potential to be an allergen itself, especially in those who suspect that they may have a pineapple allergy. It can also cause some mild gastrointestinal side effects, including heartburn and diarrhea.[8] There is some evidence that bromelain can increase the action of certain blood-thinning medications as well as antibiotics known as tetracyclines. If you are currently taking these drugs, consult with your doctor before starting a bromelain supplement.

Vitamin B_6

Vitamin B_6 (pyridoxine) is an important vitamin that helps your body make proteins, hormones, and neurotransmitters. It's particularly critical for proper functioning of your brain, nerves, and skin.[9] In your body, vitamin B_6 is absorbed in your small intestine and transported to your liver, where it is converted to its metabolically active form, pyridoxal 5'-phosphate.

HOW IT FIGHTS ALLERGY OR ASTHMA SYMPTOMS

A few studies have suggested that vitamin B_6 may help people with asthma. One study on 76 children with asthma found that kids who took a vitamin B_6 supplement for 2 months were able to reduce their doses of asthma medications.[10]

Another small study published in the *American Journal of Clinical*

Nutrition found that adult asthmatics had significantly lower levels of vitamin B_6 than controls. The study subjects with asthma were then given 50 milligrams of vitamin B_6 twice daily and noted a dramatic decrease in the frequency and severity of wheezing and asthma attacks while taking the supplement.[11]

Also, people with high levels of inflammation often have depressed vitamin B_6 levels. As discussed, inflammation sets the stage for the development of a range of diseases, from heart disease to allergies. In a 2012 study published in the *Journal of Nutrition*, researchers looked at vitamin B_6 levels and 13 different markers of inflammation in 2,229 adults. The researchers found that those with the highest levels of inflammation had the lowest levels of vitamin B_6. Conversely, those with the highest levels of B_6 had the lowest levels of inflammation.[12]

Another interesting study published in the same journal found that vitamin B_6–deficient rats had an impaired ability to convert dietary proinflammatory omega-6 fatty acids into anti-inflammatory omega-3 fats. The researchers found that the animals had an 80 percent reduction in the activity of the enzyme acyl-CoA oxidase, which is responsible for fatty acid metabolism.[13] Granted, we're not rats, but one thing is becoming clear in the medical literature: There is a definite link between vitamin B_6 deficiency and inflammation.

HOW TO GET IT

While you can get vitamin B_6 from some foods, including avocados, bananas, poultry, soybeans, sunflower seeds, and watermelon, it can also be taken as a supplement. Currently, the recommended daily allowance (RDA) of vitamin B_6 is between 1 and 2 milligrams per day. However, most of the research regarding B_6 for therapeutic purposes has used dosages ranging from 50 to 200 milligrams per day. I recommend taking 50 milligrams each day.

Vitamin B_6 is a water-soluble vitamin and is generally recognized as safe. However, in the past there has been some concern about this vitamin being neurotoxic at high doses. Most cases of neurotoxicity and vitamin B_6 have involved dosages of at least 500 milligrams per day for 2 years.[14,15]

CONTRAINDICATIONS AND THINGS TO CONSIDER

Many prescription medications have the ability to cause a deficiency in vitamin B_6. Eating a diet rich in vitamin B_6 can help to improve your body's stores. I recommend that you have your vitamin B_6 levels checked prior to taking the vitamin in large doses. Also, because vitamin B_6 has the potential to interfere with some types of medications (cycloserine, hydralazine, levodopa, isoniazid, penicillamine, and theophylline), it is a good idea to discuss taking vitamin B_6 with a physician experienced with its use.[16]

Vitamin B_{12}

Vitamin B_{12} (cobalamin) is an important cofactor in DNA synthesis, nerve health, and carbohydrate metabolism. This vitamin is found mainly in animal products such as beef liver, clams, salmon, lamb, and cheese. Nonanimal sources of vitamin B_{12} include brewer's yeast, sea vegetables, chlorella, and spirulina.[17]

HOW IT FIGHTS ALLERGY OR ASTHMA SYMPTOMS

There is some evidence that vitamin B_{12} may help with asthma. In a 2010 study published in the journal *Allergy*, researchers looked at 4,516 people ages 30 to 60. They found that those deficient in B_{12} were more likely to suffer from asthma attacks and shortness of breath over a 5-year period than people with adequate levels of the B vitamin.[18]

A smaller study published in the *Journal of Allergy and Clinical Immunology* reported that people who suffer from asthma caused by an intolerance to sulfites could be helped by vitamin B_{12}. In this study, children with confirmed sulfite intolerances were given 1,500 micrograms of vitamin B_{12} and then exposed to sulfites. The majority of children (four out of five) did not develop bronchospasm after sulfite exposure.[19] While this was a small study, it does show the potential of vitamin B_{12} in helping asthmatics.

HOW TO GET IT

The current RDA for B_{12} is up to 3 micrograms daily, whereas the dosage for clinical effect ranges from 1,500 to 6,000 micrograms per day.[20] For maintenance, you can take a dose of 1,000 micrograms daily. B_{12} comes in both chewable and sublingual forms.

CONTRAINDICATIONS AND THINGS TO CONSIDER

Vitamin B_{12} has excellent tolerability and is relatively safe. This vitamin can be administered orally, intramuscularly, or intravenously, with all routes of administration providing positive outcomes. My favorite form of vitamin B_{12} is methylcobalamin, as it appears to be better absorbed and utilized by the body.

Vitamin C

Vitamin C (ascorbic acid) is the most popular supplement in the world, and it's no wonder; it does many good things for your body. Some of vitamin C's most important actions include protecting fat-soluble vitamins from oxidative damage and producing collagen to strengthen connective tissues. Vitamin C is also a powerful antioxidant, and it helps protect against damage from free radicals. It may also prevent plaque buildup in the arteries by lowering LDL (bad) cholesterol. Vitamin C is also useful for regulating your immune system and helping your body deal with stress, and it has anticancer properties as well. One of its most well-known powers is its ability to shorten the duration of the common cold.

HOW IT FIGHTS ALLERGY OR ASTHMA SYMPTOMS

Not surprisingly, there's also evidence that vitamin C can help ease asthma and allergy symptoms.[21] Research shows that vitamin C helps prevent histamine from being released by stabilizing the membranes of mast cells. Mast cells are the storage units for histamine, and when their cell membranes rupture, histamine is released, causing allergic symptoms. Vitamin C can also break down histamine once it has started circulating in your body.[22] In a 2013 study, researchers found that when they injected allergic people with vitamin C, their blood levels of histamine went down.[23]

In another 2013 study published in *Allergy, Asthma, and Immunology*

Research, Korean children ages 6 to 12 with high intakes of vitamin C had fewer symptoms of allergic rhinitis (hay fever) than kids who did not increase their daily vitamin C intake.[24]

Vitamin C also appears to help reduce inflammation. In a 2006 cross-sectional study published in the *American Journal of Clinical Nutrition,* researchers looked at 3,258 men participating in the British Regional Heart Study and found that those with higher intakes and blood levels of vitamin C had lower levels of C-reactive protein (CRP), an important marker of inflammation.[25] The same relationship between higher vitamin C and lower CRP was noted in a National Health and Nutrition Examination Survey, which looked at data from more than 14,500 adults.[26] And yet another study found that when healthy nonsmokers took 1,000 milligrams of vitamin C for 2 months, their CRP levels dropped nearly 17 percent, compared to an 8.6 percent drop in the placebo group.[27]

HOW TO GET IT

You can easily get vitamin C from foods, and nearly everyone should try to eat some of this vitamin daily. Focus on foods like acerola berries, cauliflower, guavas, kiwis, mangoes, melons, oranges, peppers, strawberries, and tomatoes. The current RDA for vitamin C is 60 milligrams per day, and this is likely just enough to prevent a person from developing a deficiency. In my practice, I have used dosages exceeding 50,000 milligrams without adverse effects. When using vitamin C therapeutically, dosages of greater than 6 grams per day are frequently used.

There is a large variety of vitamin C supplements available, including liquid, tablet, capsule, powdered crystalline, and effervescent forms. For allergies and asthma, I generally recommend taking vitamin C in divided dosages ranging from 6 to 10 grams (6,000 to 10,000 milligrams) per day. For some people, I find that using intravenous vitamin C provides the quickest results.

CONTRAINDICATIONS AND THINGS TO CONSIDER

It is important to know that dosages of vitamin C greater than 3 to 4 grams (3,000 to 4,000 milligrams) taken at once may result in gastrointestinal discomfort and diarrhea. To help prevent this, vitamin

C can be taken in divided doses throughout the day. (For example, 2,000 milligrams, three times per day.)

While dietary intakes of vitamin C are generally safe, the use of vitamin C supplements may produce unwanted reactions when combined with certain medications. Blood-thinning medications, such as warfarin, may lose some of their effectiveness when combined with vitamin C, so people taking those medications should consult with their physicians before starting to take vitamin C or starting to take any new medications while taking vitamin C.[28,29,30]

Coenzyme Q10

First discovered by the Japanese in the 1960s, coenzyme Q10 (CoQ10) has quickly become one of the most popular supplements in the United States. CoQ10 is an enzyme found in almost every cell in your body, and it is a necessary intermediary in the production of the cellular energy molecule adenosine triphosphate (ATP). CoQ10 is also a powerful antioxidant and can buffer your body against damaging free radicals. As a result of its involvement in ATP production and as an antioxidant, CoQ10 affects the functioning of all of the cells in your body and is essential for the health of all human tissues and organs. Many diseases and health conditions—including heart disease, fibromyalgia, Parkinson's disease, diabetes, bronchitis, and allergy—have been linked with depleted levels of CoQ10.[31]

HOW IT FIGHTS ALLERGY OR ASTHMA SYMPTOMS

Research has shown that people with asthma have lower than normal levels of CoQ10, suggesting that the enzyme might help treat this condition. In a 2002 Slovakian study, researchers looked at the coenzyme Q10 levels of 56 asthmatic adults and 25 adults without asthma. They found that the asthmatics had significantly lower levels of CoQ10 than the nonasthmatic participants.[32]

CoQ10 may also work well alongside conventional asthma medications.[33] In fact, 2005 British research found that asthmatics who took CoQ10 supplements were able to reduce their dosages of the corticosteroids they took to help control asthma attacks.[34]

A more recent study examined the relationship between

antioxidant levels and airway inflammation in asthmatic children. The results of this study suggested that antioxidants positively influenced antioxidant levels and reduced airway inflammation in asthmatic children.[35]

HOW TO GET IT

CoQ10 comes in a number of forms, including chewable wafers, tablets, soft gel capsules, and powder-filled capsules. Typical dosages range from 30 to 300 milligrams in divided doses daily, although higher dosages are also used. Absorption of CoQ10 seems to improve when it's taken with food.

CONTRAINDICATIONS AND THINGS TO CONSIDER

There are several types of conventional medications that can lower CoQ10 levels in your body. These include the cholesterol-lowering drugs known as statins and blood pressure–lowering drugs like beta-blockers. People on these medications may benefit from incorporating CoQ10 into their treatment plans. CoQ10 is generally a safe supplement and adverse reactions are rare, but there are reports of doses greater than 200 milligrams per day causing nausea in some people.[36]

Vitamin E

Vitamin E is actually a family of related molecules that exhibit similar biological activity. Alpha-tocopherol causes the most actions in the body, but beta-, gamma-, and delta-tocopherols are the forms found naturally in foods. Vitamin E is one of nature's most potent antioxidants and has significant anti-inflammatory actions as well.[37]

Vitamin E seems to be particularly powerful against free radical harm to blood and tissues caused by vigorous exercise, and it may help decrease muscle injury and inflammation. It also appears to reduce the risk of some cancers, including breast, colon, prostate, liver, lung, and pancreatic.[38]

HOW IT FIGHTS ALLERGY OR ASTHMA SYMPTOMS

Some studies have shown that vitamin E can help dampen allergies by regulating the part of your immune system involved in allergic response.[39] Other research has shown that deficiencies in the vitamin can increase asthma symptoms.

In one study published in the *Annals of Allergy, Asthma, and Immunology*, researchers looked at the effects of vitamin E on 112 men and women with allergic rhinitis (hay fever). For 10 weeks, participants took either 800 international units of vitamin E per day or a placebo. At the end of the 10 weeks, the vitamin E group had significantly fewer allergy symptoms—especially nasal congestion—compared to the placebo group.[40]

Population-based British studies have also looked into the relationship between antioxidant intake and asthma and found that low levels of both vitamin C and vitamin E may increase asthma symptoms, such as wheezing.[41]

In a 2008 study published in *Free Radical Biology and Medicine*, researchers found that the gamma-tocopherol form of vitamin E helped reduce markers of inflammation and oxidative stress in people with asthma.[42]

Newer research has begun to shed light on the mechanism behind vitamin E's ability to suppress allergic symptoms. A 2013 study found that vitamin E suppressed the degranulation of mast cells and thus inhibited histamine release.[43]

HOW TO GET IT

You can get vitamin E from food, including wheat germ (the richest source), asparagus, avocados, nuts (almonds contain the most vitamin E of all nuts), and whole-grain products.[44] In addition, many different vitamin E supplements are available. These supplements come in natural (d-alpha-tocopherol) and synthetic (dl-alpha-tocopherol) forms, in capsules, soft gels, tablets, and topical oils. The natural d-alpha-tocopherol form can potentially deplete gamma-tocopherol levels in your body, so supplements containing mixed tocopherols are preferable.[45]

The recommended daily allowance for vitamin E is based solely on d-alpha-tocopherol, and no official recommendations exist for the other naturally occurring forms of vitamin E. The current RDA is 22.4 international units (IU), with a suggested upper limit of 1,490 IU daily. I recommend 400 to 800 IU, if no contraindications exist.

CONTRAINDICATIONS AND THINGS TO CONSIDER

Vitamin E has a low toxicity profile, but concerns exist regarding the influence that vitamin E may have on blood-thinning medications. Consult with your physician if you are taking any such medications.

Evening Primrose (*Oenothera biennis*)

True to its name, the flowers of the evening primrose plant open at dusk and close again at dawn. Oil from this plant (*Oenothera beinnis*) is traditionally used to help treat women's health issues such as PMS and hot flashes as well as some skin conditions like rashes, eczema, and hives.[46]

HOW IT FIGHTS ALLERGY OR ASTHMA SYMPTOMS

In addition to its other uses, evening primrose oil (EPO) has anti-inflammatory properties, which makes it a good remedy for arthritis and other inflammatory conditions.[47] More than 30 studies have shown that evening primrose oil can help ease eczema and dermatitis. One 2006 review of 26 studies that encompassed a total of 1,207 people found that EPO helped ease redness, itching, crusting, and swelling from skin conditions.[48]

HOW TO GET IT

Look for EPO that is standardized to contain 8 percent gamma-linolenic acid (GLA), and always take it with food. Studies have suggested that it is the GLA found in evening primrose oil that is responsible for most of its ability to treat atopic dermatitis.[49] Common dosages of EPO range between 2 and 6 grams per day taken in divided doses.

CONTRAINDICATIONS AND THINGS TO CONSIDER

EPO rarely causes side effects, but it may sometimes lead to headaches, nausea, and abdominal pain.[50] Also keep in mind that evening primrose oil can interfere with some medications, including antibiotics, chemotherapy drugs, nonsteroidal anti-inflammatory drugs (NSAIDS), anesthetics, anticonvulsant medications, and cyclosporine.[51]

Magnesium

This is a very important mineral involved in metabolism and energy production as well as muscle, heart, and lung function. Magnesium may help prevent or treat a whole list of other common health problems, from sleep issues to hot flashes to constipation.[52] A magnesium deficiency is quite common, as this mineral is not generally found in processed foods, which most people eat too much of.[53]

HOW IT FIGHTS ALLERGY OR ASTHMA SYMPTOMS

Magnesium can help relieve lung constriction in people who have asthma by relaxing the smooth muscles of the bronchioles, which are the airways within your lungs. One study showed that magnesium-deficient lab animals had more histamine in their blood when exposed to allergens than animals with sufficient magnesium levels.[54] Other studies have shown that magnesium may help treat acute asthma attacks and that people with asthma who have good magnesium intakes may have decreased wheezing and better lung function than asthmatics who have lower magnesium levels.[55]

HOW TO GET IT

As with most minerals, the best and safest way to get more magnesium is to eat foods containing it. Magnesium is found in many foods, including buckwheat and whole-wheat flours, almonds, avocados, bananas, beans, Brazil nuts, brown rice, cocoa, and dried figs.[56] In cases where a little extra magnesium would be helpful, a supplement can make getting magnesium easier.

The daily dose varies based on age and gender. While the RDA is 350 milligrams per day for men and 280 milligrams per day for women, the dosages used in clinical practice may be higher. Dosages as high as 1,200 milligrams in divided doses are sometimes used. Magnesium intakes greater than 800 milligrams per day are associated with a risk of diarrhea, although some people can handle these doses without a problem. To begin, I would recommend 400 milligrams per day. Magnesium may also cause a calcium deficiency, so high doses should be used with caution in people with low calcium. One study investigating magnesium's effect on allergic rhinitis found 365 milligrams per day to be an effective treatment.[57]

CONTRAINDICATIONS AND THINGS TO CONSIDER

Talk to your health-care provider before you start taking magnesium, especially if you have heart or kidney disease or are taking amiloride, tetracycline antibiotics, heart medications, or oral diabetes drugs.[58]

Probiotics

We discussed the power of probiotics in Chapter 10. I think it is worth repeating that *I believe everyone should take probiotics.*

HOW IT FIGHTS ALLERGY OR ASTHMA SYMPTOMS

Not only can probiotics such as acidophilus, bifidobacterium, and lactobacillus help strengthen your immune system but also they can help control your allergies. Research shows that probiotics may regulate the immune system overreaction that occurs in allergy sufferers.[59]

In fact, one important theory on why developed countries have higher rates of allergies is that we have fewer "good" probiotics in our flora. When you repopulate with the good guys, you can bolster your body's defenses against allergens.[60]

There's research to back up these potentially protective effects. In a 2013 review published in the journal *Current Opinion in Allergy and Clinical Immunology,* researchers found that probiotics may help prevent eczema as well as respiratory allergies.[61]

HOW TO GET IT

You can get probiotics from foods such as miso soup, some yogurts, sauerkraut, and kefir, but since you can't get too much of a good thing when it comes to probiotics, I also recommend you take supplements.

A variety of products claim to contain probiotics these days, so you have to choose carefully. Look for a probiotic supplement that needs to be refrigerated. (There are a few shelf-stable probiotic brands on the market, but most need to be refrigerated or the bacteria will die.) A quality probiotic supplement should also contain a range of different species of good bacteria, including acidophilus, bifidobacterium, and lactobacillus. Probiotics are measured in colony forming units (CFUs); look for a supplement that provides at least 5 billion CFUs. I also recommend that you switch your probiotic brand every once in a while. They all contain slightly different strains of bacteria, and it can never hurt to add fresh DNA to your beneficial bacteria gene pool.

CONTRAINDICATIONS AND THINGS TO CONSIDER

One word of caution regarding probiotics: If you have a compromised immune system, you need to exercise caution whenever you introduce any sort of bacteria into your system. Even bacterial strains that are normally found on and in us have the potential to be pathogenic in people with poorly functioning immune systems. Immunocompromised individuals can greatly benefit from taking probiotics, but they need to consult with their physicians to confirm that they're using probiotic supplements that contain no potentially pathogenic bacteria.

Pycnogenol

Pycnogenol is a registered trademark for a plant antioxidant that comes from the bark of the *Pinus pinaster* tree. It is also found in grape seed, peanut skin, and witch hazel bark.[62]

HOW IT FIGHTS ALLERGY OR ASTHMA SYMPTOMS

Some research shows that pycnogenol may help reduce allergy symptoms in people with birch allergies.[63] In a 2010 study, researchers found that pycnogenol improved symptoms of hay fever. Researchers gave 39 birch allergy sufferers pycnogenol for 5 to 8 weeks before the start of the 2009 allergy season. Once the season kicked in, participants had 35 percent lower scores for allergy symptoms pertaining to their eyes and 20.5 percent lower scores concerning their nasal allergy symptoms compared to people who took a placebo. In addition, those who took the pycnogenol had a 19.4 percent increase in their birch-specific immunoglobulin E (IgE), compared with a 31.9 percent increase in the placebo group. The participants with the best results in terms of improved allergy symptoms started taking the pycnogenol 7 to 8 weeks before the allergy season kicked in.[64]

Pycnogenol has also been shown to help people with asthma, specifically by decreasing levels of inflammatory leukotrienes. In a 2013 study published in *Food and Chemical Toxicology*, pycnogenol was reported to help protect allergic asthma sufferers from attacks.[65]

A 2002 review of studies on pycnogenol found that it may reduce symptoms and improve lung function in people with asthma. Another study found that the supplement could help children with asthma use their rescue inhalers less frequently to manage their conditions.[66]

HOW TO GET IT

To treat allergies, take 50 to 200 milligrams of pycnogenol, twice daily.[67] It's available in pill form and can be found at health food stores and online.

CONTRAINDICATIONS AND THINGS TO CONSIDER

As always, talk to your health-care provider before you start taking this supplement. Pycnogenol may cause some side effects, including headaches, stomach upset, dizziness, and mouth ulcers. It has not been proven safe during pregnancy or breastfeeding. And because it can stimulate your immune system, you should avoid taking it if you have an autoimmune disease such as multiple sclerosis, lupus, or rheumatoid arthritis. Also avoid it if you are taking an immunosuppressant medication or blood thinners.[68]

N-acetylcysteine

N-acetylcysteine (NAC) is a derivative of the amino acid cysteine. It is a powerful antioxidant itself, and it's also a precursor molecule to one of your body's strongest antioxidants, glutathione. In addition to its antioxidant abilities, it is also helpful in treating respiratory conditions due to its mucus-thinning ability. More specifically, n-acetylcysteine helps break down mucus and make it less sticky. It is commonly used to help people with cystic fibrosis, a condition in which people lack the tiny, hairlike structures called cilia that sweep mucus away from the lungs. NAC helps clear the mucus from the lungs of these people so that they can breathe more easily.[69] It can also help reduce inflammation and prevent heart disease, cancer, and other diseases related to aging.[70]

HOW IT FIGHTS ALLERGY OR ASTHMA SYMPTOMS

Research shows that n-acetylcysteine also helps prevent allergy symptoms.[71] In a 2007 study, researchers found that n-acetylcysteine inhibited eosinophils, a type of white blood cell that plays a crucial part in allergic inflammation. As a result, they concluded that n-acetylcysteine may be a useful treatment for inflammation resulting from allergic reactions.[72]

Interestingly, NAC's role as a precursor to glutathione is also likely to be helpful in addressing allergic inflammation. Recent research has found that increasing glutathione stores using NAC counteracted allergen-induced airway reactivity and inflammation and restored the balance between oxidants and antioxidants.[73]

HOW TO GET IT

In people with allergies and other respiratory problems, NAC doses range from 600 to 1,500 milligrams per day, taken in three divided doses. NAC is available in a liquid form or aerosol spray by prescription, or over the counter as tablets or capsules.[74]

CONTRAINDICATIONS AND THINGS TO CONSIDER

Side effects of NAC are rare, but they may include nausea and vomiting. Those with peptic ulcers should not take NAC. Also, talk to your health-care provider before taking NAC if you are on immunosuppressive or antifungal medications, if you are pregnant.[75]

Omega-3 Fatty Acids

Omega-3 fatty acids are essential fatty acids that help fight inflammation by balancing out their proinflammatory cousins, the omega-6 fatty acids.[76]

In a review of studies on omega-3s published in *American Family Physician*, researchers found that, when given in doses of at least

3 grams a day, omega-3 fatty acids helped lower inflammation, stiffness, and pain in people with rheumatoid arthritis. Omega-3s can also help fight heart disease and cancer and protect your brain from depression and dementia.[77,78]

HOW IT FIGHTS ALLERGY OR ASTHMA SYMPTOMS

In a 2005 German study, researchers looked at 325 women and 243 men and found that those with a high content of omega-3 fatty acids in their red blood cells—particularly eicosapentaenoic acid (EPA) and alpha-linolenic acid (ALA)—had fewer hay fever symptoms than people with lower levels of omega-3s.[79]

In a 2010 study published in *Respiratory Medicine,* researchers examined the dietary intake of fish oil in 38 people with allergic asthma and 19 people without asthma. They then exposed the participants to grass pollen. The researchers found that the asthmatics had higher ratios of omega-6 to omega-3 fatty acids than those without asthma and that those with the lowest intakes of omega-3 fatty acids had the strongest allergic reactions during the grass pollen challenge.[80]

Researchers have also found that omega-3 fatty acids seem to help prevent allergies as early as the prenatal stage. In a 2011 study published in the journal *BJOG: An International Journal of Obstetrics and Gynaecology,* researchers found that women who took omega-3 fatty acid supplements during pregnancy were less likely to have children who went on to suffer from asthma and allergies than pregnant women who did not take omega-3 supplements.[81]

HOW TO GET IT

You can get omega-3 fatty acids from foods, such as flaxseed, soybeans, spinach, walnuts, and oily fish. Anchovies, bluefish, herring, Atlantic salmon, Atlantic halibut, black cod, and sardines are the best fish sources.[82] However, there's a limit to how much fish you can eat because of the potential for mercury contamination. As discussed, limit your fish servings to one to two per week. Different species of fish are known to have higher levels of environmental contaminants; the worst offenders are shark, swordfish, king mackerel, and tilefish.[83]

Because of the possibility of mercury contamination in fresh fish, omega-3 supplements may be a better bet, as most quality fish-oil products go through a molecular distillation process to remove environmental toxins. Look for omega-3 supplements that contain both eicosapentaenoic acid (EPA) and docosahexaenoic acid (DHA). Most supplements contain 12 percent DHA and 18 percent EPA, or a total of 30 percent omega-3 fatty acids.[84] The recommended dosage of fish oil varies widely, from 1 to 10 grams daily. For most conditions, 3 grams daily is a good place to begin. You may have to swallow a lot of capsules to get this amount, so as an alternative, look for fish oil in a liquid form, where a larger dose can be achieved by taking as little as 1½ teaspoons per day.

CONTRAINDICATIONS AND THINGS TO CONSIDER

Omega-3 fatty acids are generally considered safe. The most frequently seen adverse effects are gastrointestinal upset and the notorious "fish burps" experienced by some. Some people have found that freezing fish-oil capsules or taking them prior to a meal can help reduce the incidence of burping. Additionally, research has found that fish oil has a blood-thinning effect that can compound the effects of blood-thinning medications such as warfarin and aspirin.[85]

Quercetin

A type of antioxidant called a flavonoid, quercetin is found in some fruits and vegetables, such as apples, berries, broccoli, capers, garlic, lettuce, red grapes, red onions, and tomatoes as well as in black tea and wine.

HOW IT FIGHTS ALLERGY OR ASTHMA SYMPTOMS

Quercetin is one of my favorite supplements for allergies. It seems to work as a mast cell stabilizer, blocking the histamine that unleashes the swelling and itching of allergic reactions.[86] In addition to its antihistamine properties, quercetin also appears to block tumor necrosis factor-alpha (TNF-alpha) and prostaglandins, thus fighting inflammation.[87]

With respect to allergies, in a 2012 study, researchers found that quercetin was more effective than the allergy drug cromolyn sodium in blocking mast cell cytokines and helping to prevent contact dermatitis and photosensitivity. These are two allergic skin conditions that don't usually respond well to conventional medications.[88]

In an earlier study published in the *Iranian Journal of Allergy, Asthma, and Immunology*, researchers found that quercetin may help decrease the potentially deadly anaphylactic reaction associated with peanut allergies.[89] Additionally, in a 2007 study, mice that ate a quercetin-rich diet had lower levels of inflammatory markers linked to allergies than mice who ate a standard diet.[90]

HOW TO GET IT

Quercetin typically comes in 250-, 300-, or 500-milligram capsules. For allergies, the usual dose is between 200 and 500 milligrams, three times a day.[91]

CONTRAINDICATIONS AND THINGS TO CONSIDER

There are none, so you can feel completely at ease taking this supplement, even if you're currently taking other medications. That said, always consult with an experienced physician, just to be safe.

Selenium

One of the best antioxidant minerals out there, selenium can help fight damage from free radicals, reduce inflammation, and boost your immune system. As a result, it may help prevent a number of diseases and conditions, including cancer, macular degeneration, eczema, and asthma.[92]

HOW IT FIGHTS ALLERGY OR ASTHMA SYMPTOMS

A few studies have shown that people who are deficient in selenium are more likely to suffer from asthma attacks than people with adequate levels of the mineral.[93] A 2013 German study looked at 35 asthmatic kids and 21 children without asthma and found that those with asthma had significantly lower levels of selenium as well as low levels of the antioxidants vitamin A, vitamin E, and coenzyme Q10.[94] Other research has suggested that selenium may inhibit the release of mast cells that unleash the allergic response.[95]

HOW TO GET IT

You can get selenium from some foods, including barley, Brazil nuts, brown rice, dairy, garlic, oats, orange juice, turnips, wheat germ, and seafood. The actual amount of selenium you get depends on how much of the mineral was in the soil in which your food was grown. Most crop land today is selenium-deficient, so a selenium supplement is probably the best way to go.[96]

Selenium supplements come in organic and inorganic forms, and in capsules, extended-release tablets, and regular tablets. Research shows that organic supplements may be preferred because they are easier for your body to absorb. A typical safe dose for adults is up to 200 micrograms.[97]

CONTRAINDICATIONS AND THINGS TO CONSIDER

Selenium is one of the most toxic of the essential minerals, and although doses greater than 200 micrograms per day have been used in the research setting, taking larger doses is only advisable under the care of an experienced physician.

Zinc

One of the most important trace minerals in your body, zinc is considered essential, meaning that you must get it from your diet. It's also essential for normal growth, development, and reproduction. Zinc plays a significant role in immunity, which is why zinc lozenges help fight the common cold.[98]

HOW IT FIGHTS ALLERGY OR ASTHMA SYMPTOMS

Zinc is an antioxidant that can help combat inflammation. Low levels of zinc have been linked with an increased risk of asthma symptoms, such as chest tightness, wheezing, shortness of breath, and chronic cough.[99] A 1997 study published in the journal *Thorax* linked zinc deficiency with an increased risk of asthma and allergies.[100] And a 2011 review done at the University of Edinburgh Medical School in Scotland examined 62 studies and concluded that zinc deficiency, among deficiencies of other nutrients, was associated with increased risk of asthma and allergies.[101]

Other research has shown the benefits of zinc supplementation in asthma patients. In a 2009 study published in the journal *Acta Paediatrica*, researchers gave 60 children 7 to 10 years old who had mild to moderate asthma either 1,000 milligrams of fish oil, 15 milligrams of zinc, 200 milligrams of vitamin C, a combination of all three supplements, or a placebo. After 6 weeks, the children taking the zinc, fish oil, or vitamin C all had better scores on their asthma control and standard pulmonary function tests. They also had lower levels of several markers of inflammation. The children who took the combination of all three supplements had even better results.[102]

HOW TO GET IT

Zinc sulfate is the most common zinc supplement. This is the least-expensive form of zinc, but it is also the least absorbed by the body. It can also cause nausea in some people. The better forms are zinc citrate, zinc glycerate, zinc monomethionine, and zinc acetate. For zinc-responsive conditions, dosages of 20 to 30 milligrams one to three times per day for 1 to 2 months have been used. After this initial period, the dosage should be reduced to a maintenance dose of 10 to 20 milligrams daily.[103] Zinc can also be found in foods such as grains, legumes, meats, seafood, wheat bran, wheat germ, nuts, and seeds.

CONTRAINDICATIONS AND THINGS TO CONSIDER

Potential side effects of zinc include nausea, vomiting, and a metallic taste in your mouth. Zinc can be toxic in large doses, so remember that more is not necessarily better. One concern is that taking too much zinc can deplete copper levels in your body. Zinc can also interfere with the absorption of some other minerals, such as calcium, magnesium, and iron.

Talk to your health-care provider before taking large doses of zinc through supplements, especially if you are taking blood pressure medication, hormone replacement therapy, diuretics, drugs to reduce stomach acid, immunosuppressants, nonsteroidal anti-inflammatory drugs (NSAIDS), muscle relaxants, or antibiotics.[104]

HEALING HERBS

Boswellia

Boswellia is a gummy bark from the Boswellia tree (*Boswellia serrata*), which is native to India, the Middle East, and North Africa. Boswellia has anti-inflammatory properties; some studies have shown it to be as effective as ibuprofen and aspirin at reducing swelling. It's also been used in Chinese medicine to treat pain and inflammation in the mouth, throat, and gums, and it is often used in natural mouthwashes.[105]

HOW IT FIGHTS ALLERGY OR ASTHMA SYMPTOMS

The active ingredient in boswellia is boswellic acid, which seems to reduce inflammation by inhibiting inflammatory enzymes called leukotrienes. Studies show that boswellia can help treat a number of inflammatory conditions, including osteoarthritis, Crohn's disease, tendonitis, and asthma.[106]

In a double-blind, placebo-controlled study, 40 people with asthma took 300 milligrams of boswellia three times a day for 6 weeks. At the end of the study, 70 percent of the people who took boswellia showed improvements in their lung function, compared with only 27 percent of the people who took the placebo.[107]

HOW TO GET IT

Boswellia is available in tablets and capsules. To reduce inflammation or to treat asthmatic conditions, a typical dose is 300 to 400 milligrams of a standard extract containing 60 percent boswellic acids, three times a day as needed.

CONTRAINDICATIONS AND THINGS TO CONSIDER

It's best to take boswellia with a fatty meal to maximize absorption. When taken at normal doses, as suggested above, there are no toxicity concerns.[108]

Ginkgo Biloba

Ginkgo biloba is thought to be the oldest surviving tree on Earth—around 200 million years old. Healers were using ginkgo for asthma and bronchitis as long ago as 2600 BC,[109] and gingko biloba extract (GBE) is still used today. In fact, it is one of the most popular herbal supplements in both Europe and the United States.[110]

GBE is especially used for boosting memory, but it also has a long list of other uses, from treating depression to improving vision to treating asthma. It has antioxidant effects and can therefore help buffer your body from free radical damage. It also seems to improve blood flow to the brain and boost cell metabolism.[111]

HOW IT FIGHTS ALLERGY OR ASTHMA SYMPTOMS

In a 2007 Chinese study, researchers looked at the effects of ginkgo biloba extract on asthma. They gave 75 asthmatics either fluticasone propionate (a standard glucocorticosteroid asthma treatment) for 2 weeks or 4 weeks or fluticasone propionate *plus* GBE for 2 weeks or 4 weeks. They also looked at these treatments in 15 healthy controls. At the end of the study, the researchers concluded that GBE significantly decreased the number of inflammatory cells and relieved airway inflammation. Therefore, in addition to being a good anti-inflammatory on its own, ginko may also be a good complementary treatment to glucocorticosteroid therapies for asthma.[112]

HOW TO GET IT

Ginkgo biloba is available in capsules, tablets, and tinctures, but it is most commonly used as concentrated ginkgo biloba extract (GBE) that's standardized to contain 24 percent flavonoids and 6 percent terpenoids. The dose ranges from 40 to 80 milligrams two or three times per day.[113]

CONTRAINDICATIONS AND THINGS TO CONSIDER

Talk to your health-care provider before you start taking ginkgo biloba. It's safe in small doses but can occasionally cause side effects such as stomach upset, headaches, heart palpitations, dizziness, or skin rashes. You should avoid it if you have liver or kidney problems, are pregnant or breastfeeding, or if you have a history of seizures. Ginkgo biloba can also have blood-thinning effects, so avoid taking it within 2 weeks of a scheduled surgery.[114]

Green Tea Extract

Next to water, green tea is the most popular beverage in the world. And for good reason: A rich source of antioxidants called polyphenols, green tea has a long list of health benefits. Most notably, it may help prevent certain cancers, including breast, prostate, cervical, and digestive as well as some types of leukemia. Because of its antioxidant powers, green tea may also help protect your immune system, decrease inflammation, and fight allergies.[115]

HOW IT FIGHTS ALLERGY OR ASTHMA SYMPTOMS

In a 2002 Japanese study published in the *Journal of Agriculture and Food Chemistry*, researchers found that one of the most abundant compounds in green tea—epigallocatechin gallate (EGCG)—can fight allergy symptoms, such as sneezing and runny nose. The researchers found EGCG blocked production of both histamine and IgE, two of the most important chemicals involved in allergic reactions.[116] Additionally, in a 2010 study published in the *Annals of Clinical and Laboratory Science*, researchers found that green tea extract helped suppress IgE, and the higher the dose of green tea extract, the lower the IgE levels.[117]

HOW TO GET IT

You can make green tea with dried tea leaves or tea bags, or you can buy it as capsules or in the form of an extract made from the leaves and leaf buds of the tea plant. Drinking green tea is a great way to get a nice dose of the active ingredients, but it should be noted that the levels of EGCG in decaffeinated tea are significantly less. Supplement dosages used in clinical practice range between 100 and 750 milligrams per day. If you take an extract, look for one standardized to contain a minimum of 90 percent total tea catechins and a minimum of 70 percent EGCG.[118]

CONTRAINDICATIONS AND THINGS TO CONSIDER

Green tea is generally pretty harmless, especially in people who are not sensitive to caffeine. In fact, studies show that you can safely drink as many as 20 cups a day. Most of the side effects of green tea come from the caffeine and include restlessness, insomnia, irritability, heart palpitations, and dizziness.[119]

Licorice Root

Licorice Root (Glycyrrhiza glabra) is the scientific name of the licorice plant, of which the roots and underground stems are used. Because it is at least 50 times sweeter than table sugar, licorice root has gotten the nickname "sweet root."[120]

Licorice root can help prevent and treat a number of conditions, including stomach ulcers, heartburn, gas, respiratory infections, and cough. It may also help lower cholesterol and triglycerides, lowering risk of heart disease.[121]

HOW IT FIGHTS ALLERGY OR ASTHMA SYMPTOMS

The active ingredient glycyrrhizin has been shown in studies to decrease inflammation; soothe the throat, bronchial membranes, and lungs; promote mucus secretion; and stimulate the adrenal glands.[122] In a 2010 study, 63 asthma patients took either a placebo or an herbal combination containing licorice root, turmeric, and boswellia for 4 weeks. At the end of the study, the participants taking the herbal combination containing licorice root had lower levels of inflammatory markers and improved pulmonary function than those taking the placebo.[123] In a 2007 study published in *Planta Medica*, mice given glycyrrhizin had lower levels of IgE, suggesting that the compound may help relieve IgE-induced allergies such as eczema and allergic asthma.[124]

HOW TO GET IT

You can take licorice root in a few different forms, including capsules, chewable tablets, teas, or oral drops. There are two types—whole licorice and the chemically modified form deglycyrrhizinated licorice (DGL), which doesn't contain more than 3 percent glycyrrhizin. The dosage for licorice root is 2 to 6 milliliters of a 1:1 liquid extract or 1.2 to 4.6 grams per day of DGL. The German Commission E monograph advises a dosage of 5 to 15 grams per day but states that treatment undertaken without medical supervision should be discontinued after 6 weeks due to the risk of adverse effects.[125,126] Tea is a great way to use licorice, and in addition to providing the anti-inflammatory effects, it also tastes great!

CONTRAINDICATIONS AND THINGS TO CONSIDER

Talk to your health-care provider before taking licorice. In high doses, licorice can also cause more serious side effects, including a condition called pseudoaldosteronism, which can lead to heart attack. Do not take licorice root if you have high blood pressure, kidney or liver problems, obesity, heart disease, or diabetes.

Butterbur

(*Petasites hybridus*) is a shrublike plant that grows in parts of North America, Europe, and Asia, and seems to work like a leukotriene inhibitor, blocking the chemicals that trigger nasal swelling. One of the extracts in butterbur root, Ze 339, is particularly effective when it comes to controlling coughs, asthma, and allergies.[127]

HOW IT FIGHTS ALLERGY OR ASTHMA SYMPTOMS

In a 2013 study published in the *Journal of Ethnopharmacology*, researchers looked into the anti-inflammatory and antiallergic effects of *Petasites* leaves and found that a particular compound in the leaves called bakkenolide B helped inhibit mast cell degranulation and also helped suppress the inflammatory response. The researchers concluded that it could potentially be used as an asthma treatment.[128]

In an earlier, 2010 study, Ze 339 helped prevent airway inflammation and airway hyperresponsiveness in mice exposed to allergens. More specifically, researchers found that Ze 339 produced these antiallergy effects by suppressing proinflammatory cytokines in the mice.[129]

And in a related 2005 study, 330 people with hay fever got one of three different treatments—one tablet three times a day of butterbur extract, the antihistamine drug fexofenadine (Allegra), or a placebo. The people who took the butterbur extract had the same reduction in their symptoms as the people who took the Allegra. Both treatments were more effective than the placebo. Therefore, butterbur may be as effective as taking the popular antiallergy drug, without Allegra's sedating side effects.[130]

Additionally, in another study, Ze 339 was found to help prevent allergic asthma in asthmatic mice exposed to house dust mites.[131]

HOW TO GET IT

You can find this herb in capsule form. In terms of a recommended dosage, stay between 50 and 100 milligrams per day.

CONTRAINDICATIONS AND THINGS TO CONSIDER

Talk to your health-care provider before taking butterbur. Possible side effects of butterbur extract include headaches, fatigue, indigestion, nausea, vomiting, diarrhea, and constipation. Never eat unprocessed, raw butterbur root, which can be toxic.[132]

Stinging Nettle

A plant whose leaves and stems are covered with fine hairs that contain irritating chemicals, stinging nettle (*Urtica dioica*) has been used for centuries as a diuretic and to treat joint pain. The hairs on the plant are painful to the touch, but when they come into contact with an inflamed, painful area of the body, they can actually *decrease* pain. Scientists think the plant does this by interfering with the transmission of pain signals.[133]

HOW IT FIGHTS ALLERGY OR ASTHMA SYMPTOMS

A few studies have found that stinging nettle may have antihistamine properties; therefore, it can help calm itching and sneezing in hay fever sufferers.[134] In a double-blind study done at the National College of Naturopathic Medicine in Portland, Oregon, researchers found that freeze-dried stinging nettle was as or more effective at relieving allergy symptoms than conventional allergy medications were.[135] Also in a 2009 study published in the journal *Phytotherapy Research*, researchers found that stinging nettle may help fight allergies by reducing inflammation.[136]

HOW TO GET IT

For treating allergies, typical dosages range from 200 to 800 milligrams per day of the dried herb, although dosages up to 10 grams per day have been used. For tinctures of nettle leaf, recommended dosages range from 7 to 14 milliliters per day of a 1:5 tincture. And don't forget about nettle leaf tea! Nettle tea can be found at most shops that deal in herbs. For allergies, make sure to use a product that is made up of the nettle leaf, rather than the root. (Nettle root is primarily used for treating a condition known as benign prostatic hyperplasia and is not as effective as the leaf in treating allergies.)[137]

CONTRAINDICATIONS AND THINGS TO CONSIDER

Stinging nettle is a pretty safe herb, but it may cause some side effects, such as stomach upset, diarrhea, sweating, fluid retention, or hives or rash when it is used topically. Never apply stinging nettle to an open wound.[138]

Also, talk to your health-care provider before you start using stinging nettle. The herb can interfere with several medications, including blood thinners, drugs for high blood pressure, diabetes drugs, diuretics, lithium, and nonsteroidal anti-inflammatory drugs (NSAIDs).[139]

Tylophora

Tylophora (*Tylophora indica*) is a climbing vine that grows in India. It has been used as a treatment for asthma since the 1800s. It has also been used to treat allergies, bronchitis, and the common cold as well as osteoarthritis pain, constipation, and stomach upset.[140]

HOW IT FIGHTS ALLERGY OR ASTHMA SYMPTOMS

A few studies have touted tylophora as a treatment for allergies and asthma, but most of them are old, from the 1960s and 1970s. In one of the most noteworthy, published in the *Journal of Allergy* in 1969, asthma sufferers who chewed and swallowed 150 milligrams of tylophora leaf daily in the early morning for 6 days saw moderate to total relief of their asthma symptoms.[141]

In a similar study done in 1972, 195 asthma sufferers took either

40 milligrams of tylophora alcohol extract or a placebo for 6 days. The group taking the tylophora had fewer asthma symptoms, and their symptoms remained controlled for months after they stopped taking the herb.[142] Tylophora can be found at health food stores and online.

HOW TO GET IT

The usual dose of tylophora for asthma is 250 milligrams, one to three times per day.[143]

CONTRAINDICATIONS AND THINGS TO CONSIDER

Tylophora is relatively safe, but it can have potentially serious side effects at high doses, so talk to your health-care professional before taking it. Also, keep in mind that you shouldn't take tylophora if you are pregnant or breastfeeding, or if you have high blood pressure, diabetes, or congestive heart failure.[144]

Guduchi

An herb long used in Ayurvedic medicine to treat a variety of conditions from liver disease to arthritis to diarrhea, Guduchi (*Tinospora cordifolia*) is thought to remove toxins from the body. It is still used today for its "adaptogenic" effects, meaning it can help your body adapt to stress.[145]

HOW IT FIGHTS ALLERGY OR ASTHMA SYMPTOMS

Some herbalists and naturopathic doctors, myself included, also use Guduchi to help treat allergies.[146] In a 2004 study, researchers gave 75 allergy patients either guduchi or a placebo for 8 weeks. At the end of the study, 83 percent of the participants who had taken the guduchi experienced complete relief from sneezing; 71 percent experienced relief from nasal pruritus (dry, itchy nose); 69 percent experienced relief from nasal discharge; and 61 percent experienced relief from nasal obstruction. In other words, most of the people taking the guduchi saw relief from all of their allergic rhinitis symptoms. Of the placebo group, 79 percent experienced no relief from sneezing; 85 percent had no relief from nasal discharge; 88 percent had no relief from nasal pruritus; and 83 percent had no relief from nasal obstruction.[147]

HOW TO GET IT

A typical dose of guduchi is 300 milligrams of an aqueous stem extract three times per day.[148]

CONTRAINDICATIONS AND THINGS TO CONSIDER

Talk to your health-care provider before you take guduchi for allergies. It appears to be a pretty safe herb, but it hasn't been studied thoroughly. One study suggested that it might decrease male fertility, and it has not been proven safe for pregnant or breastfeeding women.[149] It is most commonly available in pill form and can be found in most health food stores and online.

Now that you've learned about the supplements and herbs that can help treat allergies, asthma, and contributing inflammation, you are better equipped to start using one or more of them as part of The Allergy Solution Plan. Read on, and I will help you appropriately incorporate herbs and supplements into your life.

12

An Antiallergy Way of Life: The Power of the Little Things You Do Every Day

ONCE WHILE VOLUNTEERING ON A MEDICAL MISSION in Mexico, I treated an indigenous woman from the southern part of the country. Through an interpreter, she complained of having developed a rash about 3 months prior to our meeting. This rash was on her torso, upper arms, back, and legs. It was slightly raised, red, and itchy, and she had no idea what might have caused it. While I was consulting with her, I asked her if she had started eating any new foods or taking any new medications that could have contributed to the development of this rash. She had not. During the time we talked, it came to light that she had started using a new laundry detergent around the time the rash developed. As the rash was really only present on her body in areas that came in contact with her clothing, we deduced that this new detergent might be the cause. Once she stopped using the detergent, the rash went away.

The lesson here is twofold. First, it illustrates that you have to consider *everything* in your environment when you're trying to figure out what's causing an allergic reaction. Second, it's a reminder that you should stop and think about all the products and chemicals you come into contact with on a daily basis and how those substances may be affecting your health.

When it comes to the connection between lifestyle and health, it's usually not one bad habit or chemical exposure that kills us or one good habit that extends our lives. (There are a few exceptions, of course, such as heavy smoking or asbestos exposure.) It's the *collection* of good and bad habits—the things you do here and there—that add up to your total routine. Maybe you smoke a few cigarettes now and then, you have some plug-in air fresheners in your bedroom (more to come on these), and you indulge in a doughnut for breakfast on the weekends. On the flip side, you take your vitamins every day, exercise 5 days a week, and keep stress to a minimum. It's really all about balance. These little habits have a big additive effect over months, years, and your lifetime. They contribute to or improve your inflammation; they affect whether or not you will have a particularly bad allergy season; and they ultimately determine the diseases you will develop and the length and quality of your life.

My advice to you is this: Try *every single day* to make sure your good habits outweigh your bad ones. I gave you some dietary tips in Chapter 10, and we will talk about exercise in Chapter 13. In this chapter, I offer some things you can do to make your home environment less inviting to allergens and more conducive to clean, healthy living.

HOME IS WHERE THE HARM IS

No matter how much we love fresh air and the outdoors, most of us spend most of our time inside, in an office or at home. We are sometimes under the impression that our homes are healthier than they really are. The fact is, you need to think about how healthy your home really is.

As discussed in Chapter 2, outside of our homes, we are constantly surrounded by toxic fumes coming from all sorts of places, such as vehicles and factories. One of the worst offenders identified so far for asthma and allergies is diesel exhaust particulates (DEPs). But what may be even more harmful than the DEPs floating around in the outside air are the toxins you are exposed to *inside* your home on a daily basis. Yes, the place you call your sanctuary can be the

The Toxic Big Boys—Radon and Lead

When it comes to dust, dust mites, and pet dander, you can probably handle the cleaning yourself. When it comes to removing more harmful substances, such as lead and radon, you should hire a professional.

Lead is a toxic element that was used in paints until 1978 and in plumbing until 1988. It can damage your brain and nervous system and is particularly dangerous for young children, who expose themselves to it by putting paint chips in their mouths. You should have your paint tested for lead if your home was built before 1978, and you should test your water for lead if your home was built before 1988. For more information on lead, call the National Lead Information Center at 800-424-5323.[1]

Radon is an odorless, colorless gas that comes from soil and decaying rocks. It can get into your home through cracks in your basement floor. This radioactive gas can cause lung cancer in people exposed to high levels for years. In fact, it is the second leading cause of lung cancer in the United States. Luckily, even if your home has a high radon level, you can get rid of the gas by installing a radon remediation system. For more information on radon and how to get your home tested, go to epa.gov/radon/radontest.html.[2]

most poisonous of all. From the paint on the walls to the glues in the floors to the chemicals in your cleaning products, there are lots of toxic substances in your home. (See "The Toxic Big Boys—Radon and Lead.")

In addition to the toxins, there are also a number of potential allergens lurking in your home, including dust, dust mites, animal dander, cockroaches, and mold, not to mention the pollen and other outdoor allergens you bring in on your clothing and hair. In fact, according to the Environmental Protection Agency (EPA), the levels of indoor air pollutants may be two to five times higher than the levels of pollutants outside. Indoor air pollution is among the top five environmental threats to human health. Considering that most Americans spend 90 percent of their time indoors, this is a major concern.[3]

So with all of this in mind, here's some advice on how to allergy-proof your home and make it a more healthful place to be.

Filter the air you breathe. When it comes to air, quality counts. To help make your air as clean as possible, consider investing in a high-quality air filter. There are a few different kinds of air filters. It's advisable to look for one that filters out not only particulate matter, like dust and dander, but chemical matter as well. You don't have to get a complicated air filtration system. I have freestanding air filters in my office and home, and they work quite well. The best kinds of filters for people with allergies are high-efficiency particulate air (HEPA) filters, which are specially designed to remove allergens from the air.[4] The most important place to run an air filter is in your bedroom, which is where you spend most of your time and which is also frequently the most polluted room in the house. It is a good idea to try and adjust the filter so it directs clean air toward you as you sleep.[5]

You can also help remove debris from the air by installing a furnace filter, which traps pollen and dust before these allergens have a chance to circulate throughout your house. Furnace filters are easy to install and they're relatively inexpensive.[6] If you live in an arid region such as the desert Southwest, make sure that you regularly clean or replace your air duct or furnace filters. I try to change the filters in my home on a monthly or bimonthly schedule.

Another thing to keep in mind when it comes to clean air is the state of your air conditioning (AC) unit. A clean unit can act as an air filter, but a dirty one contaminated with mold or other substances in the drip tray or filter can actually pump new allergens into your home. To truly condition your air, hire a professional to inspect your AC system once a year, and have your ducts cleaned at least once every 5 years.[7]

Make your home less comfortable for pests. From mice to bats to ants, lots of creatures like to invade our homes. Some of them are just nuisances; others can cause allergy symptoms or threaten your health in other ways. You can't completely eliminate all critters from your home, but you can make it less inviting to them.

- **Deter dust mites.** Microscopic dust mites are a common asthma and allergy trigger. They feed on sloughed-off skin cells and lurk in bedding, stuffed animals, storage boxes, carpeting, and upholstered furniture. To discourage them, do the following:

- *Encase your mattresses, box springs, and pillows in allergy-proof or airtight zippered plastic covers. You can find these covers at specialty stores and online.*

- *Wash all bedding weekly in water that is at least 130°F, and dry everything on your dryer's hottest setting.*[8]

- *Keep your home cool by turning down the heat or turning up the AC; dust mites don't reproduce in temperatures colder than about 77°F.*

- *To gauge the severity of your dust mite problem, consider purchasing a dust mite detection kit, which measures the level of dust mites in your environment.*[9]

- **Kick cockroaches to the curb.** Cockroaches, whose droppings and cast-off skins can stimulate allergy symptoms and asthma, are most often a problem in densely populated areas, but they can show up almost anywhere. To make your environment less roach-friendly, do the following:

- *Block areas where roaches can come in, including windows, wall cracks, and crevices.*

- *Realize that like us, cockroaches need water, so they seek out dripping faucets and pipes. Fix and seal any leaks.*[10]

- *Keep your kitchen clean. In addition to water, cockroaches love and need food, so clean it up, put it in covered containers, and vacuum and mop any crumbs or spills quickly. Don't forget to clean the areas where crumbs hide, such as under the stove and refrigerator. Wipe down your countertops and cupboards regularly.*[11]

- *Avoid eating in rooms other than the kitchen and dining room. The more places you eat and drop crumbs, the more attractions you create for cockroaches.*

- *Change your kitty litter at least once every few days, as roaches are attracted to the droppings.*

- *Put grocery store bags outside in recycling bins as soon as you get home from food shopping. As gross as it sounds, roaches*

*often hang out in grocery stores and have been known to hitch a
ride home in shoppers' grocery bags.[12]*

- *If roaches are still present after you try these tips, install traps
from your hardware store.[13]*
- *If things get out of control, hire an exterminator. Keep in mind
that if you see one roach in your home, especially if you see it
during the day, hundreds more are probably lurking behind the
walls, so you don't want to let a roach infestation go.[14] Look
for a pest-control company that uses the least-toxic chemicals
possible to control cockroaches.*

Make your home clean and comfortable for yourself. Not only
does a clean house make for a more pleasant and enjoyable living
environment for all, it also helps keep allergens under control. If
you can, try to clean your home weekly. Mop all of your floors with
a damp mop and vacuum all carpeting and rugs with a vacuum
cleaner that has a small-particle or HEPA filter. (Don't forget to vacuum the backs of chairs and couches, where dust, dust mites, and
mold can hide.)[15] Wipe the dust from windowsills, furniture, and
other surfaces. If you have allergies, wear a dust mask while you
clean, or ask a family member who doesn't have allergies to do
these chores.[16]

Think twice about pets. No cats or dogs are completely hypoallergenic, even the hairless varieties. After all, it's not the hair that
causes allergy symptoms, but the proteins in dog and cat saliva,
urine, and dander.[17]

Also keep in mind that while dogs and cats tend to get the most
blame when it comes to pet allergies, rabbits, mice, hamsters, and
guinea pigs can also set off allergy symptoms—even Siamese fighting fish have been known to indirectly cause allergic reactions![18]
Clothing made from animal fur, such as cashmere, goat hair, mohair,
and alpaca sweaters can trigger allergies as well.[19]

If you or one of your family members has a known pet allergy,
the very best thing you can do is not get an animal in the first place.
If you already have a pet that is part of your family, try to keep that
pet outdoors as much as possible. In addition, do the following:

- Keep the animal out of your bedroom and other rooms where you spend a lot of time.

- Vacuum carpets and rugs often.

- Ask a nonallergic family member to brush the pet or clean its cage or crate.

- Bathe the pet weekly, or better yet, twice a week to minimize dander. Ask a nonallergic family member to wash the pet.

- If possible, replace carpeting with hardwood flooring, tile, or linoleum. Keep in mind that even after a pet is no longer in a house, pet dander can remain on fabrics and in carpeting, triggering allergies for up to a year or longer.[20]

Lower humidity. In general, when it comes to fostering a clean, allergy-free environment, the rule is, "the dryer, the better." Mold loves moisture, as do allergenic pests. So aim to keep the relative humidity level in your home at 30 to 50 percent or lower by running a dehumidifier.[21] On humid days, keep your windows closed and run your air conditioner. To measure the humidity in your home and make sure you're staying in the right range, you can buy a tool called a hygrometer at your local hardware store.[22]

As a side note, if you run a dehumidifier, make sure to keep it clean. Rinse and scrub the water tank at least once a week, and dust the grills with the soft brush attachment of your vacuum cleaner.[23]

Use the less-is-more style of decorating. The more knick-knacks, ornaments, books, magazines, and general clutter you have in your house, the more places there are for allergens to park themselves. So limiting the number of picture frames, figurines, and other dust traps in your home will help you breathe better.[24]

Also, keep fibers to a minimum. Cloth and carpets create surfaces for dust and allergenic critters to hide. Old shag carpeting is the worst because it not only traps dust, but it also produces new dust as the fibers break down. Remove as much wall-to-wall carpeting as possible and replace it with hardwood floors. Throw rugs are okay if you wash or dry-clean them regularly.[25] If you must have carpeting, choose low-nap instead of the high-nap variety, and vacuum it at least once a week (or daily, if you can), preferably with a vacuum that has a HEPA filter. Also, shampoo carpets regularly using a nontoxic product.

On windows, heavy drapes and horizontal blinds are additional traps for dust and other allergens. Instead, go for washable roller shades or cotton or synthetic curtains. Or better yet, forgo window treatments entirely.

In terms of furniture, upholstered pieces trap dust mites and other allergens. The best furniture materials for people with allergies are those that are easy to clean: wood, leather, metal, and plastic.[26]

Get rid of mold, pronto. Not only can mold trigger allergy symptoms such as watery eyes, runny nose, headaches, and coughing, but some forms can also release dangerous toxins. To prevent mold growth, lower the humidity in your home (run a dehumidifier to eliminate excess moisture) and fix all leaks. If you see visible mold, wash it with soap and water and, if necessary, a 5 percent bleach solution before drying the area completely. If you can't wash and dry a moldy item, throw it away. Also get rid of any old rags, carpeting, or furniture that could harbor mold. If mold covers a significant area of your home, think about hiring a mold removal specialist to get rid of it.[27]

Keep in mind that your kitchen is one of mold's favorite places to grow. To deter it, wipe up excessive moisture in your refrigerator and clean drip pans under appliances as well as rubber seals around appliances often.[28]

Mold also loves bathrooms and basements. To keep it at bay in your bathrooms, always run your exhaust fan while you take a shower or bath; don't put carpeting in your bathroom; swap out any wallpaper for tile or drywall painted with mold-resistant enamel paint; replace moldy shower curtains and bathmats; and use a bleach solution to scrub any visible mold from your toilets and sinks.[29]

In your basement, paint the walls with mold-resistant paint, which contains chemicals that help destroy any remaining mold. The paint also helps seal the area to discourage future mold growth.[30] Low volatile organic compound (low-VOC) mold-resistant paints are also available.[31] Research has shown that high levels of

VOCs, which are found in many commercial paints, have been linked to increased rates of asthma and rhinitis in adults and worsened asthma in children.[32,33]

Pay special attention to your bedroom. You spend more time in your bedroom than any other room in your house. Unfortunately, in many cases, this room is the most polluted and inviting for allergens such as mold, pollen, animal dander, dust mites, and cockroaches. So clear out knickknacks and clutter, avoid storing things under your bed, and remove drapes from your windows. Also, keep your bed away from air vents if you can, so you don't breathe in dust that comes out of them as you sleep. Get bedding and pillows you can machine wash, and avoid down pillows and comforters, which can't be washed easily. The best choices for people with allergies are hypoallergenic bedding and pillows that can be washed often without falling apart.[34]

In kids' bedrooms, keep stuffed animals to a minimum—they are dust traps. If your kids can't part with them, wash stuffed toys every so often to remove the dust. Use a damp cloth to wipe those that can't be machine-washed, and dry them on your dryer's hottest setting to kill dust mites.

Keep yourself clean. During allergy season, pollens are rampant. When you go outside, that pollen collects on your clothing and in your hair. To minimize the allergens you drag inside, change into fresh clothes as soon as you get home, and take a shower and wash your hair before you go to bed.[35]

Use plants to clean your air. Plants act like natural air filters; they produce oxygen and actually help clean the air. As a bonus, they look pretty. Some plants are better air filters than others. According to the National Institutes of Health, the top 10 air-cleaning houseplants are as follow:[36]

1. Areca palm (*Chrysalidocarpus lutescens*)

2. Lady palm (*Rhapis excelsa*)

3. Bamboo palm (*Chamaedorea erumpens*)

4. Rubber plant (*Ficus elastica*)

5. Dracaena (*Dracaena deremensis*)

6. English ivy (*Hedera helix*)

7. Pygmy date palm (*Phoenix roebelenii*)

8. Banana-leaf ficus (*Ficus maclellandii* 'Alii')

9. Boston fern (*Nephrolepis exaltata* 'Bostoniensis')

10. Peace lily (*Spathiphyllum wallisii*)

The more of these filtering plants you can put in your home and office, the healthier your air will be. Houseplants may not be a good idea if you have a mold allergy or sensitivity, however; mold can grow in moist dirt, triggering your allergy symptoms.[37] To help control mold growth in your potted plants, spread aquarium stones over the soil.[38]

Freshen your air naturally. There are lots of things people use in their homes to make the air smell good that are, ironically, quite toxic. Plug-in air fresheners, spray air fresheners, and scented candles all give off synthetic chemicals in the fragrances that permeate your home. So if you are concerned about your respiratory health, avoid any products with added fragrances or that have "fragrance" listed as an ingredient.[39]

If you want your home to smell good but you don't want the potentially poisonous effects that come with the chemicals, one option is to use essential oils. Pure essential oils are safe and come in a variety of scents, some of which are energizing or soothing, to boot. To use them, put a few drops of pure essential oil into a spray bottle filled with water and spray it on absorbent surfaces, such as the toilet paper in your bathroom. Or dip cotton balls into essential oils and place them in open jars. Or, if no one in your home has pollen allergies, simply open up the windows and let the natural breeze sweeten your air. Modern homes are very airtight. This is great for keeping heat and air conditioning in and lowering energy bills, but it also keeps allergens trapped and circulating through your indoor air.

Clean green. Many of the cleaning products we use in our homes and offices, including soaps, polishes, and personal grooming supplies, contain chemicals that can cause health problems.[40] Some of the worst ingredients in household products are the volatile organic compounds (VOCs) used in a number of products, including chlorine bleach, detergent, dishwashing liquid, dry-cleaning chemicals, rug and upholstery cleaners, furniture polishes, oven cleaners, floor polish, air fresheners, and aerosol sprays.[41] In addition to irritating your throat, nose, and eyes and worsening asthma and allergy symptoms, these VOCs may cause lung damage.[42]

Luckily, you have alternatives. There are a number of nontoxic, environmentally friendly, and hypoallergenic detergents and cleaners available for carpeting, upholstery, and other areas of your home. Some brands include Earth Friendly Products, Simple Green, and Naturally Yours.[43] Keep in mind that not all products labeled "green," "environmentally friendly," or "eco safe" are truly harmless; check the ingredients lists. Whenever possible, clean with safer, alternative cleaning solutions, such as baking soda or a mixture of vinegar and water.[44] A good place to learn about which products are safe to use and which you should avoid is the Environmental Working Group page at ewg.org. (Check out their Consumer Guides for a ranking of common cleaning products.) And no matter which cleaning products you use, always open the windows to keep the area you are cleaning well-ventilated.[45]

Minimize toxic materials. A lot of building materials off-gas, meaning they release toxic gasses into the air, which you then breathe in. One such chemical is formaldehyde, which is used as an adhesive and bonding agent in many products such as plywood, pressed wood products, and some foam insulation. Formaldehyde is classified as a volatile organic compound. Besides being toxic, VOCs are chemicals that become gasses at room temperature (in other words, they off-gas). In the short term, formaldehyde causes coughing, headaches, and irritation of the nose, eyes, and throat. Long term, the exact effects of formaldehyde aren't known, but the EPA has classified the chemical as "carcinogenic to humans."[46]

To avoid VOCs during a renovation, you can hire a "green" contractor and use all environmentally friendly materials. In our office, we have a manufactured wood floor (not real wood) that doesn't off-gas at all; there is no solvent coming out of the glue. We also painted the walls with VOC-free paint, which has virtually no odor.

Many people can't afford to use environmentally friendly building materials, since they are more expensive. An alternative to going green from the start is to open up the windows, crank up the heat, and try to bake the smell out of your house after your renovation is over but before you start living in the renovated space.

Dry your laundry the old-fashioned way. Want fresh-smelling linens? Dry them on a clothesline outside in the breeze (pollen allergies permitting, of course). Whatever you do, try to avoid using dryer sheets and scented laundry detergents. A 2011 study done at the University of Washington found more than 25 VOCs emitted from dryer vents, two of which are considered carcinogenic. The culprit:

Lifestyle Tips for Food Allergies

There's a difference between food allergies and food sensitivities. If you have a food *sensitivity*, you should avoid the food that causes symptoms, but you know it won't be the end of the world if you come in contact with it. If you have a true food allergy—particularly if it is one that can cause life-threatening anaphylactic shock—you need to be especially careful to avoid anything that may contain that food. So in keeping with this chapter full of everyday tips, here are some things you should do to protect yourself on a daily basis if you have a food allergy.[47]

- Always check ingredients lists and labels before you eat a packaged food; you may find allergenic foods where you least expect them.
- If you are eating at a restaurant, tell your server about your food allergy and stress that you cannot eat anything that contains that food.
- Avoid close contact with someone who has recently eaten the food to which you are allergic. Kissing someone who has recently eaten your food allergen is particularly dangerous.
- Do not share utensils with someone who is eating a food to which you are allergic.
- If you have a potentially serious food allergy, always wear a MedicAlert bracelet or necklace and carry an EpiPen.

the fragrances in detergents and fabric softener sheets. The study authors noted that unlike factory smokestacks or car tailpipes, emissions from dryer vents aren't regulated. Plus, companies that make household products such as laundry detergents and fabric softeners aren't required to list all of their ingredients on their labels, so it's tough to know whether or not they contain harmful chemicals. The best thing you can do to avoid toxic laundry is to go for unscented detergent and skip the dryer sheets entirely.[48]

Just say "no" to smoke. Smoke, whether it comes from tobacco products, wood-burning fireplaces, or bonfires, can worsen allergy and asthma symptoms. So go for a gas fireplace instead of a wood-burning one if you have the choice. It also goes without saying: If you smoke cigarettes or cigars, quit. If someone in your home smokes, encourage him or her to give it up, and in the meantime, ask the smoker to take their smoke outside.

Watch out for other toxins lurking in your home. In addition to VOCs in cleaning products and building materials, there are health-damaging chemicals in some of your beauty products and household containers.

- **Parabens** are synthetic preservatives found in personal-care products and cosmetics, including deodorants, skin creams, shampoo (including baby shampoo), and hair gels. Parabens have been linked to a number of conditions, including cancer, reproductive problems, skin irritation, neurotoxicity, immunotoxicity, and hormone disruption. They have also been found in breast tumors, but so far, no direct link between parabens and cancer has been established. However, it seems that parabens may act on estrogen-sensitive tissue by mimicking the action of that hormone. To avoid parabens, choose certified organic products and those without synthetic preservatives. Keep in mind that products that claim to be "natural" aren't always so. Always read labels and look out for the words "butylparaben," "ethylparaben," "propylparaben," and "methylparaben."[49]

- **Bisphenol A (BPA)** is a chemical used mainly in plastics, including food and drink packaging such as water bottles, baby bottles, and some medical devices. You can ingest BPA through air and dust, but most exposure comes through diet; BPA can seep into foods and drinks from plastic containers. Most people have been exposed to some BPA. The 2003–2004 National Health and Nutrition Examination Survey (NHANES) found BPA in 93 percent of the 2,517 people studied, including a number of children. To avoid BPA, don't microwave plastic; steer clear of plastic containers with recycle codes 3 or 7 printed on them; keep your consumption of canned foods to a minimum; and store leftovers in glass, stainless steel, or porcelain containers instead of plastic. Additionally, newer research has found that BPA exposure in utero can predispose people to food allergies later in life.[50]

Drink clean water. There isn't much of a direct connection with allergies, but in terms of promoting your overall health, clean drinking water is extremely important. After all, your body is made mostly of water, so if you put tainted water in your body, you will literally contaminate yourself. We are lucky enough to live in a country with clean drinking water devoid of pathogens that can make you acutely ill. But some of the chemicals lurking in tap water (chlorine, for example) can harm you over time. To help purify your water, and therefore your body, try the following:

- **Get a good water filter.** Water filters come in a number of forms, from pitchers you put in your fridge to full-house filtration systems. Any filter is better than nothing. I have a simple water filter under my sink at home. I installed it myself, and it works great.

- **Put a chlorine filter on your showerhead.** If you have public water, your water probably contains chlorine to kill bacteria and viruses. But chlorine's power to kill pathogens comes at a cost: The chemical dries out your skin and hair, and it is potentially toxic. Several studies have linked it to cancer. In one 2005 study published in the *Journal of Epidemiology and Community Health,* men who drank chlorinated water were found to have an increased risk of bladder cancer. A chlorine filter will help reduce your exposure.[51]

Landscape appropriately. Get rid of any weeds growing right next to your house—they are just another source of pollen and allergens. If you have pollen allergies, ask someone else to do the weeding. Also, avoid planting flowers that are relatives of ragweed—mums, sunflowers, dahlias, and zinnias.[52]

Get away from it all. If you have hay fever, try to plan a vacation in a more pollen-free area, such as the beach, at the peak of allergy season. Your body will enjoy the break.

In conclusion, remember: The chemicals and products you surround yourself with—both indoors and outdoors—play a large role in your level of inflammation, allergy risk, and general health. So minimize the potentially harmful substances in your environment; increase the number of tiny good habits you perform daily so they outnumber the bad ones; and make your environment as clean as you possibly can.

Beth's Story

Beth, a 40-year-old stay-at-home mom, was in great shape when she first visited Dr. Psenka. She was exercising, eating well, and taking beneficial supplements.

However, ever since moving to Arizona from Washington, DC, Beth had been suffering with allergy symptoms, including a runny nose, sneezing, and plugged ears—symptoms that were getting in the way of her otherwise healthy lifestyle. Beth has a child with a dairy allergy, so some genetic factors may also have been at play.

Not wanting to take synthetic drugs, Beth was interested in what Dr. Psenka could offer her in terms of natural remedies for her allergies.

"Much of what Dr. Psenka recommended I was already doing, so he added a few supplements to my regimen and recommended I try sublingual immunotherapy (SLIT)," she says.

As a result of Dr. Psenka's treatments, the next allergy season, Beth felt much better. "My family has also noticed my allergy symptoms have improved," she says.

Beth's only regret: not seeing Dr. Psenka and starting treatment earlier. "Dr. Psenka taught me natural remedies can work to treat allergies."

13 Working Out Your Allergies: Exercise and the Allergic Response

A FEW YEARS AGO, I met a woman in her early seventies who had decided it was time to make healthy changes in her life. She was moderately overweight, fatigued, and was having trouble sleeping. Her diet was poor, and she didn't exercise at all. I counseled her on healthy eating, proper hydration, and how important it is for all people, regardless of age, to find a way to incorporate exercise into their daily lives. She decided that instead of going to the gym and walking on the treadmill or lifting weights, she would like to try yoga. In a short period of time, she found that yoga not only improved her physical health but also made her feel better mentally. She no longer had trouble sleeping and she developed an overall better sense of well-being.

Now in her mid-seventies, this woman has become a yoga instructor and teaches yoga classes three or four times a week. It's been amazing to see her progress. In her seventies, she is in better physical shape than many of the 30-year-olds I see. She's also much happier and is full of vitality. This spunky lady did not have allergies or asthma, but she is a wonderful example of the importance of regular exercise for mental and physical health.

I am a firm believer in exercise, and I enjoy it myself. I try to exercise for at least an hour a day, and I think everyone, whether they have allergies or asthma or not, should exercise for 30 to 45 minutes almost every day, if possible. Exercise promotes good health and helps prevent diabetes, heart disease, cancer, and other diseases. It also promotes stress reduction and a more grounded sense of being. Anyone who has incorporated exercise into her life will tell you that she feels better and more relaxed after a workout.[1]

If you have allergies or asthma, which you probably do if you are reading this book, you still need to exercise. However, you need to be more cautious about the type of exercise you do. In most cases, exercise can be beneficial for those with allergies and asthma when the right types of exercise are chosen. I will tell you more about how to safely work out with allergies and asthma, but first let's cover some basics regarding the importance of exercise.

WE ARE MEANT TO MOVE

Regular exercise is vital to good health. Everyone needs to incorporate some kind of physical activity into his or her life. Your body is meant to run; it is meant to move. You're not meant to sit in front of a computer screen all day, which is unfortunately what many of us do. And while we can't completely remove ourselves from our computers, we can and should make the effort to go for a walk or a bike ride once we step away from them.

According to the Centers for Disease Control and Prevention (CDC), engaging in regular physical activity is one of the most important things you can do for your health. Among its most powerful effects, exercise:

- Lowers your risk of heart disease
- Reduces your chances of developing type 2 diabetes and metabolic syndrome
- Lowers your risk of some cancers
- Strengthens your bones and muscles

- Improves your chances of living longer
- Improves your ability to go through your daily activities as well as your overall quality of life
- Reduces stress and bolsters your mental health[2]

Additionally, regular exercise lowers chronic inflammation in your body, and as discussed, inflammation puts you at risk for a number of diseases and conditions. In a 2012 study published in *Current Pharmaceutical Design,* researchers found that regular exercise helped increase anti-inflammatory cytokines and chemokines, thereby reducing chronic inflammation.[3]

In another 2012 study published in the journal *Circulation,* researchers looked at the self-reported activity of 4,289 adults and measured their levels of two inflammatory markers—C-reactive protein (CRP) and interleukin-6 (IL-6)—over a 10-year period. The adults who reported exercising for at least 2.5 hours per week had lower levels of both CRP and IL-6 at the 10-year followup than those who reported lower levels of physical activity.[4]

Exercise also burns calories and helps you lose weight or maintain a healthy weight if your body mass index (BMI) is already good. (To calculate your BMI or learn more about it, see page 147.)

As noted, maintaining your BMI within the normal range is extremely important for good health. Obesity puts you at increased risk for heart disease, high blood pressure, stroke, high cholesterol and triglycerides, metabolic syndrome, cancer, osteoarthritis, gallstones, fertility issues, sleep apnea, and other potentially serious health problems.[5]

Keeping your BMI within the suggested normal range of 18.5 to 24.9 also appears to help control your risk of asthma. In a 2014 study published in the *American Journal of Epidemiology,* researchers examined the relationship between asthma and BMI. They looked at the risk of adult-onset asthma in 76,470 women without asthma who were participants in the Nurses' Health Study between 1988 and 1998. They assessed asthma risk in four different scenarios: (1) women who had no intervention, (2) women who had a 5 percent reduction in BMI over 2 years if they were overweight or obese, (3) women who exercised at a moderate or vigorous pace for at least

2.5 hours per week, and (4) women who exercised for at least 2.5 hours per week *and* reduced their BMIs by 5 percent. The researchers found that the women who exercised and lost weight had the lowest risk for asthma of all four groups.[6]

The link between asthma and BMI seems to be present early in life—as early as the preschool years. In a 2009 study published in the *Journal of Asthma,* researchers looked at BMI and the presence of asthma, allergic rhinitis, and eczema in 1,509 children who were 4 and 5 years old. They found a clear relationship between asthma symptoms and obesity in these preschool kids; those with higher BMIs were much more likely to report ever having had asthma symptoms or having had them in the past 12 months than kids whose BMIs were normal.[7]

As discussed in Chapter 10, to maintain a healthy BMI, you have to balance the calories you take in from foods and beverages with the calories you burn through physical activity.[8] The current exercise recommendations from the U.S. Department of Health and Human Services (HHS) are as follows: To maintain your weight, aim for a total of 150 minutes of moderate-intensity aerobic activity (equivalent to a brisk walk), 75 minutes of vigorous-intensity aerobic activity (equivalent to a run), or 75 to 150 minutes of a combination of moderate and vigorous activity every week. Because our bodies and metabolisms are different, you may need to do more than the recommended 75 to 150 minutes, especially if you are trying to lose and not just maintain your weight. Some people need up to 300 minutes of physical activity per week to stay slim. You may also need to combine exercise with changes in your diet in order to drop pounds.[9,10] But no matter what your weight-loss requirements, the more you exercise, the more health benefits you will reap.[11]

In addition to aerobic activity, you should also incorporate some strength training into your exercise routine. The HHS guidelines recommend that you engage in strength training 2 or more days a week and that you work all major muscle groups, including your abdomen, chest, hips, legs, back, shoulders, and arms.[12]

While I agree with the HHS recommendations, I think you should try to exercise for at least 30 minutes every day, or almost every day. A lot of people hear 30 to 45 minutes a day and their knee-jerk reaction is, "I just don't have time for that." But you do have time—you just have to make that time, and you have to realize that you don't have to exercise for 30 to 45 minutes straight. You can break it up into a few 10-minute intervals you fit in throughout your day. Go for a 10-minute walk right before breakfast in the morning; get out during your lunch hour for another 10 minutes and walk around your building or for a few blocks, if you work in town. Then walk for 10 minutes after dinner. When you break the activity down into smaller chunks, it doesn't seem so overwhelming. Once you have incorporated these activity breaks into your daily routine, you will look forward to them. After all, they are good excuses to get out of the office and into the fresh air to do something just for you.

You don't have to choose walking for your exercise—biking, swimming, spinning, aerobics, yoga, Pilates, tai chi—they are all great for you. In fact, swimming and yoga are particularly good for people with allergies and asthma.[13,14,15,16] As long as you get moving and increase your heart rate, you are doing your body good.

In addition, and this is *very* important: If you have allergies or asthma, you can exercise, but you need to be very careful and take special precautions as you start—and as you continue—your exercise routine. If you are starting an exercise program for the first time, talk to your health-care provider before you get going. Once you've gotten the green light, start slowly, especially if it has been a long time since you've exercised regularly. It's also important to realize that you can overexercise. If exercise is new for you, consider enlisting the assistance of a professional.

EXERCISING SAFELY WITH ALLERGIES AND ASTHMA

Exercising with allergies or asthma presents some unique challenges. Physical activity can be more difficult, unpleasant, and in some cases, dangerous if you have one or both of these conditions. You may also have less energy when your allergies or asthma are acting up. If your allergies or asthma are properly managed and you have the right tools, you can work out without causing your body any harm.[17]

A Warning About Exercise-Induced Anaphylaxis

People at risk for allergies should be aware of a condition called exercise-induced anaphylaxis (EIA). Anaphylaxis is a severe, life-threatening reaction that involves hives, trouble breathing, dizziness, low blood pressure, fainting, and in some cases, death. EIA is distinctly different from food allergies, but eating an allergenic food before exercise can make EIA more likely to kick in.[18] The mechanisms behind EIA aren't fully understood, but scientists know it is an anaphylactic reaction that happens as a result of physical activity, most often running, cycling, or swimming. It seems that in some people, exercise can stimulate mast cells to release IgE.

According to a 2013 study published in *Nutrition Research and Practice*, the worst offenders when it comes to EIA are wheat, eggs, shellfish, shrimp, nuts, fruits, and vegetables.[19] It doesn't occur every time a sufferer exercises, and it is sometimes linked to the exerciser having eaten a specific food before he or she started the activity. Taking certain medications, such as aspirin, together with one of these foods further increases the risk of an attack, as does high-intensity and frequent exercise. Low-intensity and less-frequent physical activities, on the other hand, are less likely to trigger EIA.[20] EIA is more likely to occur in extreme temperatures, in people with a family history of EIA, and in women who are having their menstrual periods.[21] EIA is pretty rare; some statistics say it only affects 1 to 3 people in 10,000, and other sources say between 1 and 15 percent of the population is at risk of suffering an exercise-related anaphylactic attack. The best thing to do if you have risk factors is to carry an EpiPen with you whenever you work out.[22]

If you are among the 20 million Americans who suffer from asthma, you should be aware of the possibility of exercise-induced asthma attacks. Exercise-induced asthma is just what it sounds like: asthma that is triggered specifically by exercise, usually vigorous activities such as running or fast biking. While it is common in people with asthma (in individuals with allergic asthma as well as in those with asthma that occurs separately), it can also strike people who do not have asthma under any other conditions. In these cases, it is sometimes called exercise-induced bronchoconstriction (see "A Warning About Exercise-Induced Anaphylaxis", page 219).[23]

People with asthma and parents of children with asthma may worry about exercise triggering an asthma attack, but research shows that in the long run, aerobic exercise is good for people with asthma and improves their quality of life.[24] To exercise safely with allergies or asthma, knowledge is your best tool. First, realize that there are some activities that are better than others. Running, biking, and basketball are more likely to cause exercise-induced asthma, while less-intense forms of exercise such as swimming, baseball, and resistance training are less likely to bring it on.[25] Yoga and tai chi, which we will explore later in this chapter, are also excellent options.

If you have allergies or asthma and are thinking of starting an exercise program, consult with your health-care provider first. This is vitally important. Your doctor can help you find the best activity for your condition and give you tips on how to exercise safely.

Tips for Exercising Safely with Asthma and Allergies

To exercise safely with allergies or asthma, here are some important guidelines.[26,27]

- Talk to your health-care provider first. I have repeated this a few times throughout this chapter, and that's because I truly want it to sink in: Before you make any major change in your lifestyle, whether it is taking a new supplement or starting an exercise program, talk to your health-care provider. You simply can't be too cautious.

- Take all of your allergy and asthma medications as your doctor has prescribed them. Your doctor may tell you to take your medication shortly before you start exercising. If he or she instructs you to do this, listen.

- If you have the potential for exercise-induced anaphylaxis or if you are allergic to insect stings, always exercise with a friend (never alone), wear your medical alert bracelet or necklace, and carry your EpiPen at all times.

- If you are allergic to insect stings and you plan to exercise outside, avoid wearing brightly colored clothing, perfume, cologne, or scented lotion. Also avoid areas where bees like to hide, such as trash cans and flowerbeds.

- If you have asthma, always carry your rescue inhaler with you when you exercise.

- Check the temperature before you head outside for a run or bike ride. Avoid working out in extreme heat or cold (cold is the worst, because cold, dry air can be very irritating to your bronchial tubes; the best air to exercise in is warm and moist) or when pollen counts are high (usually in the morning and the middle of the afternoon).

- If you are exercising indoors, work out on mats instead of carpeting, and keep your windows closed if pollen counts are high. Also, avoid exercising where there are fumes from recent renovations.

- If you are exercising outdoors, avoid fields, busy roads, and factories, to keep allergens and irritants out of your lungs.

- When you exercise, breathe through your nose as much as you can. Your nasal passages are natural air filters, and they trap some of the allergens, irritants, and pollutants before they have a chance to enter your lungs. Breathing through your nose also helps keep the air you breathe moist and at the proper temperature.

- If you have asthma, to prevent an exercise-induced attack, always do a long, 15-minute warmup before you start the main part of your exercise routine, and then cool down for another 15 minutes once you've finished your activity.

- Never exercise when you have a cold or respiratory infection. Wait until your symptoms have subsided to resume your routine.

- If you have allergies or asthma, don't push yourself during exercise.

Can Running Ease Allergy Symptoms?

Do you take off from exercise on the days your allergy symptoms are at their worst? You might want to think twice about that. A study done in Thailand found that running may help relieve some allergy symptoms, such as sneezing and runny nose. In a 2012 study published in the *Asian Pacific Journal of Allergy and Immunology*, after allergy sufferers ran for 30 minutes, their nasal congestion, sneezing, runny nose, and nasal itching decreased by more than 70 percent. It seems that exercise may work by calming inflammatory proteins in your nasal passages that spark allergy symptoms.

The study authors recommend exercising at a moderate pace, at 65 to 70 percent of your heart rate reserve.[28] To calculate this number, first find your maximum heart rate by multiplying your age by 0.7 and then subtracting the resulting number from 207. (For example, if you are 40, 40 x 0.7 = 28. Now, 207–28 = 179. Your maximum heart rate is 179.) Then, to find the heart rate you should aim for in order to stay within 65 to 70 percent of your heart rate reserve, subtract your resting heart rate (the number of beats per minute) from your maximum heart rate. If your resting heart rate is 60, 179–60 = 119. You would then aim for a heart rate of 119 beats per minute while you are exercising.[29]

TO CALM YOUR ALLERGIES, RELAX YOUR BODY AND MIND

Allergies and asthma not only affect how you feel physically but also they can cause emotional stress. Knowing that you will spend the whole spring sniffling and sneezing is anxiety-provoking, and to make matters worse, stress can exacerbate the allergic response. As discussed in Chapter 7, the stress hormone cortisol increases inflammation in your body and triggers the release of histamine, the chemical that brings on allergy symptoms. Conversely, when you are more relaxed, your immune system is less likely to overreact to allergens with inflammation, increased mucus, itching, and other unpleasant symptoms. In the same way that a person who is in a calm, relaxed state of mind is less likely to overreact to criticism or pick a fight, a calm, relaxed immune system is less likely to respond in an exaggerated manner when it's exposed to pollen or dust.[30]

There are a few relaxation-type exercises that can help combat the "fight-or-flight" mode we go into when we're stressed *and* fight allergies *and* help prevent asthma symptoms at the same time, thus allowing you to metaphorically kill multiple birds with one work-out.[31] Plus, as yoga is typically done indoors, you will avoid expos-ing yourself to pollen and other allergens and irritants floating in the outside air.[32]

The Benefits of Tai Chi

One form of exercise that will relax you and can help combat aller-gies and asthma is tai chi. Similar in nature, qigong and tai chi are a group of ancient exercises comprised of slow movements that specif-ically promote relaxation. Tai chi has been shown to improve immune-system function, thereby helping to prevent allergies and asthma.[33]

The goal of tai chi and qigong is to cultivate the *qi*, which is defined in Western terms as the energy found within all living things. By cultivating, nourishing, balancing, and channeling the qi in the right directions, doing these ancient forms of martial arts can help your body heal. In addition, qigong helps people who practice

Put Down the Saltshaker to Reduce Lung Constriction

Here's another benefit to a low-salt diet: a lower risk for exercise-induced asthma. In a 2010 study, researchers gave adults with asthma a low-sodium diet for 1 to 2 weeks and found that it decreased their bronchoconstriction when they exercised. So although it cannot take the place of asthma medications, a low-sodium diet may be beneficial for people who suffer from exercise-induced asthma.[34]

it to concentrate on and control their breathing. This makes it great for people with respiratory conditions, including some types of chronic allergies.[35]

In a study done in Thailand and presented at the annual meeting of the American College of Chest Physicians, researchers looked at 17 people with persistent asthma and enrolled them in a 6-week tai chi program. Participants attended a supervised tai chi class once a week and did home-based exercises using an audiovisual guide. At the end of their 6 weeks of tai chi, the participants had better oxygen consumption and exercise endurance than they did before they started.[36,37]

In a related study published in the *Journal of Microbiology, Immunology, and Infection,* researchers looked at the pulmonary function of 30 asthmatic children at rest, after exercise, and after exercise plus drinking ice water. They then enrolled half of the kids in a 12-week tai chi program. The other half made up the control group and performed no exercise routine. After 12 weeks, the children in the tai chi group had significant improvements in their overall pulmonary function compared to the control group. Under the stronger challenge of exercise plus drinking ice water, the children in the tai chi group had milder asthma symptoms than the kids in the control group did.[38]

To find a good tai chi instructor, ask your health-care provider if he or she can recommend one or consult the American Tai Chi and Qigong Association at americantaichi.net/taichiqigongclass.asp.[39]

The Benefits of Yoga

Another relaxation exercise that is good for people with allergies and asthma is yoga. In a 2012 study published in the *Indian Journal of Physiology and Pharmacology,* researchers compared lung function and diffusion capacity (how well the lungs process air) of people with asthma before and after 2 months of practicing yoga. They found that pranayama yoga breathing and stretching postures increased respiratory stamina, relaxed the chest muscles, expanded the lungs, improved energy levels, and helped calm the body.[40]

A related 2012 study published in the *Journal of Alternative and Complementary Medicine* assessed the effects of 10 weeks of yoga training on quality of life and heart rate variability (HRV), the variation in the time between heartbeats. The researchers randomly assigned 19 women with mild to moderate asthma to either a yoga group or a control group. The participants all completed quality-of-life questionnaires and underwent isometric handgrip tests to assess their HRV. After 10 weeks, the yoga group saw significant improvements in their quality of life; in fact, their quality of life was rated 45 percent higher than that of the control group. The yoga group also saw improvements in their HRV.[41]

In a 2009 randomized controlled trial, researchers looked at 57 adults with mild or moderate asthma and put them into a yoga group or a control group. The yoga group received conventional care as well as yoga instruction, and the control group just got conventional care. More specifically, the yoga group received 2 weeks of supervised training on lifestyle, medication, and stress management based on yoga, followed by a closely monitored continuation of the program at home for 6 weeks. The researchers looked at the progress of both groups at the beginning of the study and 2 weeks, 4 weeks, and 8 weeks into the study. In the yoga group, they found a steady, progressive improvement in lung function. The yoga group also saw a reduction in exercise-induced bronchoconstriction and improvements in quality of life.[42]

When you practice yoga, especially one of the less-vigorous forms, you relax your mind and your immune system. According to *Yoga Journal*, the best way to use yoga for relaxation is to perform it smoothly and slowly.[43] Further, yoga instructors discourage allergy and asthma sufferers from engaging in certain yoga forms, including Bikram or "hot yoga," which is done in a room that is at least 105°F and at 60 percent relative humidity, as well as Ashtanga yoga, which is an intense and physical yoga form.[44,45,46]

As you practice yoga, try to steer clear of forceful breathing through your nostrils, which can be uncomfortable and difficult if you are congested. Instead, do a short inhalation followed by a long, slow exhalation, which is more calming for your body and mind.[47]

THE BEST YOGA POSES FOR ALLERGY AND ASTHMA SUFFERERS

In general, standing poses that involve forward and backward bends and twists, like the Shoulder Stand Pose and the Plow Pose (described on the following pages), massage your spine and thoracic cage and help condition your lungs, thus strengthening your immune system.[48] There are also a few specific yoga poses that can help with asthma and allergy symptoms.

WARRIOR 1 POSE

This pose helps your chest and lungs to open and uses gravity to drain mucus out of your nose and lungs. To perform the pose:

1. Stand with your feet together and arms at your sides.

2. Step forward with your right foot so your feet are 3 feet apart, and bend your right knee until your thigh is parallel to the floor. Try to keep your back left heel pressed to the floor.

3. As you're bending your right knee, raise your arms above your head, keeping them shoulder-width apart, with your arms straight and your palms facing each other. (Your arms should be next to your ears.)

4. Inhale and exhale slowly. Hold this pose for 3 to 10 slow, deep breaths.

5. Come back to standing and repeat the pose on your left side.

HALF MOON POSE

This pose eases breathing by opening your rib cage and lungs, so it will help clear your head if you have hay fever symptoms such as sneezing, runny nose, and watery eyes. To perform the pose:

1. Stand with your feet shoulder-width apart and arms at your sides.

2. Place your left hand on your left hip and turn your right leg 90 degrees out to the right.

3. Extend your right arm straight out to your side at shoulder-height.

4. Bending at your waist, reach down with your right hand and place your fingertips on the floor a few inches in front of your right foot.

5. Lift your left leg straight behind you so that it is parallel to the floor, and open your hips to the left. Extend your left arm so that it is in line with your right arm. Turn your head and look up at your left hand. Hold for 3 to 5 breaths.

6. Slowly lower your left arm back to your left hip and look toward the floor. Slightly bend your right knee and gently lower your left leg. Straighten your right knee.

7. Come back to standing and repeat the pose on the opposite side.

SHOULDER STAND POSE

Both the Shoulder Stand Pose and the Plow Pose are used to open nasal passages and help drain the sinuses.[49] Fold two or more blankets into rectangles and stack them to create your support. You may want to place a sticky mat on top of the blankets to help your upper arms stay in place while you are performing the pose. To perform the pose:

1. Lie down so your head is on the floor and your shoulder blades are on the blankets. (The short edge of the blanket should be parallel to your arms.) Place your arms flat on the floor so they are parallel to your torso, bend your knees, and put your feet flat on the floor.

2. As you exhale, press your arms against the floor and push your knees away from the floor. Draw your thighs in toward your torso.

3. Continue to lift your legs upward by curling your pelvis, and push the back of your torso away from the floor so your knees come toward your face. Put your

arms out so they are parallel to the edge of the blanket, and turn them so your thumbs are behind you and your fingers press against the floor.

4. Bend your arms and draw your elbows toward each other, then place your palms flat on your lower back and the backs of your upper arms on the blanket. Raise your pelvis over your shoulders so your torso is perpendicular to the floor. Walk your hands up your back and down toward the floor, keeping your elbows shoulder-width apart.

5. As you inhale, lift your bent knees toward the ceiling, bring your thighs in line with your torso, and let your heels hang down by your buttocks. Press your tailbone toward your pubic bone and turn your upper thighs slightly inward. As you inhale, straighten your legs and press your heels up toward the ceiling. Once the backs of your legs are fully extended, push your feet upward through the balls of your big toes so your inner legs are slightly longer than your outer legs.

6. Push your shoulder blades and the backs of your arms into the blanket support and move your chin toward your sternum. In this position, your forehead should be parallel to the floor, and your chin should be perpendicular to the floor. Try to lift your upper spine away from the floor and look at your chest.

7. Hold the pose for 30 seconds. As you get stronger, gradually add 5 to 10 seconds to the pose until you can do it comfortably for 3 minutes. To exit the pose, as you exhale, bend your knees toward your torso and keep the back of your head against the floor as you roll your back slowly down onto the floor. You may also move right into the Plow Pose without exiting the Shoulder Stand Pose.

THE PLOW POSE

The Plow Pose is usually performed after the Shoulder Stand Pose, for anywhere between 1 and 5 minutes. To perform the pose:

1. From the Shoulder Stand Pose, exhale and bend from your hip joints, and slowly lower your toes to the floor so they are above and behind your head and your thighs are in front of your face. Your torso should be perpendicular to the floor and your legs should be straight and completely extended.

2. Keeping your toes on the floor, lift the top of your thighs and your tailbone toward the ceiling, drawing your inner groin into your pelvis. Imagine that your torso is hanging down from your groin. Draw your chin away from your sternum and soften your throat.

3. Press your hands against the back of your torso, pushing up toward the ceiling as you press the backs of your upper arms down onto the floor. Actively press your arms down on the floor behind your back as you lift your thighs toward the ceiling.

4. To exit the pose, bring your hands onto your back and roll out of the pose as you exhale.

MAKING EXERCISE A PART OF YOUR LIFE

The most difficult part of getting into an exercise routine is . . . getting into an exercise routine. Once you find an activity you enjoy and make it a part of your daily life, the hardest part's over. At that point, you can just have fun exercising and reap the benefits, both in terms of your health and your appearance. In the meantime, there are some things you can do to transform yourself into someone who looks forward to exercising.

Schedule your time for exercise. The excuse I hear most often when it comes to exercise is, "I don't have the time." But if you schedule exercise time like you do a half-hour business meeting, as something that cannot be overridden or removed, you will be much more likely to do it. Like most people, I am very busy. I have a business to run, I see patients every day, I do research, and I am a father of two with a wife and a house. There are not a lot of hours in the day to accomplish all of the things I need to do, but I still find time to exercise for 1 to 2 hours almost every day by scheduling time for my activity.

For example, I often keep my bike at my office. If I have a break in my day, even a short one, I often jump on the bike and go for a quick ride. Taking an exercise break not only helps to keep me physically fit but also it's a great way to stay mentally sharp throughout the day. So write "exercise" in your planner, block off time in your smart phone calendar for a yoga class, or book a date with your exercise partner— whatever you need to do to make exercise a priority in your day.

Find an activity you enjoy. When I ask patients about exercise, a lot of them tell me they have this great treadmill in their bedroom. I sometimes jokingly ask how many pieces of clothing are hanging on that treadmill. Most people chuckle and admit that their treadmill gets more use as a hanger than as a piece of exercise equipment. I think that one of the reasons bedroom treadmills don't get enough use is because they are not very exciting.

Exercise should be fun; it should be the sort of thing that you look forward to doing. For me, riding my mountain bike is fun, and I look forward to my rides. However, even biking loses some of its appeal every so often, and when it does, I simply start doing something else I enjoy, such as swimming. So if you're not exercising enough, ask yourself why not, and if you find the reason is a lack of enthusiasm about your routine, think about what you might find fun and exciting.

The best way to find an exercise you love is to try different things. Sign up for a tai chi class or two, join a friend on a hike, or pay for a few swimming sessions at your local YMCA. Chances are, when you've found a good activity for you, you'll know it. Some people (myself included) don't enjoy engaging in just one type of exercise. They run one day, hike the next, and ride their bikes the day after that. Not only does switching activities prevent boredom, it keeps your muscles challenged as well, which is great for fitness and overall health.

Find an exercise partner. This person can be a good friend, a not-so-good friend, or a personal trainer. It doesn't matter—as long as you have someone to keep you accountable. When you are only accountable to yourself, it's far too easy to make excuses, like *I'm too* *tired* or *I don't have time*, and then skip your workout. When you know your exercise partner is waiting for you on the corner at 6:00 a.m. to go for a walk, you will be a lot less likely to hit the snooze button and a lot more likely to get up and put on your shoes when the alarm goes off.

I also recommend that you consider using the services of a qualified personal trainer. Using a personal trainer has many advantages, especially when you're beginning an exercise program. A good personal trainer will encourage you to stick with your exercise routine and will be your cheerleader. Personal trainers will also keep you accountable to your workouts, as you'll likely be paying for their services. Most important, a trainer will help you work out safely. I see many people, especially men in their thirties and forties, who try to jump right into a workout routine similar to what they were doing when they were 18 years old. Unfortunately, this often results in an injury that derails the entire exercise effort. A qualified personal trainer will work with you to exercise safely, whether you have allergies or asthma or not. Consider it a smart investment in yourself.

With these tips, you have a recipe for exercise success. As we move on to The Allergy Solution Plan (see page 231), remember the importance of regular exercise, not just for allergies and asthma, but for lowering inflammation, keeping weight off, and improving your overall health.

14

Countdown to an Allergy-Free You: The 4-Week Allergy Solution Plan

A FEW YEARS AGO, I WAS TALKING WITH A FELLOW DOCTOR who is in her thirties, and she told me about her terrible allergies. She had several confirmed food allergies, significant seasonal allergies, and was allergic to cats and dogs. She knew how to deal with her food allergies and she had taken measures to clean up the environment in her home. In other words, she was doing everything in her power to control her allergies. She didn't have any pets, but she had started a serious relationship with a guy who had both cats and dogs. Because of her exposure to the pets, she had to dose herself with antihistamines multiple times a day to control her allergy symptoms.

In addition to the lifestyle factors she had already initiated, we discussed a newer treatment called sublingual immunotherapy (SLIT) as a possible treatment option. As discussed, SLIT is an allergy treatment that involves giving the allergy sufferer small doses of what he or she is allergic to in order to increase his or her tolerance to that allergen. SLIT differs from injection immunotherapy (allergy shots) in that it is given orally via a spray or a dissolvable tablet, not through an injection.[1]

I ordered some blood tests and found that she was, in fact,

severely allergic—more than 15 antigens showed up on her blood test, including those for cats and dogs, so it was no wonder she was suffering after starting her relationship with the animal lover.

The SLIT took a few months to begin alleviating her symptoms, which is typical for immunotherapy, but when it did, she experienced dramatic results. Her seasonal allergies were for the most part eliminated, and she was able to move in with her boyfriend (who is now her husband). She can tolerate the dogs and cats, so he was able to keep his pets. My patient is so happy with the results of SLIT that she now uses it in her own practice.

As we launch into the 4-week Allergy Solution Plan, I must note that this woman was a severe case, and her story illustrates that in some instances, people must try several different measures before they find the right combination of things, be they lifestyle changes or supplements, that work for them. In her situation, it was the combination of eating a healthy, noninflammatory diet; removing all feasible allergy risk factors from her home; taking specific supplements; and using SLIT that provided her allergy solution. It may seem like her plan entails quite a lot just to get rid of her allergies—especially when many take only a small number of pills to achieve similar results. However, the beauty of a natural approach to allergies is that it not only treats your allergies but, as we've discussed throughout this book, it can also dramatically improve your overall health.

Most allergy sufferers are less allergic than this patient, however, and therefore might not need to take all of the same steps as she did. Many people respond well to simple changes like eliminating certain foods and allergy-proofing their homes.

BEGINNING THE ALLERGY SOLUTION PLAN

As our journey comes to a close, the Allergy Solution Plan will put all of the knowledge and tips you've gained so far into play. The plan will tell you, step-by-step, what to do as allergy season approaches to both strengthen your body and to prevent the development of allergies. It will also instruct you on the best practices to employ at the peak of your allergy season.

Most of the advice I have given thus far involves healthy lifestyle habits you should be engaging in all of the time. It's important to incorporate these good habits into your routine all year long, and it is especially critical to make sure you practice them as much as possible heading into allergy season.

The Allergy Solution Plan is separated into 4 different weeks, with corresponding steps and phases occurring within each week. That's because a few weeks before allergy season starts—or better yet, a few months before—is the time to start reducing the inflammation in your body. You can do this by cleaning your home to lower the levels of dust mites, mold, and other allergens; by eating anti-inflammatory foods like walnuts, flax, and cold-water fish; by steering clear of proinflammatory foods like dairy and red meat; and by exercising for at least 30 minutes every day. Of course you could, and likely should, make these things part of your normal daily routine anyway, all year long.

If you're reading this book at the end of allergy season or when allergy season is still months and months away, you can still get started with the Allergy Solution Plan. That way, once allergy season does roll around, your inflammation will be even lower and you will be better armed and ready to keep your allergy symptoms at bay. Once you have this preparation underway, it will become part of your routine, and then further down the road, it will become your way of life. The best time to start using all of the tips you've learned so far is *now*.

WEEK 1: PROMOTE AN ALLERGY-FREE HOME

Two weeks before allergy season, your focus should be on allergy-proofing your home. Most of us spend the majority of our time indoors, so it's important to make this environment as pure and allergen-free as possible.

Phase 1: Clean Your In-Home Air

As noted in Chapter 12, the pollution and allergens lurking in your indoor environments can be even worse than the substances floating around in the outside air. Therefore, the cleaner you can make the air inside your home and office, the better you will breathe.

One of the best ways to purify your air is with an air filter, a mechanical device that traps and removes dust, pollen, and other particles from the air before they make their way into your lungs. In addition to removing particulate matter, high-quality air filters will also remove chemicals from the air. There are a number of different types of air filters, from whole-house filtration systems to freestanding, single-room filters. They range in price from about $50 for a freestanding air filter to thousands of dollars for whole-house filtration systems. No matter what kind you choose, look for the Underwriters Laboratories (UL) seal, which indicates that the filter is safe, as well as a statement from the FDA indicating that the filter has met the FDA's Class II approval, which means the device has a legitimate medical benefit.[2]

Personally, I use freestanding air filters in both my office and my home, and they work great. There are a few different types of single-room air filters to choose from.

- **Mechanical air cleaners.** These include fan-driven high-efficiency particulate air (HEPA) filters, which force air through a special mesh that physically traps particles such as dust, pollen, pet dander, and tobacco smoke.

- **Electronic air cleaners.** These include ion-type cleaners and use an electrical charge to attract and get rid of irritants and allergens.

- **Hybrid air cleaners.** These filters have elements of both mechanical and electronic air filters.

- **Gas-phase air cleaners.** These filters do not remove allergens, but they are good for eliminating gas pollutants such as cooking gas, perfumes, and fumes released by building materials and paint.[3]

It's particularly important to run an air filter in your bedroom and to point it toward your body as you sleep. You spend more time in your bedroom than any other room in your house, but unfortunately, this room is often the dirtiest and most laden with allergens, including dust mites, dust, and mold. In addition to running an air filter in your bedroom, go with a minimalist style of decor to reduce the number of places allergens can hide—eliminate knickknacks, picture frames, window dressings, and other clutter. Also avoid storing things under your bed, and keep your bed away from vents, so you're not breathing in particles that blow out of them as you sleep.[4]

No matter what kind of air filter you use, as allergy season approaches, kick it into high gear. If you normally only run it at night, start running it all day long. If you normally run it on low, push it to high. This is the time to pull out all the stops and make sure you are doing everything you can to clean up the air in your house.

Phase 2: Increase the Oxygen in Your Home Air

One of the best ways to increase the amount of oxygen in your home is to get air-cleaning houseplants. Because they produce oxygen, houseplants act like natural air filters and can actually help clean the air. Some can also absorb allergens.[5] Plants make great air filters because they are simple, safe, and inexpensive. Plus, they're decorative. If you or someone in your household has allergies, look for plants that are good air filters but that don't produce a lot of pollen or other allergens. For a list of air-cleaning houseplants, see page 205.

Phase 3: Minimize Your Exposure to Environmental Toxins

Aside from moving to a remote area of the country, which isn't feasible for most of us, there isn't a whole lot you can do to avoid environmental toxins that come from outside pollution—sources like vehicle exhaust and by-products from plants and factories. But there are things you can do to reduce your exposure to environmental toxins *inside* your own home. From paint to glues used in flooring and other building materials to caustic cleaning products, a number of chemicals in your indoor work and home environments can cause you harm. As you close in on allergy season, it's particularly important to minimize your exposure to these toxins because they can increase inflammation in your body and therefore make you even more vulnerable to allergy symptoms once the season kicks in.[6]

As we discussed in Chapter 12, some of the worst offenders in household products are volatile organic compounds (VOCs), which are chemicals used in detergents, dishwashing liquids, furniture polishes, rug and upholstery cleaners, floor polishes, chlorine bleach, air fresheners, and aerosol sprays.[7] To avoid VOCs, you can clean the old-fashioned way with everyday household products. Baking soda is a great carpet cleaner—just sprinkle it on your carpet and vacuum it up to eliminate odors.[8] You can also make a homemade all-purpose cleaning solution by mixing equal parts white vinegar and water.[9] Or, you can look for green cleaning products. Remember, reputable brands include Earth Friendly Products, Simple Green, and Naturally Yours.[10]

Another thing to watch out for is dry-cleaning chemicals. Most conventional dry cleaners use perchloroethylene (sometimes referred to as "perc"), which is toxic to humans and contributes to environmental pollution in the form of smog. Look for a dry cleaner who uses green methods—the two most common are a patented process called GreenEarth Cleaning and carbon dioxide cleaning. Or, if you must use a conventional dry cleaner, take your clothing out of the plastic bag as soon as you get it home, and hang it outside to air out before you wear it. This won't help with environmental pollution, but it will help keep the air in your home clean.[11]

Another way to reduce the number of toxins in your living space is to ask people to take off their shoes at the door. Along with dirt that you have to vacuum, sweep, and mop, shoes bring animal waste, particulate pollution, pollen, antifreeze, oil, and other potentially harmful chemicals into your home.[12]

If you have a home cleaning service, make sure that they are using green cleaning products in your home. If they are not, consider providing the cleaning supplies for them, or look for a service that uses them.[13]

WEEK 2: CHANGE YOUR RISK FACTORS

Make these changes beginning at least 1 week before allergy season. You can't change some of your risk factors for allergies, such as family history, but there are some risk factors for allergies that you *can* change. These include your eating habits and your level of physical activity.

Phase 1: Assess and Eliminate Dietary Offenders

If you have a food allergy, it goes without saying that you should stay away from foods to which you are allergic—not just going into allergy season, but throughout the year. This is particularly important if you have a food allergy that could cause a potentially life-threatening anaphylactic reaction.

But even if your allergies aren't food-related, you should be careful about what you eat, especially leading into allergy season. Most important, avoid foods that can increase inflammation in your body. After all, the more inflammation you have going into allergy season, the more likely you will be to react to your triggers (ragweed, pollen, dust, or another substance to which you are allergic) once they appear.

The worst foods when it comes to inflammation—and therefore, the ones you want to be most diligent about avoiding going into allergy season—are red meat, excessive sugar, and dairy products. These foods are especially bad for allergies because they contain arachidonic acid, which stimulates the production of leukotrienes, fatty molecules in your immune system that are proinflammatory. Now, I am not promoting a strict vegetarian diet. It is acceptable to have an organic carnivorous treat once in a while throughout the year. But I do think that during the few weeks before allergy season, you should completely abstain. To satisfy your meat craving, you can use substitutes like textured vegetable protein (TVP), veggie burgers, portobella mushroom burgers, and quinoa (in place of ground beef).

As allergy season approaches, you'd also be wise to avoid foods that contain excess calcium, including fortified orange juice; sardines; green, leafy vegetables; and bananas. Eating these foods can perpetuate the production of phospholipase, another enzyme that produces inflammatory enzymes in your body.

Phase 2: Start Eating an Antiallergy Diet

Just as important as avoiding proinflammatory foods at the dawn of allergy season is eating their *anti*-inflammatory counterparts. Increase your intake of foods rich in the omega-3 fatty acids EPA and DHA, such as flaxseed, walnuts, and cold-water fish like salmon. These omega-3–rich foods can help decrease the leukotrienes that contribute to the bronchoconstriction involved in some allergic reactions and allergic asthma attacks.

In addition, boost your intake of foods that contain flavonoids such as quercetin and beta-carotene as well as vitamin C. To get more flavonoids, eat more apples, berries, broccoli, celery, cranberries, endive, grapes, green beans, kale, onions, strawberries, sweet red peppers, and tomatoes.[14] To increase your intake of the flavonoid quercetin, which is a natural antihistamine, eat lots of apples (with the skin), cherries, cranberries, currants, garlic, and onions.[15] For added beta-carotene, go for apricots, broccoli, cantaloupe, carrots, mangoes, pumpkin, spinach, squash, sweet peppers, and sweet potatoes.[16] And to boost your intake of vitamin C, which is another of nature's powerful antihistamines, eat more citrus fruits, peppers, strawberries, and tomatoes.[17,18]

I have to point out that one of the most powerful foods when it comes to allergy-fighting potential is broccoli sprouts. A study published in *Food and Function* showed that broccoli sprout extract could actually lessen the impact of diesel exhaust particles (DEPs), one of the worst environmental pollutants, in people with allergies and asthma.[19] As an added bonus, broccoli sprouts are a great source of vitamin C, so this is truly a superfood when it comes to allergy and asthma prevention.[20]

If you are feeling extra gung ho, you may want to consider switching to a vegan diet in the weeks leading up to allergy season. By eliminating all animal products, you will lower your levels of proinflammatory arachidonic acid and therefore decrease the leukotrienes that get released as part of the allergic response. In a landmark Swedish study done in 1985, researchers found that asthmatics who followed a vegan diet saw a 71 percent improvement in their asthma symptoms after 4 months and a 92 percent improvement after a year.[21]

In addition to getting the right nutrients and eliminating proinflammatory foods, you should also be vigilant about staying adequately hydrated at this time. Your body is mostly made of water, so you need H_2O to keep your systems functioning smoothly. Also, staying adequately hydrated as you head into allergy season will help thin your mucus and prevent congestion. Hydration also promotes general detoxification in your body, so it will help flush out proinflammatory markers that can worsen an allergic response.[22]

To stay hydrated, I recommend that you drink water (not soda, juice, coffee, or caffeinated tea). You can substitute decaffeinated herbal tea here and there, but most of your beverages should be H_2O. You should drink half of your body weight in ounces of water a day, so if you weigh 150 pounds, drink 75 ounces of water. That's a lot, but it is doable, especially if you make it a point to keep water with you at all times and you drink it steadily throughout the day.

Phase 3: Exercise for Physical and Mental Health

As I mentioned in Chapter 13, I am a firm believer in exercise, and I think that everyone should make time for at least 30 minutes of physical activity every single day. If you have asthma or the potential for exercise-induced bronchoconstriction or exercise-induced anaphylaxis, you should still exercise, but you may need to be a little more cautious with your exercise routine. Ideal activities for you will include gentle yoga, qigong, and tai chi. As a bonus, these activities help bolster your body against allergies and asthma.[23]

By harnessing the energy, or *qi,* tai chi and qigong can improve your immune system function and help prevent allergies and asthma. Research has shown that tai chi can help improve oxygen consumption and exercise endurance as well as decrease asthma symptoms.[24,25]

Yoga is also beneficial for asthma and allergy sufferers. Studies have shown that the practice can help calm the body, increase respiratory stamina, boost energy levels, improve lung function, reduce exercise-induced bronchoconstriction, and improve overall quality of life in people with asthma and allergies.[26,27,28]

In addition to their physical benefits, yoga and tai chi are also wonderful stress-relievers. Anyone who has suffered from allergies or asthma knows how stressful these conditions can be. As allergy season looms and you anticipate the sniffling and sneezing, you may feel your anxiety building. So the more you can do to keep your body relaxed during this time, the better. We learned in Chapter 8 that stress and anxiety contribute to inflammation, so as you lower your stress levels, you will lower your inflammation levels, too, and therefore make your body less susceptible to allergy symptoms.[29]

All forms of exercise—not just yoga and tai chi—have some stress-relieving effects and are great for mental health.[30] And if you can add some meditation to your routine as allergy season approaches, even better. In a 2011 study published in *Alternative Therapies in Health and Medicine,* researchers found that individuals who meditated for 15 minutes once or twice a day for 4 weeks showed improvements in their levels of stress and anxiety as well as in their overall quality of life.[31]

WEEK 3: INCORPORATE ANTIALLERGY SUPPLEMENTS AND HERBAL MEDICINE

As allergy season begins, it is important to keep up with the lifestyle changes you've implemented—cleaning up your environment and air, eating anti-inflammatory foods, avoiding proinflammatory foods, and exercising on a regular basis, with an emphasis on stress-relieving workouts. Some people respond well to these lifestyle interventions alone; these people get substantial relief from their allergies just by lowering their inflammation levels. Others need to do more.

If you have milder allergy symptoms, I suggest that at this time you also begin taking supplements that will make your body stronger, allowing you to better stave off allergy symptoms. If you are a little more allergic, I recommend you start taking a few antiallergy herbs and maybe homeopathic treatments in addition to those basic supplements. If you are highly allergic or you know from past experience that your allergies are stubborn, you may want to consider SLIT at this point.

Everyone is different, and it takes some people longer than others to achieve the same results using lifestyle interventions. That's where supplementation, herbs, homeopathy, and SLIT can help. These remedies can lower your allergic potential and stabilize mast cells so you don't get the histamine release and resulting allergy symptoms (such as itching and sneezing) that can make the few months of allergy season so miserable for you.

All of the herbs and supplements here are generally regarded as safe. However, everyone's body is different, and herbs can interfere with some drugs and medical conditions, so you should always talk to a health-care provider experienced in prescribing supplements and herbal medicines before starting any new herb or supplement.

Supplements

At the very beginning of allergy season, you can start with the most basic supplements for improving overall health. These include the following:

Vitamin C (ascorbic acid). This is a good supplement to start right at the beginning of allergy season. Ideally, you should be taking vitamin C all year long, as it does a number of things for your body: It's a natural anti-inflammatory and it helps prevent histamine release, so it can ease asthma and allergy symptoms. Take 2 to 3 grams a day.[32,33]

B Vitamins. I recommend you take vitamin B_6 and vitamin B_{12} as part of your supplement repertoire. B_6 (pyridoxine) may help prevent inflammation and ease asthma symptoms,[34,35,36] and studies show that B_{12} can help stave off asthma attacks as well.[37]

Herbal Remedies

You can bolster your immune system at the start of allergy season by taking herbs that have antiallergic effects. If you've already started experiencing mild symptoms, these herbs can help prevent your allergies from becoming full-blown.

Here's a refresher on some of the best herbs for allergies. If you want to mix a few of these remedies, there are some products on the market that combine multiple herbs and supplements in one pill, so you don't have to purchase or swallow multiple products.

You can also make an "allergy remedy" herbal tea using a combination of the loose leaves of a few of the herbs below; drink a few cups a day starting at the beginning of allergy season. Or, if your herbal remedies are in tincture form, mix several of them together to make them easier to take.[38]

In terms of dosages of the following herbs, I've given the usual ranges, but you may want to start off with a higher loading dose and then take a lower maintenance dose for the rest of allergy season. Generally speaking, people can often find relief using only one or two of these herbs at a time. Remember, natural does not equal safe, and every person is unique, so make sure to talk to a qualified physician before taking herbal medicines. (For more detailed information on these herbs, including side effects and warnings, see Chapter 11.)

Boswellia (page 190). This bark has anti-inflammatory properties. The typical dose is 150 to 400 milligrams of a standardized extract, three times a day as needed.[39]

Butterbur (page 194). A shrublike plant, butterbur (or *Petasites*) works like a leukotriene inhibitor, blocking the chemicals that can trigger allergy symptoms such as nasal swelling.[40,41] The typical dose for treating hay fever is 50 milligrams of butterbur root extract, two times a day.[42]

Gingko biloba extract (GBE) (page 190). GBE has antioxidant properties and has been shown in some studies to help fight asthma.[43] The dose ranges from 120 to 160 milligrams per day.[44]

Green tea extract (page 192). One of the most abundant compounds in green tea, called epigallocatechin gallate (EGCG), can help fight allergy symptoms such as runny nose and sneezing. The dose is around 100 milligrams per day.

Licorice root (page 193). Licorice root, or *Glycyrrhiza glabra,* helps with allergies by fighting inflammation; soothing the throat, bronchial membranes, and lungs; and promoting mucus secretion. The dose ranges from 5 to 15 milligrams per day.[45]

Stinging nettle (page 195). A few studies have shown that stinging nettle has antihistamine properties and therefore may help ease sneezing and itching in people with hay fever.[46] The dose for treating allergies is about 500 milligrams, three times a day.[47]

Guduchi (page 197). An herb long used in Ayurvedic medicine to remove toxins from the body, guduchi can also help treat allergies, specifically hay fever.[48] The dose is about 300 milligrams, three times a day, for the course of allergy season.[49]

Tylophora (page 196). A climbing vine that grows in India, tylophora has been shown to help treat both allergies and asthma. The dose is around 250 milligrams, one to three times per day.[50]

WEEK 4: LIVE ALLERGY-FREE

At the height of allergy season, you should be doing all you can to keep your current allergy symptoms at bay as well as planning ahead for next year's allergy season. The types of remedies you try—and the dosages—will depend on your individual symptoms and the degree of your allergies. If you have a number of allergies, or if your allergies are particularly stubborn, in addition to following the lifestyle recommendations of Weeks 1 through 3, you will probably need to kick things up a notch, perhaps with SLIT.

Phase 1: Control Persistent Symptoms Using Natural Supplements

If your allergy symptoms have persisted after you have employed the basic supplements recommended during Week 3, you can try some other natural remedies with antiallergy effects. As was the case with the herbs, if you find that you have to take several different supplements, you may want to reduce the number of pills you need to swallow by looking for a supplement that combines a few different remedies. The best antiallergy supplements include the following. (For detailed information on these supplements, including side effects and warnings, see Chapter 11.)

Bromelain (see page 170). The usual dose is 3,000 milk clotting units (MCU), three times a day for a few days, then a maintenance dose of 2,000 MCU three times a day.

Coenzyme Q10 (see page 176). The recommended dose of this powerful antioxidant ranges from 30 to 300 milligrams per day, divided into two or three doses.

Evening primrose (see page 179). The dose ranges from 3 to 6 grams per day.

Magnesium (see page 180). The typical dosage range for magnesium is between 30 and 400 milligrams per day.

N-acetylcysteine (see page 183): In people with allergies and other respiratory conditions, the dose ranges from 600 to 1,500 milligrams per day, taken in three divided doses.

Omega-3 fatty acids (see page 184). I recommend taking about 3 grams each of the omega-3 fatty acids eicosapentaenoic acid (EPA) and docosahexaenoic acid (DHA). You may have to swallow a lot of capsules to get this amount, so look for it in liquid form.

Probiotics (see page 181). I have said it a few times throughout this book: I think that all people should take a probiotic supplement daily. Look for a supplement that provides at least 5 billion CFUs, and switch your brand every once in a while to keep the bacteria colonies fresh.

Pycnogenol (see page 182). For allergies, take 50 milligrams, two times a day. For asthma in children, the daily dose is 1 milligram per pound of body weight, given in two divided doses.

Quercetin (see page 186). For allergies, the dose ranges from 200 to 400 milligrams, three times a day.

Selenium (see page 187). Take about 400 micrograms of this antioxidant per day.

Vitamin E (see page 177). The dose for treating allergies and asthma is 400 international units of a natural supplement containing mixed tocopherols and d-alpha-tocopherol.

Zinc (see page 188). I recommend 10 to 15 milligrams of zinc daily for most people.

Phase 2: Keep Allergy Symptoms at Bay with Homeopathic Remedies

To control any allergy symptoms that persist into the height of allergy season, you can try some homeopathic remedies. I want to start by saying that there are two schools of thought on homeopathy. The first school includes classically trained homeopathic physicians who sit down with patients for detailed interviews to discover all of their individualized, specific symptoms so they can then prescribe very targeted homeopathy. In the second school, there are physicians like myself who prescribe homeopathic remedies acutely, based on current symptoms.

For example, if you come in with runny eyes and an acrid nasal discharge, I may say, "Try *Allium cepa*." That having been said, the following homeopathic remedies are best used to curb existing allergy symptoms or asthma symptoms you know you can expect once the season really ramps up. Here are the best homeopathic remedies for allergies and asthma, along with a list of the specific symptoms they treat.

The standard dosage for acute symptoms is three pellets of 30c every 4 hours until symptoms resolve. Stop using the remedy if you fail to notice any improvement after three doses.[51]

- *Allium cepa*: Hay fever, profusely tearing eyes, irritating and painful nasal discharge that turns skin red
- *Agaricus:* Hay fever, especially with itchy ears and mouth
- *Ammonium carbonicum:* Sneezing at night or in the morning upon waking
- *Apis:* Swelling around the eyes, swollen face that gets better with cold
- *Arsenicum album:* watery, acrid, dripping nose with nasal obstruction; swollen lower eyelids; dry, itchy eczema
- *Arundo mauritanica:* Profuse salivation with rhinitis
- *Blatta orientalis:* Trouble breathing with shortness of breath on exertion, asthma, allergy to mold and mildew

- *Causticum:* Constant desire to clear throat, hoarseness
- *Dulcamara:* Hay fever at the end of summer or beginning of fall
- *Euphrasia officinalis:* Runny nose and profusely watery eyes, burning eyes, sensitivity to light
- *Iodum:* Hay fever with acrid nasal discharge that worsens with heat
- *Kali arsenicosum:* Allergy that gets worse in the cold, asthma that gets worse at night (1:00 to 3:00 a.m.), psoriasis, eczema, burning and itching skin eruptions
- *Kali iodatum:* Swelling of the eyelids, edema of conjunctiva, thick nasal discharge, asthma in the early morning, sinusitis
- *Natrum carbonicum:* Food allergies, especially to milk and dairy; diarrhea
- *Nux vomica:* Sneezing and rhinitis upon waking, hay fever
- *Psorinum:* Hay fever, eczema with itching at night, itching until it bleeds
- *Pulsatilla:* Hay fever with rhinitis, hay fever that gets worse outside and in the evening, greenish nasal discharge
- *Sabadilla:* Hay fever, rhinitis with tremendous sneezing
- *Sanguinaria:* Hay fever; sensitivity to odors and pollens; frequent sneezing; watery rhinitis; burning nose, mouth, and throat; allergic asthma
- *Sticta:* Very stuffy nose with urge to blow that isn't productive, crusting in the nose, nasal obstruction, pain in the nose and forehead, allergic asthma
- *Sulphur:* Red, itchy eyes with the sensation of having sand in the eyes
- *Sulphicum acidum:* Aggravations from fumes or exhaust, asthma from fumes, smoke, or dust
- *Wyethia:* Hay fever; tremendous itching in the nose, throat, or palate; the urge to scratch the tongue

Phase 3: Plan Ahead to Reduce Symptoms During the Next Allergy Season with SLIT

To plan ahead for the next allergy season, you should continue eating well, exercising regularly, and keeping your environment as clean and allergen-free as possible.

You might also start receiving SLIT. Before I start SLIT, I confirm a patient's allergies with a blood test that measures levels of immunoglobulin E against specific allergens, such as pollen, dust.[52] I then custom-compound the SLIT preparation based on each patient's allergies. The first 3 months of SLIT are considered the escalation, or buildup phase; during this time, the dosage of the allergens gradually increases. After 3 months, the maintenance phase begins, and the patient takes the same dose each day.[53]

SLIT is a long-term treatment for allergies, and patients usually take a daily dose for up to 3 years to help their bodies become desensitized to their allergies. The treatment is very safe, and it is convenient; patients can take their treatment at home, instead of having to go to the doctor every week for immunotherapy injections.[54] SLIT is not just an allergy treatment—it has the potential to actually cure a person of his or her allergies. This is done by retraining the immune system to no longer produce elevated levels of IgE when it's exposed to allergens.

In the research community and in clinical practice, SLIT is showing a great deal of promise for the treatment of allergies. In a study published in the *Journal of Allergy and Clinical Immunology: In Practice*, SLIT was found to be a safe and effective treatment for people with respiratory allergies.[55]

Personally, I believe that when SLIT is used correctly and under the guidance of an experienced physician, it can wipe out allergies. SLIT is one of the areas of medicine where we can actually use the word "cure" because it does have the potential to cure, rather than just cover up the symptoms, like conventional allergy medications do.

To summarize, here are the main points of the 4-week Allergy Solution Plan.

Overall, you should incorporate the lifestyle tips you've learned into your everyday routine, including daily physical activity and healthful eating. Ideally, you will start these lifestyle changes a few months before allergy season, but if you're just picking up this book a few weeks before the season starts, that's okay, too.

- Week 1 (2 weeks before allergy season): Clean your in-home air by running an air filter, eliminate your exposure to toxic chemicals, and use air-cleaning houseplants to naturally filter your air.

- Week 2 (1 week before allergy season): Eliminate proinflammatory foods, such as red meat, dairy, and excessive sugar Boost your intake of anti-inflammatory foods, such as flaxseed, cold-water fish, and walnuts, and make sure to drink at least half your body weight in ounces of water every day. Start eating foods rich in quercetin, beta-carotene, and vitamin C. Also start engaging in exercises that boost your energy level and reduce stress, such as yoga and tai chi. If you can, start a meditation program.

- Week 3 (at the start of allergy season): Start taking antiallergy herbs, such as stinging nettle, butterbur, and boswellia as well as basic supplements that boost your health and immunity, like vitamins B_6, B_{12}, and C.

- Week 4 (during allergy season): If your symptoms have persisted despite having incorporated the recommended lifestyle interventions and taking basic supplements or antiallergy herbs, you can start using supplements with allergy-fighting properties and homeopathic remedies that combat your specific allergy symptoms. This is also the time to plan ahead for next allergy season by continuing your healthy exercise and eating plan and, if necessary, starting SLIT to build your allergen tolerance so it is extra strong the following year.

As we draw to a close, you should feel equipped with practical, effective tips that will not only fight your allergies but will also make you healthier, less inflamed, and better armed to stave off some of the other big chronic lifestyle diseases, such as type 2 diabetes, heart disease, and cancer.

My goal as a naturopathic physician and as the author of this book is to help guide you toward living a healthier life free of allergies, and to put you in better shape overall, both physically and mentally, so you have the freedom to pursue all that you enjoy. It's been my pleasure to join you on this journey. May it be just the beginning—not just of an allergy-free season, but of a happier, healthier you.

Acknowledgments

I WOULD LIKE TO SAY THANK YOU to some of the people who played a role in helping me write this book. First, to my very beautiful, very loving, and very supportive wife Missy, words cannot describe how much I love and cherish you. To my children, Illia and Rocco, who are both boundless sources of joy and inspiration. Also to my parents Joe and Alice, and my siblings Charles and Lisa, for their love and encouragement in believing that anything is possible.

I also wish to express my sincere gratitude to my agent Trina Becksted for her tireless work and also for being the one who suggested I write this book! A big thank you to my editor, Lora Sickora, for all her excellent help and guidance though the writing process (not to mention her patience!). And, a very special thank you to Elizabeth Shimer Bowers, as this book simply wouldn't have happened without her help.

I would also like to thank all the staff in my office: Katie, Sanchez, Tami, and Tracey, and the docs, Tamburri, Marchese, Retz, and DiCampli. You are all great people and I appreciate your support, help, and friendship more than you know. I would also like to say thank you to all my friends for making sure there are plenty of fun times. Lastly, a special thanks to friends Brian and Lars for igniting my interest in allergy.

Endnotes

CHAPTER 1

1 "Allergies Getting Worse?" Environmental Protection Agency, February 2011, epa.gov /research/gems/scinews_aeroallergens.htm.

2 L. F. Wang et al., "Serum 25-Hydroxyvitamin D Levels are Lower in Chronic Rhinosinusitis with Nasal Polyposis and Are Correlated with Disease Severity in Taiwanese Patients," *American Journal of Rhinology and Allergy* 27, no. 6 (November–December 2013): e162–65. doi:10.2500/ajra.2013.27.3948.

3 "Trends in Allergic Conditions among Children: United States, 1997–2011," Centers for Disease Control and Prevention, NCHS Data Brief Number 121, May 2013, cdc.gov/nchs /data/databriefs/db121.htm.

4 "Allergy Statistics," American Academy of Allergy, Asthma, and Immunology, aaaai.org /about-the-aaaai/newsroom/allergy-statistics.aspx.

5 "Allergy Facts and Figures," Asthma and Allergy Foundation of America, aafa.org /display.cfm?id=9&sub=36.

6 "Facts and Statistics," Food Allergy Research and Education, foodallergy.org/facts-and -stats.

7 Ibid.

8 C. Hadley, "Food Allergies on the Rise? Determining the Prevalence of Food Allergies, and How Quickly It Is Increasing, Is the First Step in Tackling the Problem," *EMBO Reports* 7, no. 11 (November 2006): 1080–83. ncbi.nlm.nih.gov/pmc/articles/pmc1679775/.

9 "Peanut Allergy," Food Allergy Research and Education, foodallergy.org/allergens /peanut-allergy.

10 C. Hadley, "Food Allergies on the Rise? Determining the Prevalence of Food Allergies, and How Quickly It Is Increasing, Is the First Step in Tackling the Problem," *EMBO Reports* 7, no. 11 (November 2006): 1080–83. ncbi.nlm.nih.gov/pmc/articles/pmc1679775/.

11 Ibid.

12 "Facts and Statistics," Food Allergy Research and Education, foodallergy.org/facts-and -stats.

13 C. Hadley, "Food Allergies on the Rise? Determining the Prevalence of Food Allergies, and How Quickly It Is Increasing, Is the First Step in Tackling the Problem," *EMBO Reports* 7, no. 11 (November 2006): 1080–83. ncbi.nlm.nih.gov/pmc/articles/pmc1679775/.

14 "Allergy," National Institutes of Health, nlm.nih.gov/medlineplus/allergy.html.

15 "Allergies," American Academy of Allergy, Asthma, and Immunology, aaaai.org /conditions-and-treatments/allergies.aspx.

16 "Allergy Facts and Figures," Asthma and Allergy Foundation of America, aafa.org /display.cfm?id=9&sub=30.

17 "Allergies across America: The Largest Study of Allergy Testing in the United States," Quest Diagnostics, 2011, questdiagnostics.com/dms/Documents/Other/2011_QD _AllergyReport.pdf.

18 "Trends in Allergic Conditions among Children: United States, 1997–2011," Centers for Disease Control and Prevention, NCHS Data Brief Number 121, May 2013, cdc.gov/nchs /data/databriefs/db121.htm.

19 Ibid.

20 Ibid.

21 Ibid.

22 Ibid.

23 "Allergies across America: The Largest Study of Allergy Testing in the United States," Quest Diagnostics, 2011, questdiagnostics.com/dms/Documents/Other/2011_QD _AllergyReport.pdf.

24 "Prevention of Allergies and Asthma in Children: Tips to Remember," American Academy of Allergy, Asthma, and Immunology, 2013, aaaai.org/conditions-and-treatments/library /at-a-glance/prevention-of-allergies-and-asthma-in-children.aspx.

25 "Asthma," National Institutes of Health, nlm.nih.gov/medlineplus/asthma.html.

26 "Allergies Getting Worse?" Environmental Protection Agency, February 2011, epa.gov /research/gems/scinews_aeroallergens.htm.

27 "Allergies across America: The Largest Study of Allergy Testing in the United States," Quest Diagnostics, 2011, questdiagnostics.com/dms/Documents/Other/2011_QD _AllergyReport.pdf.

28 J. Barta et al., "Air Pollution and Allergens," *Journal of Investigational Allergology and Clinical Immunology* 17, sup. 2 (2007): 3–8.

29 C. Hadley, "Food Allergies on the Rise? Determining the Prevalence of Food Allergies, and How Quickly It Is Increasing, Is the First Step in Tackling the Problem," *EMBO Reports* 7, no. 11 (November 2006): 1080–83. ncbi.nlm.nih.gov/pmc/articles/pmc1679775/.

30 "State of Air 2013: Most Polluted Cities," American Lung Association, stateoftheair .org/2013/city-rankings/mobile/most-polluted-cities.html.

31 "Allergies across America: The Largest Study of Allergy Testing in the United States," Quest Diagnostics, 2011, questdiagnostics.com/dms/Documents/Other/2011_QD _AllergyReport.pdf.

32 "Why Are Allergies Increasing?" UCLA Food and Drug Allergy Care Center, fooddrugallergy.ucla.edu/body.cfm?id=40.

33 "Allergies Getting Worse?" Environmental Protection Agency, February 2011, epa.gov /research/gems/scinews_aeroallergens.htm.

34 "The Rise of Spring Allergies: Fact or Fiction?" American College of Allergy, Asthma, and Immunology, March 6, 2014, acaai.org/allergist/news/New/Pages /TheRiseofSpringAllergiesFactorFiction.aspx.

35 S. Sausenthaler et al., "Maternal Diet during Pregnancy in Relation to Eczema and Allergic Sensitization in the Offspring at 2 y of Age," *The American Journal of Clinical Nutrition* 85, no. 2 (February 2007): 530–37, ajcn.nutrition.org/content/85/2/530.full.

36 E. Maslova et al., "Consumption of Artificially-Sweetened Soft Drinks in Pregnancy and Risk of Child Asthma and Allergic Rhinitis," *PLOS ONE* 8, no. 2 (2013): e57261. doi:10.1371 /journal.pone.0057261.

37 M. Cantorna et al., "Vitamin D Status, 1,25-Dihydroxyvitamin D_3, and the Immune System," *The American Journal of Clinical Nutrition* 80, no. 6 (December 2004): 1717S–1720S, ajcn.nutrition.org/content/80/6/1717S.full.

38 L. F. Wang et al., "Serum 25-Hydroxyvitamin D Levels are Lower in Chronic Rhinosinusitis with Nasal Polyposis and Are Correlated with Disease Severity in Taiwanese Patients," *American Journal of Rhinology and Allergy* 27, no. 6 (November– December 2013): e162-65. doi:10.2500/ajra.2013.27.3948.

CHAPTER 2

1 G. D'Amato et al., "Environmental Risk Factors and Allergic Bronchial Asthma," *Clinical and Experimental Allergy* 35, no. 9 (September 2005): 1113–24.

2 "The International Scientific Forum on Home Hygiene. Activity Review 2013," Home Hygiene and Health, ifh-homehygiene.org/public-leaflet/international-scientific-forum -home-hygiene-activity-review-2013.

3 O. Gruzieva et al., "Traffic-Related Air Pollution and Development of Allergic Sensitization in Children during the First 8 Years of Life," *Journal of Allergy and Clinical Immunology* 129, no. 1 (January 2012): 240–46. doi:10.1016/j.jaci.2011.11.001.

4 E. Levetin et al., "Environmental Contributions to Allergic Disease," *Current Allergy and Asthma Reports* 1, no .6 (November 2001): 506–14.

5 "Air Pollution and Allergies: A Connection?" Medicinenet.com, March 2007, medicinenet .com/script/main/art.asp?articlekey=17112.

6 D. Jenerowicz et al., "Environmental Factors and Allergic Diseases," *Annals of Agricultural and Environmental Medicine* 19, no. 3 (2012): 475–81.

7 G. D'Amato, "Effects of Climactic Changes and Urban Air Pollution on the Rising Trends of Respiratory Allergy and Asthma," *Multidisciplinary Respiratory Medicine* 6, no. 1 (2011): 28–37.

8 "Air Pollution and Allergies: A Connection?" Medicinenet.com, March 2007, medicinenet .com/script/main/art.asp?articlekey=17112.

9 G. D'Amato, "Outdoor Air Pollution in Urban Areas and Allergic Respiratory Diseases," *Monaldi Archives for Chest Disease* 54, no. 6 (1999): 470–74.

10 "Air Pollution and Allergies: A Connection?" Medicinenet.com, March 2007, medicinenet
    .com/script/main/art.asp?articlekey=17112.

11 "5 Things That Make Your Allergies Worse, HealthyWomen.org, healthywomen.org/print
    /node/9322.

12 "Why Is Allergy Increasing?" Allergy UK, November 2013, allergyuk.org/why-is-allergy
    -increasing.

13 T. Olszak et al., "Microbial Exposure during Early Life Has Persistent Effects on Natural
    Killer T Cell Function," *Science* 336, no. 6080 (April 27, 2012): 489–93.

14 "The Allergic March," World Allergy Organization, September 2007, worldallergy.org
    /professional/allergic_diseases_center/allergic_march.

15 R. Goldberg et al., "Intrauterine Infection and Preterm Delivery," *New England Journal of
    Medicine* 342 (May 18, 2000): 1500–507. doi:10.1056/NEJM200005183422007.

16 "The Allergic March," World Allergy Organization, September 2007, worldallergy.org
    /professional/allergic_diseases_center/allergic_march.

17 J. Davies, "Where Have All the Antibiotics Gone?" *Canadian Journal of Infectious Disease and
    Medical Microbiology* 17, no. 5 (September–October 2006): 287–90.

18 "The International Scientific Forum on Home Hygiene. Activity Review 2013," Home
    Hygiene and Health, ifh-homehygiene.org/public-leaflet/international-scientific-forum
    -home-hygiene-activity-review-2013.

19 Ibid.

20 "Why Is Allergy Increasing?" Allergy UK, November 2013, allergyuk.org/why-is-allergy
    -increasing.

21 D. Blyweiss, "The Silent Killer," *Advanced Natural Medicine Health Newsletter* 2010,
    advancednaturalmedicine.com/heart-health/the-silent-killer.html.

22 F. Sacks, "Ask The Expert: Omega-3 Fatty Acids," Harvard School of Public Health,
    The Nutrition Source. hsph.harvard.edu/nutritionsource/omega-3.

23 Ibid.

24 K. Weaver et al., "Effect of Dietary Fatty Acids on Inflammatory Gene Expression in
    Healthy Humans," *The Journal of Biological Chemistry* 284, no. 23 (June 5, 2009): 15400–407.

25 "Sugar 101," American Heart Association, 2014, heart.org/HEARTORG/GettingHealthy
    /NutritionCenter/Sugars-101_UCM_306024_Article.jsp.

26 "The Pancreas and Pancreatitis," *MIMS*, mims.co.uk/news/882288/Pancreas-Pancreatitis.

27 M. Abhilash et al., "Long-Term Consumption of Aspartame and Brain Antioxidant Defense
    Status," *Drug and Chemical Toxicology* 36, no. 2 (April 2013): 135–40. doi:10.3109/01480545.201
    2.658403.

28 J. M. Mercola, "Aspartame: Is This FDA-Approved Sweetener Causing Brain Damage?",
    March 24, 2012, articles.mercola.com/sites/articles/archive/2012/03/24/aspartame
    -affects-brain-health.aspx.

29 "Food Additive Intolerance," American College of Allergy, Asthma, and Immunology,
    2012, acaai.org/allergist/allergies/types/food-allergies/types/pages/food-additive
    -intolerance.aspx.

30 A. Aubrey, "Almost 500 Foods Contain the 'Yoga Mat' Compound. Should We Care?"
    National Public Radio, March 6, 2014, npr.org/blogs/thesalt/2014/03/06/286886095/almost
    -500-foods-contain-the-yoga-mat-compound-should-we-care-keep.

31 "Food Additives," Asthma and Allergy Foundation of America, 2005, aafa.org/display
    .cfm?id=9&sub=20&cont=285.

32 "Food Additive Intolerance," American College of Allergy, Asthma, and Immunology,
    2012, acaai.org/allergist/allergies/types/food-allergies/types/pages/food-additive
    -intolerance.aspx.

33 "Trans Fats," American Heart Association, 2014, heart.org/HEARTORG/GettingHealthy
    /FatsAndOils/Fats101/Trans-Fats_UCM_301120_Article.jsp.

34 L. G. Wood et al., "A High-Fat Challenge Increases Airway Inflammation and Impairs
    Bronchodilator Recovery in Asthma," *Journal of Allergy and Clinical Immunology* 127, no. 5
    (May 2011): 1133–40. doi:10.1016/j.jaci.2011.01.036.

35 S. Sausenthaler et al., "Maternal Diet during Pregnancy in Relation to Eczema and Allergic
    Sensitization in the Offspring at 2 y of Age," *The American Journal of Clinical Nutrition* 85,
    no. 2 (February 2007): 530–37. ajcn.nutrition.org/content/85/2/530.full.

36 "Food for Thought: Preventing Food Allergies," Kids with Food Allergies.org, December 2013, kidswithfoodallergies.org/resourcespre.php?id=108.

37 "Pregnancy and Peanuts: The End of the Avoidance Theory," Boston Children's Hospital, December 2013, childrenshospital.org/health-topics/thriving/2013/december-2013/12-23 -2013-peanuts-and-pregnancy.

38 S. Sausenthaler et al., "Maternal Diet during Pregnancy in Relation to Eczema and Allergic Sensitization in the Offspring at 2 y of Age," *The American Journal of Clinical Nutrition* 85, no. 2 (February 2007): 530–37. ajcn.nutrition.org/content/85/2/530.full.

39 E. Maslova et al., "Consumption of Artificially-Sweetened Soft Drinks in Pregnancy and Risk of Child Asthma and Allergic Rhinitis," *PLOS ONE* 8, no. 2 (2013): e57261. doi:10.1371 /journal.pone.0057261.

40 M. Frieri et al., "Vitamin D Deficiency as a Risk Factor for Allergic Disorders and Immune Mechanisms," *Allergy and Asthma Proceedings* 32, no. 6 (November–December 2011): 438–44. doi:10.2500/aap.2011.32.3485.

41 "Increasing Rates of Allergies and Asthma," American Academy of Allergy, Asthma, and Immunology, 2014, aaaai.org/conditions-and-treatments/library/allergy-library /prevalence-of-allergies-and-asthma.aspx.

42 J. W. Jung et al., "Allergic Rhinitis and Serum 25-Hydroxyvitamin D Level in Korean Adults," *Annals of Allergy, Asthma, and Immunology* 111, no. 5 (November 2013): 352–57. doi:10.1016/j.anai.2013.08.018.

43 M. Frieri et al., "Vitamin D Deficiency as a Risk Factor for Allergic Disorders and Immune Mechanisms," *Allergy and Asthma Proceedings* 32, no. 6 (November–December 2011): 438–44. doi:10.2500/aap.2011.32.3485.

44 J. Arndt et al., "Stress and Atopic Dermatitis," *Current Allergy and Asthma Reports* 8, no. 4 (July 2008): 312–17.

45 M. Gauci et al., "A Minnesota Multiphasic Personality Inventory Profile of Women with Allergic Rhinitis," *Psychosomatic Medicine* 55, no. 6 (November–December 1993): 533–40.

46 J. K. Kiecolt–Glaser et al., "How Stress and Anxiety Can Alter Immediate and Late Phase Skin Test Responses in Allergic Rhinitis," *Psychoneuroendocrinology* 34, no. 5 (June 2009): 670–80. doi:10.1016/j.psyneuen.2008.11.010.

47 Ibid.

48 "9 Habits That Make Allergies Worse," *Prevention*, 2014, prevention.com/health/health -concerns/9-habits-make-allergies-worse.

49 "A Review of the Impact of Climate Variability and Change on Aeroallergens and Their Associated Effects," United States Environmental Protection Agency, July 2009, cfpub.epa .gov/ncea/cfm/recordisplay.cfm?deid=190306.

50 "Asthma, Respiratory Allergies and Airway Diseases, and Climate Change," National Institute of Environmental Health Sciences, March 2013, niehs.nih.gov/research /programs/geh/climatechange/health_impacts/asthma/index.cfm.

51 S. Li et al., "An Australian National Panel Study of Diurnal Temperature Range and Children's Respiratory Health," *Annals of Allergy, Asthma, and Immunology* 112, no. 4 (April 2014): 348–53.e1–8. doi:10.1016/j.anai.2014.01.007.

52 C. Hadley, "Food Allergies on the Rise? Determining the Prevalence of Food Allergies, and How Quickly It Is Increasing, Is the First Step in Tackling the Problem," *EMBO Reports* 7, no.11 (November 2006):1080–83. ncbi.nlm.nih.gov/pmc/articles/pmc1679775/.

53 V. Mahillon et al., "High Incidence of Sensitization to Ornamental Plants in Allergic Rhinitis," *Allergy* 61, no. 19 (September 2006): 1138–40.

CHAPTER 3

1 J. Rao et al., "Dermatologic Manifestations of Gastrointestinal Disease," Medscape.com, November 2013, emedicine.medscape.com/article/1093801-overview.

2 "Frequently Asked Questions," American College of Allergy, Asthma, and Immunology, 2010, acaai.org/allergist/resources/pages/frequently-asked-questions.aspx.

3 "Food Allergies," The Nemours Foundation, November 2011, kidshealth.org/teen/food _fitness/nutrition/food_allergies.html.

4 Ibid.

5 "Allergic Reactions: Tips to Remember," American Academy of Allergy, Asthma, and Immunology, 2013, aaaai.org/conditions-and-treatments/library/at-a-glance/allergic -reactions.aspx.

6 "IgE's Role in Allergic Asthma," Asthma and Allergy Foundation of America, 2005, aafa
   .org/display.cfm?id=8&sub=16&cont=54.

7 Ibid.

8 P.M. Ehrlich and E.S. Bowers, *Teen Guides: Living with Allergies* (New York: Facts on File,
   2008).

9 "IgE's Role in Allergic Asthma," Asthma and Allergy Foundation of America, 2005, aafa
   .org/display.cfm?id=8&sub=16&cont=54.

10 "Frequently Asked Questions," American College of Allergy, Asthma, and Immunology,
   2010, acaai.org/allergist/resources/pages/frequently-asked-questions.aspx.

11 "Food Allergies," The Nemours Foundation, November 2011, kidshealth.org/teen/food
   _fitness/nutrition/food_allergies.html.

12 "Food Allergies," The Nemours Foundation, November 2011, kidshealth.org/teen/food
   _fitness/nutrition/food_allergies.html.

13 "Allergies: Nothing to Sneeze At," The University of Illinois McKinley Health Center, 2011,
   mckinley.illinois.edu/handouts/allergies.htm.

14 "Food Allergies," The Nemours Foundation, November 2011, kidshealth.org/teen/food
   _fitness/nutrition/food_allergies.html.

15 "FPIES: Food Protein Induced Enterocolitis Syndrome," Kids with Food Allergies.org,
   February 2008, kidswithfoodallergies.org/resourcespre.php?id=99.

16 "Blood Test: Allergen-Specific Immunoglobulin E (IgE)," The Nemours Foundation,
   February 2011, kidshealth.org/parent/system/medical/test_ige.html.

17 Ibid.

18 Ibid.

19 "Allergies: Nothing to Sneeze At," The University of Illinois McKinley Health Center, 2011,
   mckinley.illinois.edu/handouts/allergies.htm.

20 "How to Use a Rotation Diet," FoodAllergy.org, 2007, food-allergy.org/rotation.html.

21 "Food Allergies," The Nemours Foundation, November 2011, kidshealth.org/teen/food
   _fitness/nutrition/food_allergies.html.

22 "Sublingual Immunotherapy," The Johns Hopkins Sinus Center, 2008, hopkinsmedicine
   .org/sinus/allergy/sublingual_immunotherapy.html.

23 "Frequently Asked Questions," American College of Allergy, Asthma, and Immunology,
   2010, acaai.org/allergist/resources/pages/frequently-asked-questions.aspx.

24 "Food Allergies," The Nemours Foundation, November 2011, kidshealth.org/teen/food
   _fitness/nutrition/food_allergies.html.

CHAPTER 4

1 "Foods That Aggravate Allergies and Foods That Fight Allergies," AchooAllergy.com, June
   2007, achooallergy.com/foods-aggravate-fight-allergies.asp.

2 "Pollen and Mold Counts," Asthma and Allergy Foundation of America, 2005, aafa.org
   /display.cfm?id=9&sub=19&cont=264.

3 Ibid.

4 P.M. Ehrlich and E.S. Bowers, *Teen's Guides: Living with Allergies*. New York: Facts on File,
   2008.

5 "Pollen and Mold Counts," Asthma and Allergy Foundation of America, acaai.org/display
   .cfm?id=9&sub=19&cont=264.

6 P.M. Ehrlich and E.S. Bowers, *Teen's Guides: Living with Allergies*. New York: Facts on File,
   2008.

7 "Rhinitis Overview," American Academy of Allergy, Asthma, and Immunology, 2014,
   aaaai.org/conditions-and-treatments/allergies/rhinitis.aspx.

8 "Pollen and Mold Counts," Asthma and Allergy Foundation of America, acaai.org/display
   .cfm?id=9&sub=19&cont=264.

9 P.M. Ehrlich and E.S. Bowers, *Teen's Guides: Living with Allergies*. New York: Facts on File,
   2008.

10 "Pollen and Mold Counts," Asthma and Allergy Foundation of America, 2005, aafa.org
   /display.cfm?id=9&sub=19&cont=264.

11 Ibid.

12 P.M. Ehrlich and E.S. Bowers, *Teen's Guides: Living with Allergies*. New York: Fact on File, 2008.

13 "Pet Allergy Overview," American Academy of Allergy, Asthma, and Immunology, 2014, aaaai.org/conditions-and-treatments/allergies/pet-allergy.aspx.

14 "Rhinitis Overview," American Academy of Allergy, Asthma, and Immunology, 2014, acaai.org/conditions-and-treatments/allergies/rhinitus.aspx.

15 "Pollen and Mold Counts," Asthma and Allergy Foundation of America, 2005, aafa.org /display.cfm?id=9&sub=19&cont=264.

16 "Pet Allergy Overview," American Academy of Allergy, Asthma, and Immunology, 2014, aaaai.org/conditions-and-treatments/allergies/pet-allergy.aspx.

17 Ibid.

18 G. Roberts et al., "Horse Allergy in Children," *BMJ* 321, no. 7256 (July 29, 2000): 286–87.

19 Ibid.

20 "House Dust Allergy," American College of Allergy, Asthma, and Immunology, 2010, acaai.org/allergist/allergies/types/dust-allergy-information/pages/default.aspx.

21 Ibid.

22 Ibid.

23 Ibid.

24 "Skin Allergy Overview," American Academy of Allergy, Asthma, and Immunology, 2014, aaaai.org/conditions-and-treatments/allergies/skin-allergy.aspx.

25 "Allergic Conjunctivitis," National Institutes of Health, May 2014, nlm.nih.gov /medlineplus/ency/article/001031.htm.

26 P.M. Ehrlich and E.S. Bowers, *Teen's Guides: Living with Allergies*. New York: Facts on File, 2008.

27 "Skin Allergy Overview," American Academy of Allergy, Asthma, and Immunology, 2014, aaaai.org/conditions-and-treatments/allergies/skin-allergy.aspx.

28 Ibid.

29 Ibid.

30 Ibid.

31 P.M. Ehrlich and E.S. Bowers, *Teen's Guides: Living with Allergies*. New York: Facts on File, 2008.

32 "House Dust Allergy,"American College of Allergy, Asthma, and Immunology, 2010, acaai.org/allergist/allergies/types/dust-allergy-information/pages/default.aspx.

33 P.M. Ehrlich and E.S. Bowers, *Teen's Guides: Living with Allergies*. New York: Facts on File, 2008.

34 "House Dust Allergy," American College of Allergy, Asthma, and Immunology, 2010, acaai.org/allergist/allergies/types/dust-allergy-information/pages/default.aspx.

35 J. B. Price et al., "IgE against Bed Bug (Cimex lectularius) Allergens Is Common among Adults Bitten by Bed Bugs," *Journal of Allergy and Clinical Immunology* 129, no. 3 (March 2012): 863–65.e2. doi:10.1016/j.jaci.2012.01.034.

36 P.M. Ehrlich and E.S. Bowers, *Teen's Guides: Living with Allergies*. New York: Facts on File, 2008.

37 "Cockroach Allergy Information," American College of Allergy, Asthma, and Immunology, 2010, acaai.org/allergist/allergies/types/pages/cockroach-allergies.aspx.

38 Ibid.

39 P.M. Ehrlich and E.S. Bowers, *Teen's Guides: Living with Allergies*. New York: Facts on File, 2008.

40 "Peanut Allergy," Food Allergy Research and Education, 2014, foodallergy.org/allergens /peanut-allergy.

41 Ibid.

42 Ibid.

43 P.M. Ehrlich and E.S. Bowers, *Teen's Guides: Living with Allergies*. New York: Facts on File, 2008.

44 "Peanut Allergy," Food Allergy Research and Education, 2014, foodallergy.org/allergens /peanut-allergy.

45 Ibid.

46 "Tree Nut Allergies," Food Allergy Research and Education, 2014, foodallergy.org /allergens/tree-nut-allergy.

47 Ibid.

48 Ibid.

49 "Milk Allergy," Food Allergy Research and Education, 2014, foodallergy.org/allergens /milk-allergy.

50 Ibid.

51 Ibid.

52 "Egg Allergy," Food Allergy Research and Education, 2014, foodallergy.org/allergens/egg -allergy.

53 Ibid.

54 Ibid.

55 "Soy Allergy," Food Allergy Research and Education, 2014, foodallergy.org/allergens/soy -allergy.

56 "Allergic Conjunctivitis," National Institutes of Health, May 2014, nlm.nih.gov /medlineplus/ency/article/001031.htm.

57 "Soy Allergy," Food Allergy Research and Education, 2014, foodallergy.org/allergens/soy -allergy.

58 Ibid.

59 "Shellfish Allergy," American College of Allergy, Asthma, and Immunology, 2010, acaai .org/allergist/allergies/types/food-allergies/types/pages/shellfish-allergy.aspx.

60 "Fish Allergy," Food Allergy Research and Education, 2014, foodallergy.org/allergens /fish-allergy.

61 "Shellfish Allergy," American College of Allergy, Asthma, and Immunology, 2010, acaai .org/allergist/allergies/types/food-allergies/types/pages/shellfish-allergy.aspx.

62 Ibid.

63 Ibid.

64 "Wheat Allergy," Food Allergy Research and Education, 2014, foodallergy.org/allergens /wheat-allergy.

65 Ibid.

66 Ibid.

67 "Corn Allergy," American College of Allergy, Asthma, and Immunology, 2010, acaai.org /allergist/allergies/Types/food-allergies/types/Pages/corn-allergy.aspx.

68 Ibid.

69 Ibid.

CHAPTER 5

1 "Quercetin," University of Maryland Medical Center, May 2013, umm.edu/health /medical/altmed/supplement/quercetin.

2 Ibid.

3 Ibid.

4 S. R. Naik, "Inflammation, Allergy, and Asthma, Complex Immune Origin Diseases: Mechanisms and Therapeutic Agents," *Recent Patents on Inflammation and Allergy Drug Discovery* 7, no. 1 (January 1, 2013): 62–95.

5 Ibid.

6 E. Moilanen, "Two Faces of Inflammation: An Immunopharmacological View," *Basic and Clinical Pharmacology and Toxicology* 114, no. 1 (January 2014): 2–6.

7 S. R. Naik, "Inflammation, Allergy, and Asthma, Complex Immune Origin Diseases: Mechanisms and Therapeutic Agents," *Recent Patents on Inflammation and Allergy Drug Discovery* 7, no. 1 (January 1, 2013): 62–95.

8 "Phytochemicals, Antioxidants, and Omega-3 Fatty Acids," Stanford Medicine, 2014, cancer.stanford.edu/information/nutritionAndCancer/reduceRisk/phyto.htm.

9 M. Schatz et al., "Overweight/Obesity and Risk of Seasonal Asthma Exacerbations," *Journal of Allergy and Clinical Immunology: In Practice* 1, no. 6 (November–December 2013): 618–22. doi:10.1016/j.jaip.2013.07.009.

10 "Chronic Inflammation and Chronic Disease," AchooAllergy.com, February 2007, achooallergy.com/chronic-inflammation-disease.asp.

11 S. R. Naik, "Inflammation, Allergy, and Asthma, Complex Immune Origin Diseases: Mechanisms and Therapeutic Agents," *Recent Patents on Inflammation and Allergy Drug Discovery* 7, no. 1 (January 2013): 62–95.

12 "What Is Inflammation? What Causes Inflammation?" *Medical News Today*, May 2014, medicalnewstoday.com/articles/248423.php.

13 R. N. Dubois et al., "Cyclooxygenase in Biology and Disease," *FASEB Journal* 12, no. 12 (September 1998): 1063–73.

14 "Inflammation," November 2013, users.rcn.com/jkimball.ma.ultranet/BiologyPages/I /Inflammation.html.

15 M. Shih, Biocarta, "Cytokines and Inflammatory Response," biocarta.com/pathfiles /h_inflampathway.asp.

16 "Inflammation," November 2013, users.rcn.com/jkimball.ma.ultranet/BiologyPages/I /Inflammation.html.

17 "Interleukin-6—What is Interleukin-6?" News-Medical.net, 2014, news-medical.net /health/Interleukin-6-What-is-Interleukin-6.aspx.

18 P.M. Ehrlich and E.S. Bowers, *Teen's Guides: Living with Allergies*. New York: Facts on File, 2008.

19 E. Moilanen, "Two Faces of Inflammation: An Immunopharmacological View," *Basic and Clinical Pharmacology and Toxicology* 114, no .1 (January 2014): 2–6.

20 Ibid.

21 "What Is Inflammation? What Causes Inflammation?" *Medical News Today*, May 2014, medicalnewstoday.com/articles/248423.php.

22 "Natural Killer Cell," *Science Daily*, 2014, sciencedaily.com/articles/n/natural_killer_cell .htm.

23 S. R. Naik, "Inflammation, Allergy, and Asthma, Complex Immune Origin Diseases: Mechanisms and Therapeutic Agents," *Recent Patents on Inflammation and Allergy Drug Discovery* 7, no. 1 (January 2013): 62–95.

24 Ibid.

25 Ibid.

26 "Chronic Inflammation and Chronic Disease," AchooAllergy.com, February 2007, achooallergy.com/chronic-inflammation-disease.asp.

27 G. W. Canonica and E. Compalati, "Minimal Persistent Inflammation in Allergic Rhinitis: Implications for Current Treatment Strategies," *Clinical and Experimental Immunology* 158, no. 3 (December 2009): 260–71. doi:10.1111/j.1365-2249.2009.04017.x.

28 P. J. Barnes, "Pathophysiology of Allergic Inflammation," *Immunological Reviews* 242, no. 1 (July 2011): 31–50.

29 S. R. Naik, "Inflammation, Allergy, and Asthma, Complex Immune Origin Diseases: Mechanisms and Therapeutic Agents," *Recent Patents on Inflammation and Allergy Drug Discovery* 7, no. 1 (January 2013): 62–95.

30 "Immune Response," The National Institutes of Health, Medline.com, May 2012, nlm.nih .gov/medlineplus/ency/article/000821.htm.

31 "Neutrophil," *Encyclopedia Britannica*, britannica.com/EBchecked/topic/410999 /neutrophil.

32 "Eosinophil Count—Absolute," National Institutes of Health, Medline.com, May 2014, nlm.nih.gov/medlineplus/ency/article/003649.htm.

33 "Immune Response," The National Institutes of Health, Medline.com, May 2012, nlm.nih .gov/medlineplus/ency/article/000821.htm.

34 B. Ozben and O. Erdogan, "The Role of Inflammation and Allergy in Acute Coronary Syndromes," *Inflammation and Allergy-Drug Targets* 7, no. 3 (September 2008): 136–44.

35 P. J. Barnes, "Pathophysiology of Allergic Inflammation," *Immunological Reviews* 242, no. 1 (July 2011): 31–50.

36 S. Baumann et al., "Obesity: A Promoter of Allergy?" *International Archives of Allergy and Immunology* 162, no. 3 (2013): 205–13. doi:10.1159/000353972.

37 Ibid.

38 Ibid.

39 M. Schatz et al., "Overweight/Obesity and Risk of Seasonal Asthma Exacerbations," *Journal of Allergy and Clinical Immunology: In Practice* 1, no. 6 (November–December 2013): 618–22. doi:10.1016/j.jaip.2013.07.009.

40   N. M. Johannsen et al., "Association of White Blood Cell Subfraction Concentration with Fitness and Fatness," *British Journal of Sports Medicine* 44, no. 8 (June 2010): 588–93. doi:10.1136/bjsm.2008.050682.

41   S. Baumann et al., "Obesity: A Promoter of Allergy?" *International Archives of Allergy and Immunology* 162, no. 3 (2013): 205–13. doi:10.1159/000353972.

42   Ibid.

43   "Chronic Inflammation and Chronic Disease," AchooAllergy.com, February 2007, achooallergy.com/chronic-inflammation-disease.asp.

44   "What Is Inflammation? What Causes Inflammation?" *Medical News Today,* May 2014, medicalnewstoday.com/articles/248423.php.

45   Ibid.

46   Ibid.

47   Ibid.

48   "Natural Killer Cell," *Science Daily,* 2014, sciencedaily.com/articles/n/natural_killer_cell .htm.

49   S. R. Naik, "Inflammation, Allergy, and Asthma, Complex Immune Origin Diseases: Mechanisms and Therapeutic Agents," *Recent Patents on Inflammation and Allergy Drug Discovery* 7, no. 1 (January 2013): 62–95.

50   M. Wilders-Truchnig et al., "IgG Antibodies against Food Antigens are Correlated with Inflammation and Intima Media Thickness in Obese Juveniles," *Experimental and Clinical Endocrinology and Diabetes* 116, no. 4 (April 2008): 241–45.

51   Ibid.

52   G. W. Canonica and E. Compalati, "Minimal Persistent Inflammation in Allergic Rhinitis: Implications for Current Treatment Strategies," *Clinical and Experimental Immunology* 158, no. 3 (December 2009): 260–71. doi:10.1111/j.1365-2249.2009.04017.x.

53   Ibid.

54   "Leaky Gut Syndrome: Allergies," leakygut.co.uk/Allergies.htm.

55   M. Hyman, "Are Your Food Allergies Making You Fat?" 2014, drhyman.com/blog/2010 /04/20/are-your-food-allergies-making-you-fat/.

56   P. Cani et al., "Changes in Gut Microbiota Control Metabolic Endotoxemia-Induced Inflammation in High-Fat Diet–Induced Obesity and Diabetes in Mice," *Diabetes* 57, no .6 (June 2008): 1470–81. doi:10.2337/db07-1403.

57   Ibid.

58   S. Bischoff et al., "Food Allergy and the Gastrointestinal Tract," *Current Opinion in Gastroenterology* 20, no. 2 (March 2004): 156–61.

59   C. DeFilipo et al., "Impact of Diet in Shaping Gut Microbiota Revealed by a Comparative Study in Children from Europe and Rural Africa," *Proceedings of the National Academy of Sciences of the United States of America* 107, no. 33 (August 17, 2010): 14691–96. doi:10.1073 /pnas.1005963107.

60   L. Van der Poel et al., "Food Allergy Epidemic: Is It Only a Western Phenomenon?" *Current Allergy and Clinical Immunology* 22, no. 3 (August 2009): 121–26.

61   M. Hyman, "Are Your Food Allergies Making You Fat?" 2014, drhyman.com/blog/2010 /04/20/are-your-food-allergies-making-you-fat/.

62   Imayama, Y. et al., "Effects of a Caloric Restriction Weight Loss Diet and Exercise on Inflammatory Biomarkers in Overweight/Obese Postmenopausal Women: A Randomized Controlled Trial," *Cancer Research* 72, no. 9 (May 1, 2012): 2314–26. doi:10.1158/0008-5472. CAN-11-3092.

63   "Allergies, Inflammation, and Weight Control," Food Allergy Research and Education, 2011, food-allergy.org/inflammation.html.

64   "Natural Killer Cell," *Science Daily,* 2014, sciencedaily.com/articles/n/natural_killer_cell .htm.

65   M. Hyman, "Are Your Food Allergies Making You Fat?" 2014, drhyman.com/blog/2010 /04/20/are-your-food-allergies-making-you-fat/.

CHAPTER 6

1   "Link between Omega-3 Fatty Acids and Increased Prostate Cancer Risk Confirmed," Fred Hutchinson Cancer Research Center, *Science Daily,* July 10, 2013, sciencedaily.com /releases/2013/07/130710183637.htm.

2 H. Eyre et al., "Preventing Cancer, Cardiovascular Disease, and Diabetes," *Diabetes Care* 27, no. 7 (July 2004): 1812–24.

3 "Hypothalamus and Aging," Albert Einstein College of Medicine, 2014, einstein.yu.edu /news/releases/894/brain-region-may-hold-key-to-aging/.

4 T. W. McDade et al., "Psychosocial and Behavioral Predictors of Inflammation in Middle-Aged and Older Adults: The Chicago Health, Aging, and Social Relations Study," *Psychosomatic Medicine* 68, no. 3 (May–Jun 2006): 376–81.

5 J. Woods et al., "Exercise, Inflammation, and Aging," *Aging and Disease* 3, no. 1 (February 2012): 130–40.

6 T. W. McDade et al., "Psychosocial and Behavioral Predictors of Inflammation in Middle-Aged and Older Adults: The Chicago Health, Aging, and Social Relations Study," *Psychosomatic Medicine* 68, no. 3 (May–Jun 2006): 376–81.

7 J. Woods et al., "Exercise, Inflammation, and Aging," *Aging and Disease* 3, no. 1 (February 2012): 130–40.

8 T. N Akbaraly, "Chronic Inflammation as a Determinant of Future Aging Phenotypes," *CMAJ* 185, no. 16 (November 5, 2013): E763–70. doi:10.1503/cmaj.122072.

9 T. W. McDade et al., "Psychosocial and Behavioral Predictors of Inflammation in Middle-Aged and Older Adults: The Chicago Health, Aging, and Social Relations Study," *Psychosomatic Medicine* 68, no. 3 (May–Jun 2006): 376–81.

10 Ibid.

11 Ibid.

12 T. N Akbaraly, "Chronic Inflammation as a Determinant of Future Aging Phenotypes," *CMAJ* 185, no. 16 (November 5, 2013): E763–70. doi:10.1503/cmaj.122072.

13 J. Woods et al., "Exercise, Inflammation, and Aging," *Aging and Disease* 3, no. 1 (February 2012): 130–40.

14 Ibid.

15 Ibid.

16 "Hypothalamus and Aging," Albert Einstein College of Medicine, 2014, einstein.yu.edu /news/releases/894/brain-region-may-hold-key-to-aging/.

17 Ibid.

18 "What is Metabolic Syndrome?" National Heart, Lung and Blood Institute, November 2011, nhlbi.nih.gov/health/health-topics/topics/ms/.

19 "Hypothalamus and Aging," Albert Einstein College of Medicine, 2014, einstein.yu.edu /news/releases/894/brain-region-may-hold-key-to-aging/.

20 P. Tak et al., "NF-KB: A Key Role in Inflammatory Diseases," *Journal of Clinical Investigation* 107, no. 1 (January 1, 2001): 7–11. doi:10.1172/JCI11830.

21 "Antioxidants and Free Radicals," Rice University, June 1996, rice.edu/~jenky/sports /antiox.html.

22 N. Khansari et al., "Chronic Inflammation and Oxidative Stress as a Major Cause of Age-Related Diseases and Cancer," *Recent Patents on Inflammatory and Allergy Drug Discovery* 3, no. 1 (January 2009): 73–80.

23 J. Woods et al., "Exercise, Inflammation, and Aging," *Aging and Disease* 3, no. 1 (February 2012): 130–40.

24 "Septic Shock," National Institutes of Health, Medline.com, May 2014, nlm.nih.gov /medlineplus/ency/article/000668.htm.

25 "T Cells," National Institute of Allergy and Infectious Diseases, October 2008, niaid.nih .gov/topics/immunesystem/immunecells/pages/tcells.aspx.

26 D. H. Josephs et al., "Epidemiological Associations of Allergy, IgE, and Cancer," *Clinical and Experimental Allergy* 43, no. 10 (October 2013): 1110–23. doi:10.1111/cea.12178.

27 J. Woods et al., "Exercise, Inflammation, and Aging," *Aging and Disease* 3, no. 1 (February 2012): 130–40.

28 "Key Gene Found Responsible for Chronic Inflammation, Accelerated Aging and Cancer," NYU Langone, May 2012, communications.med.nyu.edu/media-relations/news/key-gene -found-responsible-chronic-inflammation-accelerated-aging-and-cancer.

29 "Septic Shock," National Institutes of Health, Medline.com, May 2014, nlm.nih.gov /medlineplus/ency/article/000668.htm.

30 "Key Gene Found Responsible for Chronic Inflammation, Accelerated Aging and Cancer," NYU Langone, May 2012, communications.med.nyu.edu/media-relations/news/key-gene -found-responsible-chronic-inflammation-accelerated-aging-and-cancer.

31 S. K. Mathur, "Allergy and Asthma in the Elderly," *Seminars in Respiratory and Critical Care Medicine* 31, no. 5 (October 2010): 587–95. doi:10.1055/s-0030-1265899.

32 J. M. Pinto, "Rhinitis in the Geriatric Population," *Allergy, Asthma, and Clinical Immunology* 6, no .1 (May 13, 2010):10. doi:10.1186/1710-1492-6-10.

33 S. K. Mathur, "Allergy and Asthma in the Elderly," *Seminars in Respiratory and Critical Care Medicine* 31, no. 5 (October 2010): 587–95. doi:10.1055/s-0030-1265899.

34 J. M. Pinto, "Rhinitis in the Geriatric Population," *Allergy, Asthma, and Clinical Immunology* 6, no .1 (May 13, 2010):10. doi:10.1186/1710-1492-6-10.

35 S. K. Mathur, "Allergy and Asthma in the Elderly," *Seminars in Respiratory and Critical Care Medicine* 31, no. 5 (October 2010): 587–95. doi:10.1055/s-0030-1265899.

36 "Older-Adults and Asthma," Allergy and Asthma Foundation of America, 2005, aafa.org /display.cfm?id=8&sub=17&cont=173.

37 J. Graham, "Allergies—At Your Age?" *Better Homes and Gardens*, 2014, bhg.com/health -family/conditions/allergies/adult-allergies/.

38 M. D. D'Arcy Little, "Allergies in the Aging," *Geriatrics and Aging* 8, no. 5 (2005): 52–53.

39 V. Cardona et al., "Allergic Diseases in the Elderly," *Clinical and Translational Allergy* 1 (2011): 11.

40 "Older-Adults and Asthma," Allergy and Asthma Foundation of America, 2005, aafa.org /display.cfm?id=8&sub=17&cont=173.

41 M. D. D'Arcy Little, "Allergies in the Aging," *Geriatrics and Aging* 8, no. 5 (2005): 52–53.

42 J. M. Pinto, "Rhinitis in the Geriatric Population," *Allergy, Asthma, and Clinical Immunology* 6, no. 1 (May 13, 2010): 10. doi:10.1186/1710-1492-6-10.

43 "Older-Adults and Asthma," Allergy and Asthma Foundation of America, 2005, aafa.org /display.cfm?id=8&sub=17&cont=173.

44 J. Graham, "Allergies—At Your Age?" *Better Homes and Gardens*, 2014, bhg.com/health -family/conditions/allergies/adult-allergies/.

45 S. K. Mathur, "Allergy and Asthma in the Elderly," *Seminars in Respiratory and Critical Care Medicine* 31, no. 5 (October 2010): 587–95. doi:10.1055/s-0030-1265899.

46 J. Graham, "Allergies—At Your Age?" *Better Homes and Gardens*, 2014, bhg.com/health -family/conditions/allergies/adult-allergies/.

47 S. K. Mathur, "Allergy and Asthma in the Elderly," *Seminars in Respiratory and Critical Care Medicine* 31, no. 5 (October 2010): 587–95. doi:10.1055/s-0030-1265899.

48 Ibid.

49 L. Hand et al., "Older Adult Asthma Patients Often Also Have Allergies," *Annals of Allergy, Asthma, and Immunology* 110 (2013): 247–52.

50 P. J. Busse et al., "Characteristics of Allergic Sensitization among Asthmatic Adults Older Than 55 Years: Results from the National Health and Nutrition Examination Survey, 2005-2006," *Annals of Allergy, Asthma, and Immunology* 110, no. 4 (April 2013): 247–52. doi:10.1016/j.anai.2013.01.016.

51 "What Is Inflammation? What Causes Inflammation?" *Medical News Today*, May 2014, medicalnewstoday.com/articles/248423.php.

52 J. Woods et al., "Exercise, Inflammation, and Aging," *Aging and Disease* 3, no. 1 (February 2012): 130–40.

53 Ibid.

54 Ibid.

55 B. J. Niklas, "Exercise Training and Plasma C-Reactive Protein and Interleukin-6 in Elderly People," *Journal of the American Geriatrics Society* 56, no. 11 (November 2008): 2045–52. doi:10.1111/j.1532-5415.2008.01994.x.

56 "Green Tea," University of Maryland Medical Center, July 2013, umm.edu/health/medical /altmed/herb/green-tea.

57 Ibid.

58 S. Y Wu et al., "Green Tea (*Camellia sinensis*) Mediated Suppression of IgE Production by Peripheral Blood Mononuclear Cells of Allergic Asthmatic Humans," *Scandinavian Journal of Immunology* 76, no. 3 (September 2012): 306–10. doi:10.1111/j.1365-3083.2012.02729.x.

59 M. El Assar et al., "Oxidative Stress and Vascular Inflammation in Aging," *Free Radical Biology in Medicine* 65 (December 2013): 380–401. doi:10.1016/j.freeradbiomed.2013.07.003.

60 M. Masternak et al., "Growth Hormone, Inflammation, and Aging," *Pathobiology of Aging and Age-Related Diseases* (2012): 2. doi:10.3402/pba.v2i0.17293.

61 "Topics of Interest: Calorie Restriction," National Institute on Aging, nia.nih.gov /newsroom/topics/calorie-restriction.

62 J. Woods et al., "Exercise, Inflammation, and Aging," *Aging and Disease* 3, no. 1 (February 2012): 130–40.

63 "Coenzyme Q10," Mayo Clinic, 2014, mayoclinic.org/drugs-supplements/coenzyme-q10 /background/hrb-20059019.

64 Ibid.

CHAPTER 7

1 N. Khansari et al., "Chronic Inflammation and Oxidative Stress as a Major Cause of Age-Related Diseases and Cancer," *Recent Patents on Inflammation and Allergy Drug Discovery* 3, no. 1 (January 2009): 73–80.

2 "Beyond Allergens and Triggers: Getting to the Root Cause of Allergies and Asthma," *Total Health Magazine,* April 2009, totalhealthmagazine.com/articles/allergies-asthma /beyond-allergens-and-triggers-getting-to-the-root-cause-of-allergies-and-asthma.html.

3 "Euphrasia/Eyebright," Herbwisdom.com, 2014, herbwisdom.com/herb-euphrasia.html.

4 M. Gurven et al., "Aging and Inflammation in Two Epidemiological Worlds," *Journals of Gerontology Series A: Biological Sciences and Medical Sciences* 63, no. 2 (February 2008): 196–99.

5 D. Johnson, *The Optimal Health Revolution* (Dallas: BenBella Books, 2009), 38, 39.

6 "What is a C-Reactive Protein (CRP) Blood Test?" MD Junction, May 2014, mdjunction .com/forums/chronic-pain-discussions/general-support/247023-what-is-a-creactive -protein-crp-blood-test.

7 M. Gurven et al., "Aging and Inflammation in Two Epidemiological Worlds," *Journals of Gerontology Series A: Biological Sciences and Medical Sciences* 63, no. 2 (February 2008): 196–99.

8 Ibid.

9 Ibid.

10 Ibid.

11 A. Bhatnagar et al., "Studying Mechanistic Links between Pollution and Heart Disease," *Circulation Research* 99 (2006). 692–705.

12 "Obesity and Overweight," Centers for Disease Control and Prevention, May 2014, cdc.gov/nchs/fastats/obesity-overweight.htm.

13 Ibid.

14 "Overweight and Obesity Statistical Fact Sheet 2013," American Heart Association, heart .org/idc/groups/heart-public/@wcm/@sop/@smd/documents/downloadable/ucm _319588.pdf.

15 A. Ruperez et al., "Genetics of Oxidative Stress in Obesity," *International Journal of Molecular Sciences* 15, no. 2 (February 20, 2014): 3118–44. doi:10.3390/ijms15023118.

16 G. W. Canonica, "Minimal Persistent Inflammation in Allergic Rhinitis: Implications for Current Treatment Strategies," *Clinical and Experimental Immunology* 158, no. 3 (December 2009): 260–71. doi:10.1111/j.1365-2249.2009.04017.x.

17 "Allergies, Inflammation, and Weight Control," Food Allergy Research and Education, 2011, food-allergy.org/inflammation.html.

18 Ibid.

19 Ibid.

20 Ibid.

21 "What is Metabolic Syndrome?" National Heart, Lung, and Blood Institute, November 2011, nhlbi.nih.gov/health/health-topics/topics/ms/.

22 "Physical Activity and Hypokinetic Disease," Western Washington University, wwu.edu /depts/healthyliving/PE511info/infection/Diseases.html.

23 "Heart Disease," Centers for Disease Control and Prevention, May 2014, cdc.gov/nchs /fastats/heart-disease.htm.

24 "Inflammation and Heart Disease," American Heart Association, September 2013, heart .org/HEARTORG/Conditions/Inflammation-and-Heart-Disease_UCM_432150_Article.jsp.

25 "What is Atherosclerosis?" National Heart, Lung, and Blood Institute, July 2011, nhlbi.nih .gov/health/health-topics/topics/atherosclerosis/.

26 "Inflammation and Heart Disease," American Heart Association, September 2013, heart .org/HEARTORG/Conditions/Inflammation-and-Heart-Disease_UCM_432150_Article.jsp.

27 Ibid.

28 J. Kim et al., "Relation between Common Allergic Symptoms and Coronary Heart Disease among NHANES III Participants," *American Journal of Cardiology* 106, no. 7 (October 1, 2010): 984–87. doi:10.1016/j.amjcard.2010.05.029.

29 B. Ozben, "The Role of Inflammation and Allergy in Acute Coronary Syndromes," *Inflammation and Allergy-Drug Targets* 7, no. 3 (September 2008): 136–44.

30 "The Facts about Diabetes: A Leading Cause of Death in the US," National Diabetes Education Program, ndep.nih.gov/diabetes-facts/.

31 H. Cucak et al., "Macrophage Contact Dependent and Independent TLR4 Mechanisms Induce β-Cell Dysfunction and Apoptosis in a Mouse Model of Type 2 Diabetes," *PLOS ONE* 9, no. 3 (March 3, 2014): e90685. doi:10.1371/journal.pone.0090685.

32 C. B. Nemeroff et al., "Differential Responses to Psychotherapy versus Pharmacotherapy in Patients with Chronic Forms of Major Depression and Childhood Trauma," *Proceedings of the National Academy of Sciences of the United States of America* 100, no. 24 (November 25, 2003): 14293–96.

33 "Vitamin C (Ascorbic acid)," University of Maryland Medical Center, June 2013, umm.edu /health/medical/altmed/supplement/vitamin-c-ascorbic-acid.

34 P. S. Marshall et al., "Effects of Seasonal Allergic Rhinitis on Fatigue Levels and Mood," *Psychosomatic Medicine* 64, no. 4 (July–August 2002): 684–91.

35 J. Engelman, "Cytokines—A Missing Link in Internal Diseases?" 2006, serendip .brynmawr.edu/bb/neuro/neuro06/web1/jengelman.html.

36 S. M. Collins et al., "The Putative Role of Inflammation in the Irritable Bowel Syndrome," *Gut* 49 (2001): 743–745. doi:10.1136/gut.49.6.743.

37 "What Is Irritable Bowel Disease?" Everydayhealth.com, 2014, everydayhealth.com /digestive-health/ibs/index.aspx.

38 S. M. Collins et al., "The Putative Role of Inflammation in the Irritable Bowel Syndrome," *Gut* 49 (2001): 743–745. doi:10.1136/gut.49.6.743.

39 E. Isolauri et al., "Food Allergy in Irritable Bowel Syndrome: New Facts and Old Fallacies," *Gut* 53, no. 10 (October 2004): 1391–93.

40 M. C. Tobin et al., "Atopic Irritable Bowel Syndrome: A Novel Subgroup of Irritable Bowel Syndrome with Allergic Manifestations," *Annals of Allergy, Asthma, and Immunology* 100, no. 1 (January 2008): 49–53. doi:10.1016/S1081-1206(10)60404-8.

41 S. Rakoff-Nahoum, "Why Cancer and Inflammation?" *Yale Journal of Biology and Medicine* 79, no. 3–4 (December 2006): 123–30.

42 S. Seethaler, "Molecular Link between Inflammation and Cancer Discovered," University of California, San Diego, January 2007, ucsdnews.ucsd.edu/archive/newsrel/science /cancer07.asp.

43 D. H. Josephs et al., "Epidemiological Associations of Allergy, IgE, and Cancer," *Clinical and Experimental Allergy* 43, no. 10 (October 2013): 1110-23. doi:10.1111/cea.12178.

CHAPTER 8

1 "Stressed in America," American Psychological Association, 2011, apa.org monitor /2011/01/ stressed-america.aspx.

2 N. Vogelzangs et al., "Anxiety Disorders and Inflammation in a Large Adult Cohort," *Translational Psychiatry* 3 (April 23, 2013): e249. doi:10.1038/tp.2013.27.

3 B. Sears, "Anxiety and Omega-3 Fatty Acids," Psychologytoday.com, January 2012, psychologytoday.com/blog/in-the-zone/201201/anxiety-and-omega-3-fatty-acids.

4 Ibid.

5 "What Is Anxiety Disorder?" National Institute of Mental Health, nimh.nih.gov/health /topics/anxiety-disorders/index.shtml.

6 B. Sears, "Anxiety and Omega-3 Fatty Acids," Psychologytoday.com, January 2012, psychologytoday.com/blog/in-the-zone/201201/anxiety-and-omega-3-fatty-acids.

7 "What Is Depression?" National Institute of Mental Health, nimh.nih.gov/health /publications/depression/index.shtml.

8 B. Sears, "Anxiety and Omega-3 Fatty Acids," Psychologytoday.com, January 2012, psychologytoday.com/blog/in-the-zone/201201/anxiety-and-omega-3-fatty-acids.

9 "Q&A on Stress for Adults: How It Affects Your Health and What You Can Do about It," National Institute of Mental Health, nimh.nih.gov/health/publications/stress/index .shtml.

10 Ibid.

11 "Stressed in America," American Psychological Association, 2011, apa.org monitor /2011/01/ stressed-america.aspx.

12 N. Volgelzangs et al., "Anxiety Disorders and Inflammation in a Large Adult Cohort," *Translational Psychiatry* 3 (April 23, 2013): e249. doi:10.1038/tp.2013.27.

13 W. Cole, "Is Your Mood Suffering because Your Brain Is Inflamed?" Mindbodygreen.com, December 2013, mindbodygreen.com/0-12037/is-your-mood-suffering-because-your-brain-is-inflamed.html.

14 B. Sears, "Anxiety and Omega-3 Fatty Acids," *Psychology Today,* January 2012, psychologytoday.com/blog/in-the-zone/201201/anxiety-and-omega-3-fatty-acids.

15 N. D. Powell et al., "Social Stress Up-Regulates Inflammatory Gene Expression in the Leukocyte Transcriptome via β-Adrenergic Induction of Myelopoiesis," *Proceedings of the National Academy of Sciences* 110, no. 41 (October 8, 2013): 16574-9. doi:10.1073/pnas .1310655110.

16 Ibid.

17 "Effects of Chronic Stress Can Be Traced to Your Genes," Ohio State University, November 2013, researchnews.osu.edu/archive/stressgenes.htm.

18 Ibid.

19 N. D. Powell et al., "Social Stress Up-Regulates Inflammatory Gene Expression in the Leukocyte Transcriptome via β-Adrenergic Induction of Myelopoiesis," *Proceedings of the National Academy of Sciences* 110, no. 41 (October 8, 2013): 16574-9. doi:10.1073/pnas .1310655110.

20 "Effects of Chronic Stress Can be Traced to Your Genes," Ohio State University, November 2013, researchnews.osu.edu/archive/stressgenes.htm.

21 S. Cohen et al., "Chronic Stress, Glucocorticoid Receptor Resistance, Inflammation, and Disease Risk," *Proceedings of the National Academy of Sciences of the United States of America* 109, no. 16 (April 17, 2012): 5995–99. doi:10.1073/pnas.1118355109.

22 Ibid.

23 Ibid.

24 "How Stress Influences Disease: Study Reveals Inflammation as the Culprit," Carnegie Mellon University, April 2012, sciencedaily.com/releases/2012/04/120402162546.htm.

25 S. Cohen et al., "Chronic Stress, Glucocorticoid Receptor Resistance, Inflammation, and Disease Risk," *Proceedings of the National Academy of Sciences of the United States of America* 109, no. 16 (April 17, 2012): 5995–99. doi:10.1073/pnas.1118355109.

26 "How Stress Influences Disease: Study Reveals Inflammation as the Culprit," Carnegie Mellon University, April 2012, sciencedaily.com/releases/2012/04/120402162546.htm.

27 "Women and Depression," National Alliance on Mental Illness, October 2009, nami.org /Template.cfm?Section=Women_and_Depression&Template=/ContentManagement /ContentDisplay.cfm&ContentID=89194.

28 N. Vogelzangs et al., "Anxiety Disorders and Inflammation in a Large Adult Cohort," *Translational Psychiatry* 3 (April 23, 2013): e249. doi:10.1038/tp.2013.27.

29 M. Danner et al., "Association between Depression and Elevated C-Reactive Protein," *Psychosomatic Medicine* 65, no. 3 (May–June 2003): 347–56.

30 S. Toker et al., "The Association between Burnout, Depression, Anxiety, and Inflammation Biomarkers: C-Reactive Protein and Fibrinogen in Men and Women," *Journal of Occupational Health Psychology* 10, no 4 (October 2005): 344–62.

31 N. Vogelzangs et al., "Anxiety Disorders and Inflammation in a Large Adult Cohort," *Translational Psychiatry* 3 (April 23, 2013): e249. doi:10.1038/tp.2013.27.

32 "Dwelling on Stressful Events Can Increase Inflammation in the Body, Study Finds," Ohio University, March 2013, ohio.edu/research/communications/zoccola.cfm.

33 D. Johnson, *The Optimal Health Revolution* (Dallas: BenBella Books, 2009), 24.

34 "Dwelling on Stressful Events Can Increase Inflammation in the Body, Study Finds," Ohio University, March 2013, ohio.edu/research/communications/zoccola.cfm.

35 "Depression Increases Stress Inflammation Response," *FuturePundit,* September 2006, futurepundit.com/archives/003698.html.

36 J. Barth et al., "Depression As a Risk Factor for Mortality in Patients with Coronary Heart Disease: A Meta-Analysis," *Psychosomatic Medicine* 66, no. 6 (November–December 2004): 802–13.

37 R. Sansone et al., "Allergic Rhinitis: Relationships with Anxiety and Mood Syndromes," *Innovations in Clinical Neuroscience* 8, no. 7 (July 2011): 12–17.

38 "Vitamin B₆ (Pyridoxine)," University of Maryland Medical Center, June 2013, umm.edu /health/medical/altmed/supplement/vitamin-b6-pyridoxine.

39 Ibid.

40 A. M. Hvas et al., "Vitamin B₆ Level is Associated with Symptoms of Depression," *Psychotherapy and Psychosomatics* 73, no. 6 (November–December 2004): 340–43.

41 R. Sansone et al., "Allergic Rhinitis: Relationships with Anxiety and Mood Syndromes," *Innovations in Clinical Neuroscience* 8, no. 7 (July 2011): 12–17.

42 M. Alevizos, "Stress Triggers Coronary Mast Cells Leading to Cardiac Events," *Annals of Allergy, Asthma & Immunology* 112, no. 4 (April 2014): 309–16. doi:10.1016/j.anai.2013.09.017.

43 R. Sansone et al., "Allergic Rhinitis: Relationships with Anxiety and Mood Syndromes," *Innovations in Clinical Neuroscience* 8, no. 7 (July 2011): 12–17.

44 Ibid.

45 B. Cuffel et al., "Economic Consequences of Comorbid Depression, Anxiety, and Allergic Rhinitis," *Psychosomatics* 40, no. 6 (November–December 1999): 491–96.

46 S. B. Patten et al., "Allergies and Major Depression: A Longitudinal Community Study," *Biopsychosocial Medicine* 3 (January 26, 2009): 3. doi:10.1186/1751-0759-3-3.

47 E. Gada et al., "The Relationship between Asthma and Self-Reported Anxiety in a Predominantly Healthy Adult Population," *Annals of Allergy, Asthma, and Immunology* 112, no. 4 (April 2014): 329–32. doi:10.1016/j.anai.2013.08.027.

48 B. Sears, "Anxiety and Omega-3 Fatty Acids," Psychologytoday.com, January 2012, psychologytoday.com/blog/in-the-zone/201201/anxiety-and-omega-3-fatty-acids.

49 Ibid.

50 L. Buydens-Branchey et al., "Associations between Increases in Plasma n-3 Polyunsaturated Fatty Acids Following Supplementation and Decreases in Anger and Anxiety in Substance Abusers," *Progress in Neuro-Psychopharmacology and Biological Psychiatry* 32, no. 2 (February 15, 2008): 568–75.

51 F. Lespérance et al., "The Efficacy of Omega-3 Supplementation for Major Depression: A Randomized Controlled Trial," *Journal of Clinical Psychiatry* 72, no. 8 (August 2011): 1054– 62. doi:10.4088/JCP.10m05966blu.

52 Y. Osher et al., "Omega-3 Fatty Acids in Depression: A Review of Three Studies." *CNS Neuroscience and Therapeutics* 15, no. 2 (Summer 2009): 128–33.

53 J. K. Kiecolt-Glaser et al., "Omega-3 Supplementation Lowers Inflammation and Anxiety in Medical Students: A Randomized Controlled Trial," *Brain, Behavior, and Immunity* 25, no. 8 (November 2011): 1725–34. doi:10.1016/j.bbi.2011.07.229.

54 Ibid.

55 J. K. Kiecolt-Glaser et al., "Omega-3 Supplementation Lowers Inflammation and Anxiety in Medical Students: A Randomized Controlled Trial," *Brain, Behavior, and Immunity* 25, no. 8 (November 2011): 1725–34. doi:10.1016/j.bbi.2011.07.229.

56 "Impact of Stress," American Psychological Association, 2012, apa.org/news/press /releases/stress/2012/impact.aspx.

57 "Insomnia Information," Stanford University, 1999, stanford.edu/~dement/insomnia.html.

58 "Extent and Health Consequences of Chronic Sleep Loss and Sleep Disorders," National Institutes of Health, 2006, ncbi.nlm.nih.gov/books/NBK19961/.

59 Ibid.

60 W. Cole, "Is Your Mood Suffering because Your Brain is Inflamed?" Mindbodygreen.com, December 2013, mindbodygreen.com/0-12037/is-your-mood-suffering-because-your -brain-is-inflamed.html.

61 G. Tett, "Stressed? It's the New Normal." *FT Magazine,* January 27, 2012. FT.com/cms /s/2/18cc0240-47cc-11e1-b646-00144feabdc0.html#axzz3G2VP1g08.

62 D. Johnson, *The Optimal Health Revolution,* (Dallas: BenBella Books, 2009), 24.

63 J. K. Kiecolt-Glaser et al., "Omega-3 Supplementation Lowers Inflammation and Anxiety in Medical Students: A Randomized Controlled Trial," *Brain, Behavior, and Immunity* 25, no. 8 (November 2011): 1725–34. doi:10.1016/j.bbi.2011.07.229.

CHAPTER 9

1 M. Edelson, "Take Two Carrots and Call Me in the Morning," Hopkins Medicine, Winter 2010, hopkinsmedicine.org/hmn/w10/feature2.cfm.

2 S. Bunyavanich et al., "Peanut, Milk, and Wheat Intake during Pregnancy Is Associated with Reduced Allergy and Asthma in Children," *Journal of Allergy and Clinical Immunology* 133, no. 5 (May 2014): 1373–82. doi:10.1016/j.jaci.2013.11.040.

3 B. Nwaru et al., "Maternal Intake of Fatty Acids during Pregnancy and Allergies in the Offspring," *British Journal of Nutrition* 108, no. 4 (August 2012): 720–32. doi:10.1017 /S0007114511005940.

4 C. Ronduit et al., "Increased Food Diversity in the First Year of Life Is Inversely Associated with Allergic Diseases," *Journal of Allergy and Clinical Immunology* 133, no. 4 (April 2014): 1056–64. doi:10.1016/j.jaci.2013.12.1044.

5 "Allergies, Inflammation, and Weight Control," Food Allergy and Research Education, 2011, food-allergy.org/inflammation.html.

6 "Nonalcoholic Steatohepatitis," National Digestive Diseases Information Clearinghouse, May 2014, digestive.niddk.nih.gov/ddiseases/pubs/nash/.

7 M. Covington, "Omega-3 Fatty Acids," *American Family Physician* 70, no. 1 (July 1, 2004): 133–140.

8 "Licorice," University of Maryland Medical Center, May 2013, umm.edu/health/medical /altmed/herb/licorice.

9 Ibid.

10 M. Saeedi et al., "The Treatment of Atopic Dermatitis with Licorice Gel," *Journal of Dermatological Treatment* 14, no. 3 (September 2003): 153–57.

11 "Balancing Omega-3 and Omega-6?," Dr. Weil.com, February 2007, drweil.com/drw/u /QAA400149/balancing-omega-3-and-omega-6.html.

12 Ibid.

13 Ibid.

14 M. Edelson, "Take Two Carrots and Call Me in the Morning," Hopkins Medicine, Winter 2010, hopkinsmedicine.org/hmn/w10/feature2.cfm.

15 Ibid.

16 Ibid.

17 Ibid.

18 "The Benefits of Berries," Arthritis Foundation, 2014, arthritistoday.org/what-you-can-do /eating-well/benefits-of-eating-well/berries-benefits.php.

19 "Dark Green Leafy Vegetables," United States Department of Agriculture, March 2013, ars usda.gov/News/docs.htm?docid=23199.

20 "ORAC: Scoring Antioxidants?" Dr.Weil.com, December 2010, drweil.com/drw/u /QAA400852/ORAC-Scoring-Antioxidants.html.

21 D. Reilly, "Is Homoeopathy a Placebo Response? Controlled Trial of Homoeopathic Potency, with Pollen in Hayfever as Model," *The Lancet* (October 18, 1986): 885.

22 Ibid.

23 "Bromelain," American Cancer Society, April 2011, cancer.org/treatment /treatmentsandsideeffects/complementaryandalternativemedicine /herbsvitaminsandminerals/bromelain.

24 "Researchers Say Tart Cherries Have 'The Highest Anti-Inflammatory Content of Any Food,'" May 2012, eurekalert.org/pub_releases/2012-05/wsw-rst052912.php.

25 E. A. Droke et al., "Soy Isoflavones Avert Chronic Inflammation-Induced Bone Loss and Vascular Disease," *Journal of Inflammation* 4 (September 7, 2007): 17.

26 J. Salas-Salvado, "The Effect of Nuts on Inflammation," *Asia Pacific Journal of Clinical Nutrition* 17, sup. 1 (2008): 333–36.

27 "Olive Oil Reduces Inflammation," Arthritis Foundation, 2014, arthritistoday.org/what -you-can-do/eating-well/arthritis-diet/olive-oil-inflammation.php.

28 Ibid.

29 L. Lucas et al., "Molecular Mechanisms of Inflammation. Anti-Inflammatory Benefits of Virgin Olive Oil and the Phenolic Compound Oleocanthal," *Current Pharmaceutical Design* 17, no. 8 (2011): 754–68.

30 J. H. Shin et al., "Short-Term Heating Reduces the Anti-Inflammatory Effects of Fresh Raw Garlic Extracts on the LPS-Induced Production of NO and Pro-Inflammatory Cytokines by Downregulating Allicin Activity in RAW 264.7 Macrophages," *Food and Chemical Toxicology* 58 (August 2013): 545–51. doi:10.1016/j.fct.2013.04.002.

31 R. Grzanna et al., "Ginger—An Herbal Medicinal Product with Broad Anti-Inflammatory Actions," *Journal of Medicinal Food* 8, no. 2 (Summer 2005): 125–32.

32 Y. Fu et al., "Curcumin Attenuates Inflammatory Responses by Suppressing TLR4-
    Mediated NF-κB Signaling Pathway in Lipopolysaccharide-Induced Mastitis in
    Mice," *International Immunopharmacology* 20, no. 1 (May 2014): 54–58. doi:10.1016/j.
    intimp.2014.01.024.

33 N. S. Mashhadi et al., "Influence of Ginger and Cinnamon Intake on Inflammation and
    Muscle Soreness Endued by Exercise in Iranian Female Athletes," *International Journal of
    Preventive Medicine* 4, sup. 1 (April 2013): S11–15.

34 J. K. Kiecolt-Glaser et al., "Depressive Symptoms, Omega-6:Omega-3 Fatty Acids, and
    Inflammation in Older Adults," *Psychosomatic Medicine* 69, no. 3 (April 2007): 217–24.

35 "Foods That Fight Inflammation," Arthritis Foundation, 2014, arthritistoday.org/what
    -you-can-do/eating-well/arthritis-diet/eat-to-beat-inflammation.php.

36 M. Edelson, "Take Two Carrots and Call Me in the Morning," Hopkins Medicine, Winter
    2010, hopkinsmedicine.org/hmn/w10/feature2.cfm.

37 "Fructose Attacks Your Liver Like Alcohol—Is This What's Making You Flabby and Sick?"
    May 2012, articles.mercola.com/sites/articles/archive/2012/05/07/the-sweetener-that-is
    -more-dangerous-than-alcohol.aspx.

38 Ibid.

39 H. Parker, "A Sweet Problem: Princeton Researchers Find That High-Fructose Corn Syrup
    Prompts Considerably More Weight Gain," News at Princeton, March 2010, princeton.edu
    /main/news/archive/S26/91/22K07/.

40 Ibid.

41 Ibid.

42 Ibid.

43 "Fructose Attacks Your Liver Like Alcohol—Is This What's Making You Flabby and Sick?"
    May 2012, articles.mercola.com/sites/articles/archive/2012/05/07/the-sweetener-that-is
    -more-dangerous-than-alcohol.aspx.

44 I. Aeberli et al., "Low to Moderate Sugar-Sweetened Beverage Consumption Impairs
    Glucose and Lipid Metabolism and Promotes Inflammation in Healthy Young Men: A
    Randomized Controlled Trial," *American Journal of Clinical Nutrition* 94, no. 2 (August 2011):
    479–85. doi:10.3945/ajcn.111.013540.

45 "What You Eat Can Fuel or Cool Inflammation, a Key Driver of Heart Disease, Diabetes,
    and Other Chronic Conditions," The Harvard Medical School Family Health Guide,
    February 2007, health.harvard.edu/fhg/updates/What-you-eat-can-fuel-or-cool
    -inflammation-a-key-driver-of-heart-disease-diabetes-and-other-chronic-conditions.shtml.

46 A. Buyken et al., "Carbohydrate Nutrition and Inflammatory Disease Mortality in Older
    Adults," *American Journal of Clinical Nutrition* 92, no. 3 (September 2010): 634–43.

47 Y. Nakanishi et al., "Monosodium Glutamate (MSG): A Villain and Promoter of Liver
    Inflammation and Dysplasia," *Journal of Autoimmunity* 30, no. 1–2 (February–March 2008):
    42–50. doi:10.1016/j.jaut.2007.11.016.

48 A. K. Bauer et al., "Butylated Hydroxytoluene (BHT) Induction of Pulmonary
    Inflammation: A Role in Tumor Promotion," *Experimental Lung Research* 27, no. 3 (April–
    May 2001): 197–216.

49 "Iron Rich Foods," American Red Cross, 2014, redcrossblood.org/learn-about-blood
    /health-and-wellness/iron-rich-foods.

50 M. Edelson, "Take Two Carrots and Call Me in the Morning," Hopkins Medicine, Winter
    2010, hopkinsmedicine.org/hmn/w10/feature2.cfm.

51 Ibid.

52 Ibid.

53 Ibid.

54 S. Yeager and the editors of *Prevention*, *The Doctors Book of Food Remedies* (Emmaus, PA:
    Rodale Inc., 2008).

55 Ibid.

56 V. Konakovsky,. "Levels of Histamine and Other Biogenic Amines in High-Quality Red
    Wines," *Food Additives and Contaminants: Part A: Chemistry, Analysis, Control, Exposure, and
    Risk Assessment* 28, no .4 (April 2011): 408–16. doi:10.1080/19440049.2010.551421.

57 S. Yeager and the editors of *Prevention*, *The Doctors Book of Food Remedies* (Emmaus, PA:
    Rodale Inc., 2008).

CHAPTER 10

1 "Obesity and Overweight," Centers for Disease Control and Prevention, May 2014, cdc .gov/nchs/fastats/obesity-overweight.htm.

2 "Obesity," National Institutes of Health, MedlinePlus.com, May 2014, nlm.nih.gov /medlineplus/obesity.html.

3 Ibid.

4 Ibid.

5 Ibid.

6 "BMI," Centers for Disease Control and Prevention, December 2013, cdc.gov /healthyweight/assessing/bmi/index.html.

7 F. Huang, "Endothelial Activation and Systemic Inflammation in Obese Asthmatic Children," *Allergy and Asthma Proceedings* 29, no. 5 (September–October 2008): 453–60. doi:10.2500/aap.2008.29.3149.

8 M. Schatz, "Overweight/Obesity and Risk of Seasonal Asthma Exacerbations," *Journal of Allergy and Clinical Immunology* 1, no. 6 (November–December 2013): 618–22. doi:10.1016/j. jaip.2013.07.009.

9 S. Baumann, "Obesity—A Promoter of Allergy?" *International Archives of Allergy and Immunology* 162, no. 3 (2013): 205–13. doi:10.1159/000353972.

10 "Adult BMI Calculator: English," Centers for Disease Control and Prevention, May 2011, cdc.gov/healthyweight/assessing/bmi/adult_bmi/english_bmi_calculator/bmi _calculator.html.

11 Ibid.

12 "Mediterranean Diet," National Institutes of Health, MedlinePlus.com, May 2014, nlm.nih .gov/medlineplus/ency/patientinstructions/000110.htm.

13 L. Chatzi et al., "Protective Effect of Fruits, Vegetables, and the Mediterranean Diet on Asthma and Allergies among Children in Crete," *Thorax* 62 (2007): 677–83. doi:10.1136 /thx.2006.069419.

14 Ibid.

15 Ibid.

16 D. Grigoropoulou, "Urban Environment Adherence to the Mediterranean Diet and Prevalence of Asthma Symptoms among 10- to 12-Year-Old Children: The Physical Activity, Nutrition, and Allergies in Children Examined in Athens Study," *Allergy and Asthma Proceedings* 32, no. 5 (September–October 2011): 351–58. doi:10.2500 /aap.2011.32.3463.

17 P. Sexton et al., "Influence of Mediterranean Diet on Asthma Symptoms, Lung Function, and Systemic Inflammation: A Randomized Controlled Trial," *Journal of Asthma* 50, no. 1 (February 2013): 75–81. doi:10.3109/02770903.2012.740120.

18 D. Sewell et al., "Investigating the Effectiveness of the Mediterranean Diet in Pregnant Women for the Primary Prevention of Asthma and Allergy in High-Risk Infants: Protocol for a Pilot Randomised Controlled Trial," *Journal of Animal Science and Biotechnology* 14 (2013): 173. doi:10.1186/1745-6215-14-173.

19 L. Chatzi et al., "Mediterranean Diet in Pregnancy Is Protective for Wheeze and Atopy in Childhood," *Thorax* 63, no. 6 (June 2008): 507–13. doi:10.1136/thx.2007.081745.

20 S. Yeager and the editors of *Prevention, The Doctor's Book of Food Remedies* (Emmaus, PA: Rodale Inc., 2008).

21 Ibid.

22 "Vitamin C," National Institutes of Health, MedlinePlus.com, February 2013, nlm.nih.gov /medlineplus/ency/article/002404.htm.

23 "GMO Alert: Top 10 Genetically Modified Foods to Avoid Eating," May 2012, naturalnews .com/035734_GMOs_foods_dangers.html.

24 E. R. Secor, Jr., et al., "Bromelain Limits Airway Inflammation in an Ovalbumin-Induced Murine Model of Established Asthma," *Alternative Therapies in Health and Medicine* 18, no. 5 (September–October 2012): 9–17.

25 "GMO Alert: Top 10 Genetically Modified Foods to Avoid Eating," May 2012, naturalnews .com/035734_GMOs_foods_dangers.html.

26 D. Herber et al., "Sulforaphane-Rich Broccoli Sprout Extract Attenuates Nasal Allergic Response to Diesel Exhaust Particles," *Food and Function* 5, no. 1 (January 2014): 35–41. doi:10.1039/c3fo60277j.

27 S. Y. Han et al., "Resveratrol Inhibits IgE-Mediated Basophilic Mast Cell Degranulation and Passive Cutaneous Anaphylaxis in Mice," *Journal of Nutrition* 143, no. 5 (May 2013): 632–39. doi:10.3945/jn.112.173302.

28 L. C. Hazelwood et al., "Dietary Lycopene Supplementation Suppresses Th2 Responses and Lung Eosinophilia in a Mouse Model of Allergic Asthma," *Journal of Nutritional Biochemistry* 22, no. 1 (January 2011): 95–100. doi:10.1016/j.jnutbio.2009.12.003.

29 G. Riccioni,. "Plasma Lycopene and Antioxidant Vitamins in Asthma: The PLAVA Study," *Journal of Asthma* 44, no. 6 (July–August 2007): 429–32.

30 S. Baumann, "Obesity—A Promoter of Allergy?" *International Archives of Allergy and Immunology* 162, no. 3 (2013): 205–13. doi:10.1159/000353972.

31 C. M. Clemens et al., "The Effect of Perinatal Omega-3 Fatty Acid Supplementation on Inflammatory Markers and Allergic Diseases: A Systematic Review," *BJOG* 118, no. 8 (July 2011): 916–25. doi:10.1111/j.1471-0528.2010.02846.x.

32 "What You Need to Know about Mercury in Fish and Shellfish," United States Environmental Protection Agency, November 2013, water.epa.gov/scitech/swguidance /fishshellfish/outreach/advice_index.cfm.

33 R. Barros et al., "Dietary Intake of α-Linolenic Acid and Low Ratio of n-6:n-3 PUFA are Associated with Decreased Exhaled NO and Improved Asthma Control," *British Journal of Nutrition* 106, no. 3 (August 2011): 441–50. doi:10.1017/S0007114511000328.

34 "What Is the Recommended Intake of DHA + EPA per Day?" DHA EPA Institute, 2013, dhaomega3.org/FAQ/WHat-is-the-recommended-intake-of-DHA+EPA-per-day.

35 "Olive Oil Reduces Inflammation," Arthritis Foundation, 2014, arthritistoday.org/what -you-can-do/eating-well/arthritis-diet/olive-oil-inflammation.php.

36 "How to Choose a Quality Olive Oil," Dr.Weil.com, 2014, drweil.com/drw/u/ART02970 /Olive-Oil.html.

37 "12 Things You Shouldn't Be Cooking with Olive Oil," BuzzFeed Food, August 2013, buzzfeed.com/christinebyrne/things-you-shouldnt-be-cooking-with-olive-oil ?bffbfood#1t5duqn.

38 M. Edelson, "Take Two Carrots and Call Me in the Morning," Hopkins Medicine, Winter 2010, hopkinsmedicine.org/hmn/w10/feature2.cfm.

39 "Can Antioxidants in Fruits and Vegetables Protect Your Heart?" American Heart Association, February 2014, heart.org/HEARTORG/GettingHealthy/NutritionCenter /HealthyEating/Can-antioxidants-in-fruits-and-vegetables-protect-you-and-your-heart _UCM_454424_Article.jsp.

40 S. Yeager and the editors of *Prevention, The Doctor's Book of Food Remedies* (Emmaus, PA: Rodale Inc., 2008).

41 Naturopathic Family Care News March Newsletter, February 24, 2009, naturopathicfamilycare.blogspot.com/2009/02/nfc-march-newsletter.html.

42 S. Bushwick, "Fiber-Munching Mice Avoid Asthma," *Scientific American,* January 2014, scientificamerican.com/podcast/episode/fiber-munching-mice-avoid-asthma-14-01-08/.

43 S. Yeager and the editors of *Prevention, The Doctor's Book of Food Remedies* (Emmaus, PA: Rodale Inc., 2008).

44 J. Brusco, "What Foods Mixed with Lentils Provide a Complete Source of Amino Acids?" SF Gate, healthyeating.sfgate.com/foods-mixed-lentils-provide-complete-source-amino -acids-1195.html.

45 "Genetically Engineered Foods," The National Institutes of Health, MedlinePlus.com, May 2014, nlm.nih.gov/medlineplus/ency/article/002432.htm.

46 Ibid.

47 Ibid.

48 "GMO Alert: Top 10 Genetically Modified Foods to Avoid Eating," May 2012, naturalnews .com/035734_GMOs_foods_dangers.html.

49 B. Buchanan, "Genetic Engineering and the Allergy Issue," *Plant Physiology* 126, no. 1 (May 2001): 5–7. plantphysiol.org/content/126/1/5.full.

50 EWG's Shopper's Guide to Pesticides in Produce. ewg.org/foodnews/summary.php.

51 B. Björkstén, "Evidence of Probiotics in Prevention of Allergy and Asthma," *Current Drug Targets—Inflammation and Allergy* 4, no. 5 (October 2005): 599–604.

52 "The Allergic March," World Allergy Organization, September 2007, worldallergy.org /professional/allergic_diseases_center/allergic_march/.

53 "The International Scientific Forum on Home Hygiene. Activity Review 2013," Home Hygiene and Health, February 2013, ifh-homehygiene.org/public-leaflet/international -scientific-forum-home-hygiene-activity-review-2013.

54 M. Kuitunen, "Probiotics and Prebiotics in Preventing Food Allergy and Eczema," *Current Opinion in Allergy and Clinical Immunology* 13, no. 3 (June 2013): 280–86. doi:10.1097 /ACI.0b013e328360ed66.

55 I. Eliaz, "Are You Chronically Dehydrated?" Rodale News, August 2012, rodalenews.com /chronic-dehydration.

56 Ibid.

57 ibid.

58 Ibid.

59 Naturopathic Family Care News, February 2010, naturopathicfamilycare.blogspot.com /2010_02_01_archive.html

60 I. Eliaz, "Are You Chronically Dehydrated?" Rodale News, August 2012, rodalenews.com /chronic-dehydration.

61 Ibid.

62 G. P. Curatola, "Top Tips to Smile through Spring Allergy Season!" *The Dr. Oz Show*, April 2011, doctoroz.com/blog/gerald-p-curatola-dds/top-tips-smile-through-spring-allergy -season.

63 I. Eliaz, "Are You Chronically Dehydrated?" Rodale News, August 2012, rodalenews.com /chronic-dehydration.

64 T. Harlan, "What Can I Substitute for Fish and Shellfish, if I Am Allergic to Them?" Ask Dr. Gourmet, drgourmet.com/askdrgourmet/foods/fishsubstitute.shtml#.VDL-c2d0y70.

CHAPTER 11

1 K. McCoy, "Vitamins and Supplements for Allergy Treatment: Do They Work?" Everydayhealth.com, October 2012, everydayhealth.com/allergies/vitamins-and -supplements.aspx.

2 R. Schulman, *Solve It with Supplements* (Emmaus, PA: Rodale Inc., 2007).

3 Ibid.

4 Ibid.

5 J. M. Braun, "Therapeutic Use, Efficiency, and Safety of the Proteolytic Pineapple Enzyme Bromelain-POS in Children with Acute Sinusitis in Germany," *In Vivo* 19, no. 2 (March–April 2005): 417–21.

6 Ibid.

7 R. Schulman, *Solve It with Supplements* (Emmaus, PA: Rodale Inc., 2007).

8 Ibid.

9 "Vitamin B6 (Pyridoxine)," University of Maryland Medical Center, June 2013, umm.edu /health/medical/altmed/supplement/vitamin-b6-pyridoxine.

10 "Vitamin B6," NYU Langone Medical Center, August 2013, med.nyu.edu/content ?ChunkIID=21852#REF43.

11 R. D. Reynolds et al., "Depressed Plasma Pyridoxal Phosphate Concentrations in Adult Asthmatics," *American Journal of Clinical Nutrition* 41, no. 4 (April 1985): 684–88.

12 L. Sakakeeny et al., "Plasma Pyridoxal-5-Phosphate Is Inversely Associated with Systemic Markers of Inflammation in a Population of US Adults," *Journal of Nutrition* 142, no. 7 (July 2012): 1280–85. doi:10.3945/jn.111.153056.

13 H. Tsuge et al., "Effects of Vitamin B-6 on (n-3) Polyunsaturated Fatty Acid Metabolism," *Journal of Nutrition* 130, no. 2 (February 1, 2000): 333.

14 "Pyridoxine (Vitamin B6)," National Institutes of Health, MedlinePlus.com, July 2011, nlm.nih.gov/medlineplus/druginfo/natural/934.html.

15 A. Bendich et al., "Vitamin B6 Safety Issues," *Annals of the New York Academy of Sciences* 585 (1990): 321–30.

16 "Vitamin B6 (Pyridoxine)," University of Maryland Medical Center, June 2013, umm.edu /health/medical/altmed/supplement/vitamin-b6-pyridoxine.

17 R. Schulman, *Solve It with Supplements* (Emmaus, PA: Rodale Inc., 2007).

18 B. H. Theusen et al., "Atopy, Asthma, and Lung Function in Relation to Folate and Vitamin B(12) in Adults," *Allergy* 65, no. 11 (November 2010): 1446–54. doi:10.1111/j.1398 -9995.2010.02378.x.

19 B. Añíbarro et al., "Asthma with Sulfite Intolerance in Children: A Blocking Study with Cyanocobalamin," *Journal of Allergy and Clinical Immunology* 90, no. 1 (July 1992): 103–9.

20 R. Schulman, *Solve It with Supplements* (Emmaus, PA: Rodale Inc., 2007).

21 "Vitamin C (Ascorbic Acid)," University of Maryland Medical Center, June 2013, umm .edu/health/medical/altmed/supplement/vitamin-c-ascorbic-acid.

22 J. Galloway, "Natural Solutions Let You Breathe Deeply, without Sneezing or Side Effects," The American Association of Naturopathic Physicians, 2012, naturopathic.org /pdf/757_111105934.pdf.

23 A. F. Hagel et al., "Intravenous Infusion of Ascorbic Acid Decreases Serum Histamine Concentrations in Patients with Allergic and Nonallergic Diseases," *Naunyn-Schmiedeberg's Archives of Pharmacology* 386, no. 9 (September 2013): 789–93. doi:10.1007/s00210-013-0880-1.

24 J. H. Seo et al., "Association of Antioxidants with Allergic Rhinitis in Children from Seoul," *Allergy, Asthma, and Immunology Research* 5, no. 2 (March 2013): 81–87. doi:10.4168 /aair.2013.5.2.81.

25 S. G. Wannamethee et al., "Associations of Vitamin C Status, Fruit and Vegetable Intakes, and Markers of Inflammation and Hemostasis," *American Journal of Clinical Nutrition* 83, no. 3 (March 2006): 567–74; quiz 726–27.

26 E. S. Ford et al., "C-Reactive Protein Concentration and Concentrations of Blood Vitamins, Carotenoids, and Selenium among United States Adults," *European Journal of Clinical Nutrition* 57, no. 9 (September 2003): 1157–63.

27 G. Block et al., "Vitamin C Treatment Reduces Elevated C-Reactive Protein," *Free Radical Biology and Medicine* 46, no. 1 (January 2009): 70–77. doi:10.1016/j.freeradbiomed.2008.09.030.

28 R. Schulman, *Solve It with Supplements* (Emmaus, PA: Rodale Inc., 2007).

29 "3 Supplements for Allergies," *Prevention,* November 2011, prevention.com/health/health -concerns/3-supplements-allergies.

30 A. Satar et al., "Possible Warfarin Resistance Due to Interaction with Ascorbic Acid: Case Report and Literature Review," *American Journal of Health-System Pharmacy* 70, no. 9 (May 1, 2013): 782–86. doi:10.2146/ajhp110704.

31 R. Schulman, *Solve It with Supplements* (Emmaus, PA: Rodale Inc., 2007).

32 F. Gazdik, "Levels of Coenzyme Q10 in Asthmatics," *Bratislava Medical Journal* 103, no. 10 (2002): 353–56.

33 R. Schulman, *Solve It with Supplements* (Emmaus, PA: Rodale Inc., 2007).

34 A. Gvozdjáková et al., "Coenzyme Q10 Supplementation Reduces Corticosteroids Dosage in Patients with Bronchial Asthma," *BioFactors* 25, no. 1–4 (2005): 235–40.

35 E. Fabian et al., "Nutritional Supplements and Plasma Antioxidants in Childhood Asthma," *Wiener Klinische Wochenschrift* 125, no. 11–12 (June 2013): 309–15. doi:10.1007 /s00508-013-0359-6.

36 R. Schulman, *Solve It with Supplements* (Emmaus, PA: Rodale Inc., 2007).

37 Ibid.

38 Ibid.

39 "Fight Allergies with Vitamin E," Bastyr Center for Natural Health, 2014, bastyrcenter.org /content/view/319/.

40 E. Shahar et al., "Effect of Vitamin E Supplementation on the Regular Treatment of Seasonal Allergic Rhinitis," *Annals of Allergy, Asthma, and Immunology* 92, no. 6 (June 2004): 654–58.

41 R. Schulman, *Solve It with Supplements* (Emmaus, PA: Rodale Inc., 2007).

42 "Study Suggests Vitamin E May Help People with Asthma," National Center for Complementary and Alternative Medicine, July 2008, nccam.nih.gov/research/results /spotlight/070208.htm.

43 T. Tsuduki et al., "Tocotrienol (Unsaturated Vitamin E) Suppresses Degranulation of Mast Cells and Reduces Allergic Dermatitis in Mice," *Journal of Oleo Science* 62, no. 10 (2013): 825–34.

44 R. Schulman, *Solve It with Supplements* (Emmaus, PA: Rodale Inc., 2007).

45 Ibid.

46 Ibid.

47 Ibid.

48 N. L. Morse et al., "A Meta-Analysis of Randomized, Placebo-Controlled Clinical Trials of Efamol Evening Primrose Oil in Atopic Eczema. Where Do We Go from Here in Light of More Recent Discoveries?" *Current Pharmaceutical Biotechnology* 7, no. 6 (December 2006): 503–24.

49 D. Simon et al., "Gamma-Linolenic Acid Levels Correlate with Clinical Efficacy of Evening Primrose Oil in Patients with Atopic Dermatitis," *Advances in Therapy* 31, no. 2 (February 2014): 180–88. doi:10.1007/s12325-014-0093-0.

50 R. Schulman, *Solve It with Supplements* (Emmaus, PA: Rodale Inc., 2007).

51 Ibid.

52 Ibid.

53 Ibid.

54 "3 Supplements for Allergies," *Prevention*, November 2011, prevention.com/health/health-concerns/3-supplements-allergies.

55 R. Schulman, *Solve It with Supplements* (Emmaus, PA: Rodale Inc., 2007).

56 Ibid.

57 C. Cipolla et al., "Magnesium Pidolate in the Treatment of Seasonal Allergic Rhinitis. Preliminary Data," *Magnesium Research* 3, no. 2 (June 1990): 109–12.

58 R. Schulman, *Solve It with Supplements* (Emmaus, PA: Rodale Inc., 2007).

59 J. Galloway, "Natural Solutions Let You Breathe Deeply, without Sneezing or Side Effects," The American Association of Naturopathic Physicians, 2012, naturopathic.org/pdf/757_111105934.pdf.

60 B. Björkstén, "Evidence of Probiotics in Prevention of Allergy and Asthma," *Current Drug Targets—Inflammation and Allergy* 4, no. 5 (October 2005): 599–604.

61 M. Kuitunen, "Probiotics and Prebiotics in Preventing Food Allergy and Eczema," *Current Opinion in Allergy and Clinical Immunology* 13, no. 3 (June 2013): 280–86. doi:10.1097/ACI.0b013e328360ed66.

62 "Pycnogenol," The National Institutes of Health, MedlinePlus.com, August 2011, nlm.nih.gov/medlineplus/druginfo/natural/1019.html.

63 Ibid.

64 D. Wilson et al., "A Randomized, Double-Blind, Placebo-Controlled Exploratory Study to Evaluate the Potential of Pycnogenol for Improving Allergic Rhinitis Symptoms," *Phytotherapy Research* 24, no. 8 (August 2010): 1115–19. doi:10.1002/ptr.3232.

65 I. S. Shin et al., "Inhibitory Effects of Pycnogenol (French Maritime Pine Bark Extract) on Airway Inflammation in Ovalbumin-Induced Allergic Asthma," *Food and Chemical Toxicology* 62 (December 2013): 681–86. doi:10.1016/j.fct.2013.09.032.

66 "Asthma," University of Maryland Medical Center, June 2013, umm.edu/health/medical/altmed/condition/asthma.

67 "Pycnogenol," The National Institutes of Health, MedlinePlus.com, August 2011, nlm.nih.gov/medlineplus/druginfo/natural/1019.html.

68 Ibid.

69 R. Schulman, *Solve It with Supplements* (Emmaus, PA: Rodale Inc., 2007).

70 Ibid.

71 M. Martinez-Losa et al., "Inhibitory Effects of N-Acetylcysteine on the Functional Responses of Human Eosinophils in Vitro," *Clinical and Experimental Allergy* 37, no. 5 (May 2007): 714–22.

72 Ibid.

73 A. Nadeem et al., "Glutathione Modulation during Sensitization as well as Challenge Phase Regulates Airway Reactivity and Inflammation in Mouse Model of Allergic Asthma," *Biochimie* 103 (August 2014): 61–70. doi:10.1016/j.biochi.2014.04.001.

74 R. Schulman, *Solve It with Supplements* (Emmaus, PA: Rodale Inc., 2007).

75 Ibid.

76 P. C. Calder, "n-3 Polyunsaturated Fatty Acids, Inflammation, and Inflammatory Diseases," *American Journal of Clinical Nutrition* 83, sup. 6 (June 2006): 1505S–1519S.

77 R. Schulman, *Solve It with Supplements* (Emmaus, PA: Rodale Inc., 2007).

78 M. Covington et al., "Omega-3 Fatty Acids," *American Family Physician* 70, no. 1 (July 1, 2004): 133–140.

79 S. Hoff et al., "Allergic Sensitisation and Allergic Rhinitis Are Associated with n-3 Polyunsaturated Fatty Acids in the Diet and in Red Blood Cell Membranes," *European Journal of Clinical Nutrition* 59, no. 9 (September 2005): 1071–80.

80 R. Kitz et al., "Omega-3 Polyunsaturated Fatty Acids and Bronchial Inflammation in Grass Pollen Allergy after Allergen Challenge," *Respiratory Medicine* 104, no. 12 (December 2010): 1793–98. doi:10.1016/j.rmed.2010.06.019.

81 C. M. Klemens et al., "The Effect of Perinatal Omega-3 Fatty Acid Supplementation on Inflammatory Markers and Allergic Diseases: A Systematic Review," *BJOG* 118, no. 8 (July 2011): 916–25. doi:10.1111/j.1471-0528.2010.02846.x.

82 R. Schulman, *Solve It with Supplements* (Emmaus, PA: Rodale Inc., 2007).

83 "What You Need to Know about Mercury in Fish and Shellfish," United States Environmental Protection Agency, November 2013, water.epa.gov/scitech/swguidance /fishshellfish/outreach/advice_index.cfm.

84 R. Schulman, *Solve It with Supplements* (Emmaus, PA: Rodale Inc., 2007).

85 C. Wong, ND, "Natural Allergy Remedies," About.com, May 2011, altmedicine.about.com /od/healthconditionsatod/a/allergies.htm.

86 R. Schulman, *Solve It with Supplements* (Emmaus, PA: Rodale Inc., 2007).

87 L. Bielory, "Complementary and Alternative Therapies for Allergic Rhinitis and Conjunctivitis," Uptodate.com, May 2014, uptodate.com/contents/complementary-and -alternative-therapies-for-allergic-rhinitis-and-conjunctivitis.

88 Z. Weng et al., "Quercetin Is More Effective Than Cromolyn in Blocking Human Mast Cell Cytokine Release and Inhibits Contact Dermatitis and Photosensitivity in Humans," *PLOS ONE* 7, no. 3 (2012): e33805. doi:10.1371/journal.pone.0033805.

89 F. Shishehbor et al., "Quercetin Effectively Quells Peanut-Induced Anaphylactic Reactions in the Peanut Sensitized Rats," *Iranian Journal of Allergy, Asthma, and Immunology* 9, no. 1 (March 2010): 27–34. doi:09.01/ijaai.2734.

90 A. P. Rogerio et al., "Anti-Inflammatory Activity of Quercetin and Isoquercitrin in Experimental Murine Allergic Asthma," *Inflammation Research* 56, no. 10 (October 2007): 402–8.

91 C. Wong, ND, "Natural Allergy Remedies," About.com, May 2011, altmedicine.about.com /od/healthconditionsatod/a/allergies.htm.

92 R. Schulman, *Solve It with Supplements* (Emmaus, PA: Rodale Inc., 2007).

93 M. F. Carneiro,. "Low Concentrations of Selenium and Zinc in Nails Are Associated with Childhood Asthma," *Biological Trace Element Research* 144, no. 1–3 (December 2011): 244–52. doi:10.1007/s12011-011-9080-3.

94 E. Fabian et al., "Nutritional Supplements and Plasma Antioxidants in Childhood Asthma," *Wiener Klinische Wochenschrift* 125, no. 11–12 (June 2013): 309–15. doi:10.1007 /s00508-013-0359-6.

95 R. Safaralizadeh,. "Influence of Selenium on Mast Cell Mediator Release," *Biological Trace Element Research* 154, no. 2 (August 2013): 299–303. doi:10.1007/s12011-013-9712-x.

96 R. Schulman, *Solve It with Supplements* (Emmaus, PA: Rodale Inc., 2007).

97 Ibid.

98 Ibid.

99 P. Bass, MD, "Zinc and Asthma," About.com, October 2011, asthma.about.com/od /preventioncontrol/a/Zinc-And-Asthma.htm.

100 A. Soutar et al., "Bronchial Reactivity and Dietary Antioxidants," *Thorax* 52, no. 2 (February 1997): 166–70.

101 U. Nurmatov et al., "Nutrients and Foods for the Primary Prevention of Asthma and Allergy: Systematic Review and Meta-Analysis," *Journal of Allergy and Clinical Immunology* 127, no. 3 (March 2011): 724–33.e1-30. doi:10.1016/j.jaci.2010.11.001.

102 M. A. Biltagi et al., "Omega-3 Fatty Acids, Vitamin C, and Zn Supplementation in Asthmatic Children: A Randomized Self-Controlled Study," *Acta Paediatrica* 98, no. 4 (April 2009): 737–42.

103 A. Gaby, *Nutritional Medicine* (Concord: Fritz Perlberg Publishing, 2011).

104 R. Schulman, *Solve It with Supplements* (Emmaus, PA: Rodale Inc., 2007).

105 Ibid.

106 Ibid.

107 I. Gupta et al., "Effects of Boswellia Serrata Gum Resin in Patients with Bronchial Asthma: Results of a Double-Blind, Placebo-Controlled, 6-Week Clinical Study," *European Journal of Medical Research* 3, no. 11 (November 17, 1998): 511–14.

108 R. Schulman, *Solve It with Supplements* (Emmaus, PA: Rodale Inc., 2007).

109 "Gingko," National Institutes of Health, MedlinePlus.com, August 2013, nlm.nih.gov /medlineplus/druginfo/natural/333.html.

110 R. Schulman, *Solve It with Supplements* (Emmaus, PA: Rodale Inc., 2007).

111 Ibid.

112 Y. Tang et al., "The Effect of Ginkgo Biloba Extract on the Expression of PKCalpha in the Inflammatory Cells and the Level of IL-5 in Induced Sputum of Asthmatic Patients," *Journal of Huazhong University of Science and Tecnholog [Medical Sciences]* 27, no. 4 (August 2007): 375–80.

113 R. Schulman, *Solve It with Supplements* (Emmaus, PA: Rodale Inc., 2007).

114 Ibid.

115 Ibid.

116 "Green Tea May Fight Allergies," ScienceDaily.com, September 2002, sciencedaily.com /releases/2002/09/020919071413.htm.

117 E. Hassanain et al., "Green Tea (*Camellia sinensis*) Suppresses B Cell Production of IgE without Inducing Apoptosis," *Annals of Clinical and Laboratory Science* 40, no. 2 (Spring 2010): 135–43.

118 R. Schulman, *Solve It with Supplements* (Emmaus, PA: Rodale Inc., 2007).

119 Ibid.

120 Ibid.

121 Ibid.

122 Ibid.

123 M. Houssen et al., "Natural Anti-Inflammatory Products and Leukotriene Inhibitors as Complementary Therapy for Bronchial Asthma," *Clinical Biochemistry* 43, no. 10–11 (July 2010): 887–90. doi:10.1016/j.clinbiochem.2010.04.061.

124 Y. W. Shin et al., "In Vitro and in Vivo Antiallergic Effects of *Glycyrrhiza glabra* and Its Components," *Planta Medica* 73, no. 3 (March 2007): 257–61.

125 R. Schulman, *Solve It with Supplements* (Emmaus, PA: Rodale Inc., 2007).

126 K. Bone and S. Mills, *Principles and Practice of Phytotherapy* (London: Churchill Livingstone, 2000).

127 C. Wong, ND, "Natural Allergy Remedies," About.com, May 2011, altmedicine.about.com /od/healthconditionsatod/a/allergies.htm.

128 K. P. Lee et al., "Anti-Allergic and Anti-Inflammatory Effects of Bakkenolide B Isolated from *Petasites japonicus* Leaves," *Journal of Ethnopharmacology* 148, no. 3 (July 30, 2013): 890–94. doi:10.1016/j.jep.2013.05.037.

129 A. Brattstrom et al., "Petasites Extract Ze 339 (PET) Inhibits Allergen-Induced Th2 Responses, Airway Inflammation, and Airway Hyperreactivity in Mice," *Phytotherapy Research* 24, no. 5 (May 2010): 680–85. doi:10.1002/ptr.2972.

130 A. Schapowal et al., "Treating Intermittent Allergic Rhinitis: A Prospective, Randomized, Placebo and Antihistamine-Controlled Study of Butterbur Extract Ze 339," *Phytotherapy Research* 19, no. 6 (June 2005): 530–37.

131 J. S. Lee et al., "Suppressive Effect of *Petasites japonicus* Extract on Ovalbumin-Induced Airway Inflammation in an Asthmatic Mouse Model," *Journal of Ethnopharmacology* 133, no. 2 (January 27, 2011): 551–57. doi:10.1016/j.jep.2010.10.038.

132 C. Wong, ND, "Natural Allergy Remedies," About.com, May 2011, altmedicine.about.com /od/healthconditionsatod/a/allergies.htm.

133 "Stinging Nettle," University of Maryland Medical Center, May 2011, umm.edu/health /medical/altmed/herb/stinging-nettle.

134 B. Roschek, Jr, et al., "Nettle Extract (*Urtica dioica*) Affects Key Receptors and Enzymes Associated with Allergic Rhinitis," *Phytotherapy Research* 23, no. 7 (July 2009): 920–26. doi:10.1002/ptr.2763.

135 P. Mittlman, "Randomized, Double-Blind Study of Freeze-Dried *Urtica dioica* in the Treatment of Allergic Rhinitis," *Planta Medica* 56, no. 1 (February 1990): 44–47.

136 B. Roschek, Jr, et al., "Nettle Extract (*Urtica dioica*) Affects Key Receptors and Enzymes Associated with Allergic Rhinitis," *Phytotherapy Research* 23, no. 7 (July 2009): 920–26. doi:10.1002/ptr.2763.

137 Kerry Bone and Simon Mills, *Principles and Practice of Phytotherapy* (London: Churchill Livingstone, 2000).

138 "Stinging Nettle," University of Maryland Medical Center, May 2011, umm.edu/health /medical/altmed/herb/stinging-nettle.

139 Ibid.

140 "Tylophora," NYU Langone Medical Center, August 2013, med.nyu.edu/content ?ChunkIID=21875.

141 "Tylophora," 2001 (information unlikely to change) ip.aaas.org/tekindex .nsf/2a9c4e44835b04ea85256a7200577a64/75641188d67fb97685256c33004fbd79/Body /M1?OpenElement.

142 "Tylophora," NYU Langone Medical Center, August 2013, med.nyu.edu/content ?ChunkIID=21875.

143 "Asthma," University of Maryland Medical Center, June 2013, umm.edu/health/medical /altmed/condition/asthma.

144 Ibid.

145 *Tinospora cordifolia,*" NYU Langone Medical Center, med.nyu.edu/content?ChunkIID =111811.

146 Ibid.

147 V. A. Badar, "Efficacy of *Tinospora cordifolia* in Allergic Rhinitis," *Journal of Ethnopharmacology* 96, no. 3 (January 15, 2005): 445–49.

148 Ibid.

149 *Tinospora cordifolia,*" NYU Langone Medical Center, med.nyu.edu/content?ChunkIID =111811.

CHAPTER 12

1 P. Greco, "How to Detox Your House," *Good Housekeeping*, 2014, goodhousekeeping.com /home/cleaning-organizing/house-cleaning-hazards-apr07?click=main_sr.

2 Ibid.

3 "Questions about Your Community: Indoor Air," United States Environmental Protection Agency, September 2013, epa.gov/region1/communities/indoorair.html.

4 "7 Tips for an Allergy-Proof Bedroom," WebMD.com, October 2012, webmd.com/allergies /tips-for-an-allergy-proof-bedroom.

5 "Diseases and Conditions: Allergies," Mayo Clinic, April 2014, mayoclinic.org/diseases -conditions/allergies/in-depth/allergy/art-20049365?pg=2.

6 P. M. Ehrlich and E. S. Bowers, *Living with Allergies* (New York: Facts on File, 2008).

7 P. Greco, "How to Detox Your House," *Good Housekeeping*, 2014, goodhousekeeping.com /home/cleaning-organizing/house-cleaning-hazards-apr07?click=main_sr.

8 "The Allergen-Free Bedroom," Green America, January/February 2006, greenamerica.org /livinggreen/bedrooms.cfm.

9 P. M. Ehrlich and E. S. Bowers, *Living with Allergies* (New York: Facts on File, 2008).

10 "Indoor Allergens: Tips to Remember," American Academy of Allergy, Asthma, and Immunology, 2013, aaaai.org/conditions-and-treatments/library/at-a-glance/indoor -allergens.

11 Ibid.

12 P. M. Ehrlich and E. S. Bowers, *Living with Allergies* (New York: Facts on File, 2008).

13 "Indoor Allergens: Tips to Remember," American Academy of Allergy, Asthma, and Immunology, 2013, aaaai.org/conditions-and-treatments/library/at-a-glance/indoor -allergens.

14 Ibid.

15 P. Greco, "How to Detox Your House," *Good Housekeeping*, 2014, goodhousekeeping.com /home/cleaning-organizing/house-cleaning-hazards-apr07?click=main_sr.

16 "Indoor Allergens: Tips to Remember," American Academy of Allergy, Asthma, and Immunology, 2013, aaaai.org/conditions-and-treatments/library/at-a-glance/indoor -allergens.

17 Ibid.

18 Ibid.

19 P. M. Ehrlich and E. S. Bowers, *Living with Allergies* (New York: Facts on File, 2008).

20   "The Allergen-Free Bedroom," Green America, January/February 2006, greenamerica.org
     /livinggreen/bedrooms.cfm.

21   "Indoor Allergens: Tips to Remember," American Academy of Allergy, Asthma, and
     Immunology, 2013, aaaai.org/conditions-and-treatments/library/at-a-glance/indoor
     -allergens.

22   P. Greco, "How to Detox Your House," *Good Housekeeping*, 2014, goodhousekeeping.com
     /home/cleaning-organizing/house-cleaning-hazards-apr07?click=main_sr.

23   Ibid.

24   "7 Tips for an Allergy-Proof Bedroom," WebMD.com, October 2012, webmd.com/allergies
     /tips-for-an-allergy-proof-bedroom.

25   "Indoor Allergens: Tips to Remember," American Academy of Allergy, Asthma, and
     Immunology, 2013, aaaai.org/conditions-and-treatments/library/at-a-glance/indoor
     -allergens.

26   "Diseases and Conditions: Allergies," Mayo Clinic, April 2014, mayoclinic.org/diseases
     -conditions/allergies/in-depth/allergy/art-20049365?pg=2.

27   "Indoor Allergens: Tips to Remember," American Academy of Allergy, Asthma, and
     Immunology, 2013, aaaai.org/conditions-and-treatments/library/at-a-glance/indoor
     -allergens.

28   "Diseases and Conditions: Allergies," Mayo Clinic, April 2014, mayoclinic.org/diseases
     -conditions/allergies/in-depth/allergy/art-20049365?pg=2.

29   Ibid.

30   S. McEvoy, "Mold-Resistant Paint," HGTV, hgtvremodels.com/interiors/mold-resistant
     -paint/index.html.

31   "Interior Paint Problems: Mold and Mildew," benjaminmoore.com/en-us/for-contractors
     /mildew-paint-problem.

32   C. Billionnet, "Quantitative Assessments of Indoor Air Pollution and Respiratory Health in
     a Population-Based Sample of French Dwellings," *Environmental Research* 111, no. 3 (April
     2011): 425–34. doi:10.1016/j.envres.2011.02.008.

33   C. M. Robroeks, "Exhaled Volatile Organic Compounds Predict Exacerbations of
     Childhood Asthma in a 1-Year Prospective Study," *European Respiratory Journal* 42, no. 1
     (July 2013): 98–106. doi:10.1183/09031936.00010712.

34   P. M. Ehrlich and E. S. Bowers, *Living with Allergies* (New York: Facts on File, 2008).

35   Ibid.

36   L. Claudio, "Planting Healthier Indoor Air," *Environmental Health Perspectives* 119, no. 10
     (October 2011): a426–a427. doi:10.1289/ehp.119-a426.

37   "The Allergen-Free Bedroom," Green America, January/February 2006, greenamerica.org
     /livinggreen/bedrooms.cfm.

38   "Diseases and Conditions: Allergies," Mayo Clinic, April 2014, mayoclinic.org/diseases
     -conditions/allergies/in-depth/allergy/art-20049365?pg=2.

39   B. Burmeier, "Natural Ways to Freshen Your Home," Everyday Health, January 2012,
     everydayhealth.com/asthma-pictures/natural-ways-to-freshen-your-home.aspx.

40   "Cleaning Supplies and Household Chemicals," American Lung Association, 2014, lung
     .org/healthy-air/home/resources/cleaning-supplies.html.

41   Ibid.

42   P. Greco, "How to Detox Your House," *Good Housekeeping*, 2014, goodhousekeeping.com
     /home/cleaning-organizing/house-cleaning-hazards-apr07?click=main_sr.

43   N. Martin, "Better Sleep Strategies for Asthma Sufferers," *Real Simple*, 2014, realsimple.com
     /health/better-sleep-strategies-for-allergy-sufferers.

44   "Cleaning Supplies and Household Chemicals," American Lung Association, 2014, lung
     .org/healthy-air/home/resources/cleaning-supplies.html.

45   Ibid.

46   "Formaldehyde in Your Home," Minnesota Department of Health, health.state.mn.us
     /divs/eh/indoorair/voc/formaldehyde.htm.

47   P. M. Ehrlich and E. S. Bowers, *Living with Allergies* (New York: Facts on File, 2008).

48   H. Hickey, "Scented Laundry Products Emit Hazardous Chemicals through Dryer Vents,"
     University of Washington, August 2011, washington.edu/news/2011/08/24/scented
     -laundry-products-emit-hazardous-chemicals-through-dryer-vents/.

49   "Use Precaution with Parabens," Healthy Child Healthy World, January 30, 2013,
     healthychild.org/easy-steps/use-precaution-with-parabens/.

50   "Bisphenol A (BPA)," National Institute of Environmental Health Sciences, niehs.nih.gov /health/topics/agents/sya-bpa/.

51   C. M. Villanueva, "Meta-Analysis of Studies on Individual Consumption of Chlorinated Drinking Water and Bladder Cancer," *Journal of Epidemiology and Community Health* 57, no. 3 (March 2003): 166–73.

52   P. M. Ehrlich and E. S. Bowers, *Living with Allergies* (New York: Facts on File, 2008).

CHAPTER 13

1   "Physical Activity and Health," Centers for Disease Control and Prevention, February 2011, cdc.gov/physicalactivity/everyone/health/index.html.

2   Ibid.

3   A. Pinto et al., "Effects of Physical Exercise on Inflammatory Markers of Atherosclerosis," *Current Pharmaceutical Design* 18, no. 28 (2012): 4326–49.

4   M. Hamer et al., "Physical Activity and Inflammatory Markers Over 10 Years: Follow-Up in Men and Women from the Whitehall II Cohort Study," *Circulation*, published electronically August 13, 2012. doi:10.1161/ CIRCULATIONAHA.112.103879.

5   "What Are the Health Risks of Overweight and Obesity?" National Heart, Lung, and Blood Institute, July 2012, nhlbi.nih.gov/health/health-topics/topics/obe/risks.html.

6   J. Garcia-Aymerich et al., "Incidence of Adult-Onset Asthma after Hypothetical Interventions on Body Mass Index and Physical Activity: An Application of the Parametric G-Formula," *American Journal of Epidemiology* 179, no. 1 (January 1, 2014): 20–26. doi:10.1093 /aje/kwt229.

7   A. Tai et al., "Association between Asthma Symptoms and Obesity in Preschool (4–5 Year Old) Children," *Journal of Asthma* 46, no. 4 (May 2009): 362–65. doi:10.1080/02770900902759260.

8   "Physical Activity and Health," Centers for Disease Control and Prevention, February 2011, cdc.gov/physicalactivity/everyone/health/index.html.

9   Ibid.

10   "Dietary Guidelines for Americans, 2010," United States Department of Health and Human Services, June 2014, health.gov/dietaryguidelines/2010.asp.

11   "2008 Physical Activity Guidelines for Americans Summary," United States Department of Health and Human Services, June 2014, health.gov/paguidelines/guidelines/summary .aspx.

12   "Physical Activity: Frequently Asked Questions," Centers for Disease Control and Prevention, February 2011, cdc.gov/physicalactivity/growingstronger/faq/index.html

13   "Exercising with Allergies and Asthma," The American College of Sports Medicine, acsm.org/docs/current-comments/allergiesandasthmatemp.pdf.

14   A. Mantica, "Attack Allergies with Yoga," *Prevention*, November 2011, prevention.com /fitness/yoga/yoga-hay-fever-and-allergies.

15   S. Singh et al., "Effect of Yoga Practices on Pulmonary Function Tests Including Transfer Factor of Lung for Carbon Monoxide (TLCO) in Asthma Patients," *Indian Journal of Physiology and Pharmacology* 56, no. 1 (January–March 2012): 63–68.

16   A. J. Bidwell et al., "Yoga Training Improves Quality of Life in Women with Asthma," *Journal of Alternative and Complementary Medicine* 18, no. 8 (August 2012): 749–55. doi:10.1089/acm.2011.0079.

17   "Exercising with Allergies and Asthma," The American College of Sports Medicine, acsm.org/docs/current-comments/allergiesandasthmatemp.pdf.

18   "Physical Activity and Health," Centers for Disease Control and Prevention, February 2011, cdc.gov/physicalactivity/everyone/health/index.html.

19   C. W. Kim, "Combined Effects of Food and Exercise on Anaphylaxis," *Nutrition Research and Practice* 7, no. 5 (October 2013): 347–51.

20   Ibid.

21   "Exercising with Allergies and Asthma," The American College of Sports Medicine, acsm.org/docs/current-comments/allergiesandasthmatemp.pdf.

22   Ibid.

23   "Exercising with Allergies and Asthma," The American College of Sports Medicine, acsm.org/docs/current-comments/allergiesandasthmatemp.pdf.

24   D. Silva et al., "Physical Training Improves Quality of Life Both in Asthmatic Children and Their Caregivers," *Annals of Asthma, Allergy, and Immunology* 111, no. 5 (November 2013): 427–28. doi:10.1016/j.anai.2013.08.016.

25 "Exercising with Allergies and Asthma," The American College of Sports Medicine, acsm.org/docs/current-comments/allergiesandasthmatemp.pdf.

26 Ibid.

27 "Exercising with Allergies and Asthma," American College of Allergy, Asthma, and Immunology, 2010, acaai.org/allergist/asthma/asthma-treatment/management/pages /exercising-with-allergies-asthma.aspx.

28 W. Tontako, "The Effect of Acute Exhaustive and Moderate Intensity Exercises on Nasal Cytokine Secretion and Clinical Symptoms in Allergic Rhinitis Patients," *Asian Pacific Journal of Allergy and Immunology* 30, no. 3 (September 2012): 185–92.

29 J. Stewart, "Run Away from Your Allergies," *Men's Health*, March 2013, menshealth.com /health/run-away-from-your-allergies.

30 A. Pirisi, "Calming Yoga for Allergies," *Yoga Journal*, 2014, yogajournal.com/article/health /allergy-antidote/.

31 Ibid.

32 A. Mantica, "Attack Allergies with Yoga," *Prevention*, November 2011, prevention.com /fitness/yoga/yoga-hay-fever-and-allergies.

33 "Qi Gong and Tai Chi for Allergies," 2014, altmd.com/Articles/Qi-Gong-and-Tai-Chi-for -Allergies.

34 T. D. Mickleborough, "Salt Intake, Asthma, and Exercise-Induced Bronchoconstriction: A Review," *The Physician and Sportsmedicine* 38, no 1 (April 2010): 118–31. doi:10.3810 /psm.2010.04.1769.

35 "Qi Gong and Tai Chi for Allergies," 2014, altmd.com/Articles/Qi-Gong-and-Tai-Chi-for -Allergies.

36 T. Neale, "CHEST: Asthma Patients May Derive Extra Benefit from Tai Chi," MedPageToday, October 2008, medpagetoday.com/MeetingCoverage/CHEST/11533.

37 B. Hendrick, "Tai Chi May Help Control Asthma," October 2008, webmd.com/asthma /news/20081028/tai-chi-may-help-control-asthma.

38 Y. F. Chang et al., "Tai Chi Chuan Training Improves the Pulmonary Function of Asthmatic Children," *Journal of Microbiology, Immunology, and Infection* 41, no. 1 (February 2008): 88–95.

39 Supreme Chi Living: An Online Journal by American Tai Chi and Qigong Association. Locate Tai Chi or Qigong Classes. americantaichi.net/TaiChiQigongClass.asp.

40 S. Singh et al., "Effect of Yoga Practices on Pulmonary Function Tests Including Transfer Factor of Lung for Carbon Monoxide (TLCO) in Asthma Patients." *Indian Journal of Physiology and Pharmacology* 56, no. 1 (January–March 2012): 63–68.

41 A. J. Bidwell et al., "Yoga Training Improves Quality of Life in Women with Asthma," *Journal of Alternative and Complementary Medicine* 18, no. 8 (August 2012): 749–55. doi:10.1089/acm.2011.0079.

42 R. Vempati et al., "The Efficacy of a Comprehensive Lifestyle Modification Programme Based on Yoga in the Management of Bronchial Asthma: A Randomized Controlled Trial," *BMC Pulmonary Medicine* 9 (July 30, 2009): 37. doi:10.1186/1471-2466-9-37.

43 A. Pirisi, "Calming Yoga for Allergies," *Yoga Journal*, 2014, yogajournal.com/article/health /allergy-antidote/.

44 Ibid.

45 S. Waxman, "6 Tips to Stay Safe in Hot Yoga," *Yoga Journal*, 2007, yogajournal.com/article /yoga-101/facing-the-heat/.

46 *Yoga Journal*, "Style Profile: Ashtanga Yoga," yogajournal.com/article/beginners/spotlight -on-ashtanga-yoga/.

47 A. Pirisi, "Calming Yoga for Allergies," *Yoga Journal*, 2014, yogajournal.com/article/health /allergy-antidote/.

48 Ibid.

49 Ibid.

CHAPTER 14

1 "Sublingual Immunotherapy," The John Hopkins Sinus Center, 2008, hopkinsmedicine .org/sinus/allergy/sublingual_immunotherapy.html.

2 "Portable Air Cleaners," Asthma and Allergy Foundation of America, aafa.org/display .cfm?id=8&sub=17&cont=158.

3   Ibid.

4   P. M. Ehrlich and E. S. Bowers, *Living with Allergies* (New York: Facts on File, 2008).

5   "Five Best Allergy Friendly House Plants," Zyrtec.com, 2014, zyrtec.com/passion/gardening/allergy-friendly-house-plants.

6   "Cleaning Supplies and Household Chemicals," American Lung Association, lung.org/healthy-air/home/resources/cleaning-supplies.html

7   Ibid.

8   "How to Green Your Cleaning Routine," Treehugger, June 27, 2014, treehugger.com/htgg/how-to-go-green-cleaning.html.

9   "95+ Household Uses for Vinegar," *Reader's Digest,* rd.com/home/150-household-uses-for-vinegar/.

10 N. Martin, "Better Sleep Strategies for Allergy Sufferers," *Real Simple,* realsimple.com/health/better-sleep-strategies-for-allergy-sufferers.

11 "How to Green Your Cleaning Routine," Treehugger, June 27, 2014, treehugger.com/htgg/how-to-go-green-cleaning.html.

12 Ibid.

13 Ibid.

14 S. Yeager and the editors of *Prevention, The Doctors' Book of Food Remedies* (Emmaus, PA: Rodale, 2008).

15 Ibid.

16 Ibid.

17 Ibid.

18 "Vitamin C," National Institutes of Health, MedlinePlus.com, May 2014, nlm.nih.gov/medlineplus/ency/article/002404.htm.

19 D. Heber et al., "Sulforaphane-Rich Broccoli Sprout Extract Attenuates Nasal Allergic Response to Diesel Exhaust Particles," *Food and Function* 5, no. 1 (January 2014): 35–41. doi:10.1039/c3fo60277j.

20 "What's New and Beneficial about Broccoli," World's Healthiest Foods, 2014, whfoods.com/genpage.php?tname=foodspice&dbid=9.

21 O. Lindahl, "Vegan Regimen with Reduced Medication in the Treatment of Bronchial Asthma," *Journal of Asthma* 22, no. 1 (1985): 45–55.

22 I. Eliaz, "Are You Chronically Dehydrated?", Rodale News, 2012, rodalenews.com/chronic-dehydration.

23 "Qi Gong and Tai Chi for Allergies," 2014, altmd.com/Articles/Qi-Gong-and-Tai-Chi-for-Allergies.

24 T. Neale, "CHEST: Asthma Patients May Derive Extra Benefit from Tai Chi," MedPageToday, October 2008, medpagetoday.com/MeetingCoverage/CHEST/11533.

25 Y. F. Chang et al., "Tai Chi Chuan Training Improves the Pulmonary Function of Asthmatic Children," *Journal of Microbiology, Immunology, and Infection* 41, no. 1 (February 2008): 88–95.

26 A. Tai, "Association between Asthma Symptoms and Obesity in Preschool (4–5 Year Old) Children," *Journal of Asthma* 46, no. 4 (May 2009): 362–65. doi:10.1080/02770900902759260.

27 "Physical Activity: Frequently Asked Questions," Centers for Disease Control and Prevention, February 2011, cdc.gov/physicalactivity/growingstronger/faq/index.html.

28 "Dietary Guidelines for Americans, 2010," United States Department of Health and Human Services, 2010, health.gov/dietaryguidelines/2010.asp.

29 S. Cohen et al., "Chronic Stress, Glucocorticoid Receptor Resistance, Inflammation, and Disease Risk," *Proceedings of the National Academy of Sciences of the United States of America* 109, no. 16 (April 17, 2012): 5995–99. doi:10.1073/pnas.1118355109.

30 "Physical Activity and Health," Centers for Disease Control and Prevention, February 2011, cdc.gov/physicalactivity/everyone/health/index.html.

31 K. Prasad et al., "Effect of a Single-Session Meditation Training to Reduce Stress and Improve Quality of Life among Health Care Professionals: A "Dose-Ranging" Feasibility Study," *Alternative Therapies in Health and Medicine* 17, no. 3 (May–June 2011): 46–49.

32 "Vitamin C (Ascorbic acid)," University of Maryland Medical Center, June 2013, umm.edu/health/medical/altmed/supplement/vitamin-c-ascorbic-acid.

33 A. F. Hagel et al., "Intravenous Infusion of Ascorbic Acid Decreases Serum Histamine Concentrations in Patients with Allergic and Non-Allergic Diseases," *Naunyn-Schmiedeberg's Archives of Pharmacology* 386, no. 9 (September 2013): 789–93. doi:10.1007 /s00210-013-0880-1.

34 "Vitamin B6," NYU Langone Medical Center, August 2013, med.nyu.edu/content ?ChunkIID=21852.

35 L. Sakakeeny et al., "Plasma Pyridoxal-5-Phosphate Is Inversely Associated with Systemic Markers of Inflammation in a Population of US Adults," *Journal of Nutrition* 142, no. 7 (July 2012): 1280–85. doi:10.3945/jn.111.153056.

36 "Pyridoxine (Vitamin B6)," National Institutes of Health, MedlinePlus.com, March 2014, nlm.nih.gov/medlineplus/druginfo/natural/934.html.

37 B. H. Thuesen, "Atopy, Asthma, and Lung Function in Relation to Folate and Vitamin B(12) in Adults," *Allergy* 65, no. 11 (November 2010): 1446–54. doi:10.1111/j.1398-9995.2010.02378.x.

38 L. Lewis, ND, "Natural Treatments for Your Seasonal Allergies," The American Association of Naturopathic Physicians, 2014, naturopathic.org/content.asp?contentid=117.

39 R. Schulman, *Solve It with Supplements* (Emmaus, PA: Rodale Inc., 2007).

40 "Butterbur," National Center for Complementary and Alternative Medicine, April 2012, nccam.nih.gov/health/butterbur.

41 C. Wong, "Natural Allergy Remedies," altmedicine.about.com/od/healthconditionsatod /a/allergies.htm.

42 "Find a Vitamin or Supplement: Butterbur," 2014, webmd.com/vitamins-supplements /ingredientmono-649-butterbur.aspx?activeIngredientId=649&activeIngredientName =butterbur.

43 Y. Tang, "The Effect of Ginkgo Biloba Extract on the Expression of PKCalpha in the Inflammatory Cells and the Level of IL-5 in Induced Sputum of Asthmatic Patients," *Journal of Huazhong University of Science and Technology*, 27, no. 4 (August 2007): 375–80.

44 R. Schulman, *Solve It with Supplements* (Emmaus, PA: Rodale Inc., 2007).

45 Ibid.

46 B. Roschek, Jr, et al., "Nettle Extract (*Urtica dioica*) Affects Key Receptors and Enzymes Associated with Allergic Rhinitis," *Phytotherapy Research* 23, no. 7 (July 2009): 920–26. doi:10.1002/ptr.2763.

47 Editors of *Reader's Digest. 1,801 Home Remedies*. New York: Reader's Digest, 2004.

48 V. A. Badar et al., "Efficacy of *Tinospora cordifolia* in Allergic Rhinitis," *Journal of Ethnopharmacology* 96, no. 3 (January 15, 2005): 445–49.

49 "Tinospora Cordifolia," RXList, 2014, rxlist.com/tinospora cordifolia/supplements.htm

50 "Tylophora," NYU Langone Medical Center, August 2013, med.nyu.edu/content ?ChunkIID=21875.

51 L. Lewis, ND, "Natural Treatments for Your Seasonal Allergies," The American Association of Naturopathic Physicians, 2014, naturopathic.org/content.asp?contentid=117.

52 J. Sun et al., "Efficacy of Allergen-Specific Immunotherapy for Peanut Allergy: A Meta-Analysis of Randomized Controlled Trials," *Allergy and Asthma Proceedings* 35, no. 2 (March–April 2014): 171–77. doi:10.2500/aap.2014.35.3730.

53 "Sublingual Immunotherapy," The Johns Hopkins Sinus Center, 2008, hopkinsmedicine .org/sinus/allergy/sublingual_immunotherapy.html.

54 Ibid.

55 P. Moingeon, "Update on Immune Mechanisms Associated with Sublingual Immunotherapy: Practical Implications for the Clinician," *Journal of Allergy and Clinical Immunology: In Practice 1*, no. 3 (May–June 2013): 228–41. doi:10.1016/j.jaip.2013.03.013.

Index

Underscored page references indicate sidebars and tables.